OXFORD MEDICAL PUB

Paediatrics

Key questions answered

More key questions answered:

Clinical Medicine
Wai-Ching Leung

Endocrinology
John Laycock and Peter Wise

Paediatrics
Jonathan Round

Paediatrics

Key questions answered

Jonathan Round

*Lecturer, Department of Child Health,
St George's Hospital Medical School, London*

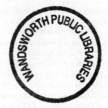

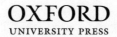

OXFORD
UNIVERSITY PRESS

OXFORD
UNIVERSITY PRESS

Great Clarendon Street, Oxford OX2 6DP

Oxford University Press is a department of the University of Oxford
and furthers the University's aim of excellence in research, scholarship,
and education by publishing worldwide in

Oxford New York

Athens Auckland Bangkok Bogota Buenos Aires Calcutta
Cape Town Chennai Dar es Salaam Delhi Florence Hong Kong Istanbul
Karachi Kuala Lumpur Madras Madrid Melbourne Mexico City Mumbai
Nairobi Paris São Paulo Singapore Taipei Tokyo Toronto Warsaw
and associated companies in
Berlin Ibadan

Oxford is a registered trade mark of Oxford University Press

Published in the United States
by Oxford University Press Inc., New York

British Library Cataloguing in Publication Data
Data available

Library of Congress Cataloging in Publication Data
Round, Jonathan.
Paediatrics : key questions answered / Jonathan Round.
p. cm. – (Oxford medical publications) (Oxford core texts)
1. Pediatrics—Examinations, questions, etc. I. title.
II. Series. III. series: Oxford core texts.
[DNLM: 1. Pediatrics examination questions. Not Acquired]
RJ80.R68 1999 618.92′00076—dc21 98-41105
ISBN 0 19 262904 2

Typeset by Downdell, Oxford
Printed in Great Britain by
Biddles Ltd, Guildford & King's Lynn

Preface

Aim and layout of book

We cannot avoid examinations, so this book was written to help those studying paediatrics to have some practise with paediatric examinations, to identify deficient areas of knowledge, and to overcome technical inefficiency that repeatedly costs intelligent and well prepared students marks. I began writing after several years teaching paediatrics to graduates and undergraduates. A common complaint is that there are not enough practise questions available. Also, many courses, although teaching a comprehensive syllabus, do not focus on the examination itself. The majority of courses have multiple choice questions (MCQs) as part of the assessment, and performance in this mode of testing is particularly dependent on technique. Furthermore, MCQs with extensive answers can be an interesting and challenging way of preparing for exams. I hope this will be the case to all those who use this book.

The book starts (as usual) with an introduction, which is probably the most important chapter if you want to increase your score. Here MCQs are reviewed, words explained and techniques for maximizing your score are covered. After that are chapters by subject, covering the range of topics that will come up in a paediatric exam. In each, questions are divided into those that test knowledge ('Do you know this fact?') and those that test reasoning and data interpretation ('Which do you think is most likely, given this information'). For each question, answers are given with extensive explanation. This will cover the answers and also any related issues. Complicated concepts and terminology are explained.

Clinical medicine is all about linking knowledge together from different fields at the same time. Therefore, the same topic may come up in different areas and no apology is made for repetition of similar information in different chapters, as this aids retention and helps link together symptoms and diseases from different systems.

The advantages of paediatrics

Paediatrics is perhaps the most diverse of all the specialities. The paediatrician must be competent at managing problems from all the different systems and experienced at assessing and treating both an adolescent weighing 70 kg and an infant born at 25 weeks weighing 700 g. Social interactions between parents, children, and the doctor are important. Diseases are often dramatic and children may present extremely ill but by the next morning be playing normally.

This does not mean that paediatrics is easy to become familiar with. People experience problems with changing normal ranges, development and the change in emphasis away from investigation results towards clinical assessment. There are also diseases that are only found in paediatrics and those that seem similar to adult diseases but are managed very differently.

All these factors should make paediatrics interesting and challenging for those willing to do more than just cram for an exam, and makes it a good career choice.

Studying paediatrics

To prepare for any exam, you cannot avoid knowing a number of facts. Modern exams aim to test more than just factual recall and try to cover higher levels of reasoning. Time on wards and in the community with children allows an appreciation of the normal, how children respond to diseases, and the paediatric approach. As more children are born and become sick at night, time shadowing the paediatric staff is needed.

A good textbook is also needed. There are several on the market at the moment. The most exhaustive are *Nelson's textbook of pediatrics* (Behrman and Kleigman) or Forfar and Arneil's *Textbook of paediatrics*, but these are for reference only. A good compromise for candidates studying for higher exams is *Nelson—essentials of pediatrics* (Behrman and Kleigman), better known as baby Nelson. For SHOs and residents this is also good choice or Lissauer and Clayden's *Illustrated textbook of paediatrics*. For undergraduates *Essential paediatrics* (Johnston and Hull) has stood the test of time, but many find this too long winded. *Manual of hospital paediatrics* (Hambleton) is good if you like lists, and *Paediatrics—understanding child health* (Waterston, Helms, and Platt) gives an excellent account of paediatrics in its social context. This book also has the advantage of a large number of example cases. Many students are also using Lissauer and Clayden, as this has a good balance of text, pictures, lists, and practise cases.

This MCQ book is not a textbook even though it covers all of the paediatric syllabus except child psychiatry. It is written to be a useful adjunct to these books and help learn and revise paediatrics.

Paediatrics in examinations

Paediatrics for examinations is different to paediatrics for clinicians. There are diseases that often come up and these are brought out in this book. The examiner will try to see if you know what is different to adult practice.

There is no perfect test of ability. The MCQ has been used as a moderately good way of testing knowledge acquisition. This format can be adapted to test interpretation, and other forms (e.g. extended matching questions or EMQs) are being developed to be more relevant to medicine. Unfortunately, much of medicine is not true or false but more or less likely, and the EMQ enables testing of this. However, only a few universities are using these at present.

OSCE (objective structured clinical examinations) are also gaining favour, and seem to be a better test of ability than other forms. However, they are difficult and labour intensive to organize.

Types of questions

MCQs are composed of a stem and usually five branches. These branches each should make statements with the stem and each one should be assessed separately by the candidate. Such statements associate at least two facts or situations (e.g. a *child with asthma* will often have *wheeze*). Here a specific child and a situation are linked with a conditional clause. More complex questions may link a child with a detailed history and a balance of probabilities. For example, a 4 year old with a past history of nocturnal cough but no family history of atopy presents short of breath. The finding of wheeze makes asthma a more likely diagnosis than pneumonia.

You will almost never be sure about all of the answers in a question. Some may be deliberately harder than the others to test the better candidates.

A good MCQ question is difficult to write. The first problem is with the language—it is easy to give away the answer in the question. It then becomes a problem avoiding ambiguity and misunderstanding. Once the writer has sorted out these problems, the question may still be too easy or too difficult.

In this question:

A male infant of 3 days is found to be cyanosed centrally. This boy

    a will always have a high level of deoxyhaemoglobin
    b may have a congenital heart disease
    c has a 3% chance of having transposition of the great arteries
    d should never be given oxygen
    e a chest X-ray should be performed and is unlikely to not demonstrate an 'egg-on-side' appearance

Some of these problems are illustrated. As all candidates know, 'may' is almost always true and 'always' or 'never' are almost always false. 'May' can only be false if the association in the branch has never been reported in the literature. Similarly 'always' and 'never' implies an invariable association, which is rare in medicine. The only time always or never will be true is when the association is part of the definition or diagnostic criteria. In part (a), 'always' turns out to be true because central cyanosis is defined as the appearance caused by a high level of arterial deoxyhaemoglobin. On the other hand in (d), 'never' is used and so the branch is false as there are bound to be some conditions in which cyanosis is not dangerous. In (b), 'may' is used and it is so obviously true that this branch will not discriminate between the good and poor candidate. In part (c), the opposite is true. The branch is so specific that it is almost certainly false. For undergraduate exams, values given will either be normal or very abnormal. Part (e) is a poor branch for several reasons. First, it asks three questions at once—should you do a chest film (yes), is transposition of the great arteries 'not an unlikely' diagnosis and does this produce an 'egg-on-side' appearance. Also there is the double negative and lastly the question has already partly been asked in part (c). The answer is false—transposition of the great arteries is not a likely diagnosis in this situation.

So the question could be improved by changing it to:

A male infant of 3 days is found to be cyanosed centrally. This boy

    a will have a level of deoxyhaemoglobin over 2 g/dl
    b is likely to have congenital heart disease
    c may have transposition of the great arteries
    d should not be given oxygen if he has a duct dependent heart malformation
    e a chest X-ray might demonstrate an 'egg-on-side' appearance

The majority of the questions in this book have already been tried out by undergraduate students. This has enabled further development of the questions to avoid these pitfalls.

Confusing words and their meanings

Here is a selection of words used in the conditional clause linking the stem and branch. The response hinges on these.

May/might—this means it is possible even if incredibly rare. A statement with these words will almost always be true unless the associations are mutually exclusive. For instance, the statement 'a child with an urinary tract infection (UTI) may have no organisms grown from a urine specimen' is true but 'a child with a UTI may have no organisms in his urinary tract' is false.

Can/could—is very similar in its meaning to may/might.

Should/ought—this means that in the vast majority of cases such a course of action has to be taken to correctly manage the child.

Must—this is stronger than should/ought, and implies that such a course of action is imperative to avoid harm to the child. It also implies that there is no controversy concerning the suggested manoeuvre. In an MCQ question, it is like 'always' and so is usually only true when it directly affects diagnosis or outcome.

For instance 'In a child unconscious after a head injury, an urgent CT scan should be performed' is true. If 'must' was used instead of 'should', then the answer would be false as there might be other priorities (airways, breathing, and circulation) and other investigations may be more appropriate first.

On the other hand 'In a child unconscious after a head injury, the airway must first be secured, would be true.

Never—this means the association has never been reported and so is usually false unless it is mutually exclusive (e.g. children with Fallot's tetralogy never have a normal right ventricle).

Always—this is the opposite of never in meaning.

Often/frequently—these words cannot be tied down to a precise percentage, but it will be a percentage well over 10%.

Usually/probably—these two words mean a percentage over 50% (i.e. more usual or more frequent than not).

Commonly—this means it is often encountered, or the association is not a surprise for the doctor. For instance 'a child presenting with a headache is commonly diagnosed as having a brain tumour' is false, but 'in a child with an intra-cranial mass a glioma is a common cause' is true.

Rarely—here the association is well recognized but uncommon.

Diagnostic—the interpretation of this word is that such a feature makes all other diagnoses very unlikely. 'a high sweat sodium is diagnostic of cystic fibrosis'.

Pathopnemonic—this means that a feature is so closely associated with a disease and no other that no other cause is possible. 'Fraying and cupping of the epiphysis of the distal radius is pathopnemonic of rickets'.

The exam

The exam usually consists of 50–60 questions each of which has a stem and five possible answers (branches), each of which may be true or false. Almost all examinations are now negatively marked, which means that you lose a mark for each incorrect answer.

There rarely is a pass mark before the marks are compiled as the examiner will not know exactly how hard the paper is so a few past questions are usually put into the paper to allow year-on-year comparison.

The exam is a fairly reproducible test of factual knowledge and to a lesser extent understanding, so you cannot avoid reading widely around the subject, and spending time with sick children and in the community. Beyond this there is some advantage to be gained by technique and practise. In undergraduate paediatrics there are only so many things that can be asked so the more questions you have done the more likely you are to see the same one again.

Many candidates wonder if they should guess. The simple answer is that one must, as one cannot be sure about enough answers to pass. The 'technique' of MCQ exams is all to do with knowing when to guess.

Guessing technique

Answering a negatively marked MCQ randomly, one would on average score zero, in that one is just as likely to gain as to lose a mark. So if someone answering randomly attempt more or less questions he or she will not improve or worsen their score. Similarly, if you come to a branch you know nothing about, on average you will not lose out by answering it, but nor will you gain. If you know anything about the question, and most students after 5 years of medical education know something, a 'guess' is usually a little more likely to be right than wrong, and so will on average improve your overall mark.

Occasionally, some candidates are bad guessers and the guessing in this way lowers their mark. To find out if this technique benefits you or not, take about 10 questions that you have not seen. First, go through the set of questions and answer the questions you are positive about and fairly sure about. Leave all those you have no idea about and those you only vaguely know something about, but not enough to feel confident of answering in a real exam. Now, in a different column, go back and answer the ones you have left that you have a vague idea about. There is no point in attempting ones you haven't a clue about. Hopefully, you will now have answered about 90% of the questions. Finally, tot up the marks separately for each column.

Most people find that they gain marks overall with their second pass through the questions, answering questions they only vaguely know the answer to, and increase their mark by about 5–10% doing this, which is an important margin.

This technique has been validated in several studies[†] where it has been shown that those randomly selected to answer all of the branches obtained higher overall marks than those who were selected to chose which branches they would like to answer.

Final pitfalls

Candidates unwittingly also reduce their own marks by several bad practices:

Panicking if they are not answering many branches. A good MCQ paper is one that discriminates between good and bad, so everyone will be unable to answer some of the questions. Also the paper may be unusually difficult for everyone.

Expecting true or false answers Candidates should remember that all the branches are independent of each other and in fact five true or false answers will usually come up at least twice in a 60 question paper.

Reading too much into the question The correct answer is usually your first impression and one tends to become less sure as you think about it more. However, marks are thrown away by not reading carefully all the words.

Carelessness Mistakes are easy to make and expensive. Always check that you have put down the response you wanted after you have done the test as there is usually plenty of time.

So, after these few pointers that hopefully are of some use, the rest of the book is questions and answers. They are designed to be negatively marked and any one of the five branches could be true or false.

[†] HARDEN R.M., BROWN R.A., BIRAN L.A., DALLAS ROSS W.P., and WAKEFORD R.E. (1976) Multiple choice questions: to guess or not to guess. *Medical Education*, 10, 27–32.
FLEMING P.R. (1988) The profitability of 'guessing' in mulitple choice question papers. *Medical Education*, 22, 509–513.

Acknowledgements

This book is written and finished with the generous support of Jane, my wife, and daughter Antonia who have provided me with time and their practical support. Also I appreciate the encouragement offered at the beginning of the project from Dafydd Walters, the students at St George's, Tooting, and OUP. I would also like to thank those who looked at the questions with me, especially Mudit Jindal, who was both critical and honest.

Contents

1 The newborn

Knowledge — questions

1 *Respiratory distress syndrome*
   a affects only infants born under 34 weeks
   b typically causes lobar collapse on chest X-ray
   c is prevented by surfactant therapy
   d usually presents before 5 days of age
   e maternal steroid therapy improves outcome

2 *Infants born prematurely are more likely to*
   a die from sudden infant death syndrome
   b have a spastic diplegia
   c develop laryngomalacia
   d have fractures
   e develop right heart failure

3 *These features increase the suspicion of sepsis in a neonate*
   a maternal fever (>38.5) during labour
   b frequent short apnoeas
   c temperature instability
   d vomiting
   e antenatal membrane rupture for 21 h

4 *The following definitions are correct*
   a the neonatal period is from birth to 1 month of age
   b the perinatal period is from 28 weeks gestation to 1 month after birth
   c the infant mortality rate is the number of deaths in the first year per 1000
      live births
   d preterm refers to infants born before their due date
   e intrauterine growth retardation means the weight of the newborn infant
      is below the 3rd percentile for gestational age

5 *The following statements are correct*
   a infant mortality rate is a marker of socio-economic deprivation
   b cerebral palsy is mainly caused by perinatal events

c gestational age at delivery is a better predictor of outcome than birth weight

d home births have been shown to be statistically more hazardous for the infant than hospital births

e an infant born at 28 weeks has about a 50% chance of survival

6 *In the first 10 min following birth in a healthy term neonate*

a pulmonary vasodilation occurs

b surfactant synthesis begins

c the ductus arteriosus closes

d arterial blood pressure rises

e right to left shunts are reduced

7 *During neonatal resuscitation*

a sodium bicarbonate can be given by an endotracheal tube

b atropine is used as the first measure to treat a bradycardia

c wrapping the infant is vital to the resuscitation

d any meconium should be sucked out of the trachea

e a heart rate of 90 is abnormally low

8 *Common indications that an infant has suffered intrapartum hypoxia include*

a hypotonia with absent reflexes

b poor feeding

c seizures

d excessive crying

e oliguria

9 *During intrauterine life the healthy fetus normally*

a makes urine

b swallows and sucks

c has regular breathing movements

d can move its limbs by 20 weeks gestation

e opens its bowels

10 *The following findings can be regarded as normal when found as part of a newborn examination on day 3*

a respiratory rate 35 breaths/min when settled

b marked jaundice

c milky discharge from the nipple

d asymmetric tonic neck reflex

e a well demarcated bluish discoloration over the buttocks

11   *When initiating feeding in a newborn infant*
   a   formula milk should be used before the mother's milk 'comes in'
   b   feeding more often than every 4 h should be discouraged
   c   colostrum provides little immunoglobulin A for the infant
   d   the sucking reflex is not present in infants born at 37 weeks
   e   fluid requirements on the first day are about 200 ml for a 3.5 kg baby

12   *These congenital infections commonly cause the associated feature in the newborn*
   a   toxoplasmosis—microcephaly
   b   rubella—cataracts
   c   cytomegalovirus—hydrocephalus
   d   chicken pox—scarring
   e   chlamydia—pneumonitis

13   *These are features commonly found in newborn term infants with uncomplicated Down's syndrome*
   a   hypertonia
   b   poor feeding
   c   asymmetrical growth retardation
   d   brachycephaly
   e   downslanting palpebral fissures

14   *A infant born at 26 weeks*
   a   has less little fat per kilogram than a term neonate
   b   requires less fluid per kilogram than a more mature infant
   c   should not be given milk until it reaches a corrected age of 34 weeks
   d   is at high risk of necrotizing enterocolitis
   e   is at high risk of subdural haemorrhage

15   *A baby born at 26 weeks*
   a   is more likely to die from sudden infant death syndrome
   b   is more likely to die from bronchiolitis
   c   has a mortality over 80% in England
   d   is more likely to have parents in low socio-economic groups
   e   has a 70% chance of developing cerebral palsy

16   *These injuries are common following an assisted delivery*
   a   fracture of the clavicle
   b   dislocation of the hip
   c   pulmonary contusion

    d subconjunctival haemorrhage
    e seventh cranial nerve palsy

Reasoning and data interpretation—questions

17   *A male infant is born after an uneventful pregnancy at*
     41 weeks gestation by emergency Caesarean section. The indication
     for this was a prolonged fetal bradycardia. The mother had previously
     had one Caesarean for breech presentation. There was thick
     meconium present in the liquor and a fresh bleed per vaginum. The
     infant was noted to have a heart rate of 40 beats/min, was pale,
     apnoeic, floppy, and unresponsive.
     a this infant has an Apgar score of 4
     b external cardiac compressions should be started
     c intravenous atropine would be useful
     d an arterial blood gas will help in the immediate management of the child
     e adrenaline can be given via the umbilical artery

18   *An infant age 2 h, born at 32 weeks gestation is in 50% oxygen. He*
     has moderate chest recession and a respiratory rate of 60 per min. He
     has had several apnoeas and bradycardias in the last hour. This is his
     arterial blood gas
     pH 7.19
     pCO$_2$ 7.5 kPa
     pO$_2$ 8.1 kPa
     base excess — 5.1 mmol/l
     a he has a partially compensated metabolic acidosis
     b intubation and ventilation is indicated
     c following stabilization the first intervention should be surfactant admin-
        istration
     d antibiotics should be given
     e his recurrent apnoeas can be treated with caffeine or a theophylline.

19   *A full-term female infant is mechanically ventilated in 50% oxygen*
     following a surgical procedure for duodenal atresia. Before operation
     she was self-ventilating in air. An arterial blood gas now shows the
     following
     pH 7.51
     pCO$_2$ 2.4 kPa

pO_2 18.0 kPa

BE -1.4 mmol/l

a she is at risk of retinopathy
b her minute volume is too high
c she has a respiratory alkalosis
d she should now be extubated
e her inspired oxygen should be reduced

20(i) *An infant is seen on day 3 for a routine postnatal check. The mother says he has not been breastfeeding well. The SHO examines him and finds he is centrally pink, with a good heart rate, but that he is sleepy, floppy, peripherally cold, and cyanosed. His fontanelle is slightly sunken. His temperature is 36.6 °C and respiratory rate 65 breaths/ min with no recession*

a infection is unlikely with a normal temperature
b respiratory illness can be ruled out clinically
c cardiac disease is a likely cause of his signs
d meningitis can be ruled out
e acidosis may explain the respiratory rate

20(ii) *in the above scenario the following test results rapidly become available*

blood glucose 0.3 mmol/l

arterial blood gas

pH 7.12

pCO_2 3.1 kPa

pO_2 10.2 kPa

BE -17.5 mmol/l

a he has a metabolic acidosis
b ventilation is not needed at this stage based on these results
c ornithine transcarbamylase deficiency may be responsible
d a bolus of feed is required
e glucagon is a recognized treatment of resistant hypoglycaemia

21 *A woman has delivered at 23 weeks gestation following premature labour and rupture of membranes, which occurred 13 days previously*

a if the baby is born dead, it is a stillbirth
b no resuscitation should be offered unless the infant is vigorous
c if the baby is born dead, the parents should not see it
d survival in this group is above 25%
e adrenaline should be given in the resuscitation

22   *A term female infant is found by a midwife on day 2 to be feeding poorly, have a temperature of 37.3°C and is floppy and difficult to wake. The infant is admitted to the neonatal unit and some investigations performed*
      CSF RBC 200/mm^3 Hb 17.1 g/dl
      WCC 5/mm^3 WCC 2.3 × 10^3/mm^3
      no organisms seen   platelets 15 × 10^3/mm^3
      a   this result rules out meningitis
      b   the temperature is diagnostic of infection
      c   the platelet count suggests platelet consumption
      d   the WCC suggests severe infection
      e   antibiotics should be started as soon as culture results are available

23   *A baby of 36 h age, having been born at 27 weeks has the following results*
      Na$^+$ 127 mmol/l
      K$^+$ 3.2 mmol/l
      urea 1.2 mmol/l
      a   these could be explained by a low urine water output
      b   fluid restriction will help to correct the problem
      c   these results can be explained by a high evaporative loss from the skin
      d   inadequate sodium in the fluids is a likely cause
      e   these results may simply reflect the mothers blood electrolytes

24   *A term male is vomiting on day 2. The pregnancy and delivery have been entirely normal. On direct questioning, he has yet to pass meconium*
      a   the presence of abdominal distension is suggestive of bowel obstruction
      b   a small amount of milky vomiting soon after the feed over his face is normal, in the absence of any other findings
      c   a family history of coeliac disease is relevant to this case
      d   bilious vomiting rules out Hirschsprung's disease
      e   a PR examination would be indicated

25   *A female infant is seen for a discharge examination on day 4. She is said to be feeding well and there is no relevant antenatal, family or birth history. The doctor examining her finds an ejection systolic murmur loudest at the lower left sternal edge, grade III. She has a liver palpable at 1.5 cm below the costal margin, and is not cyanosed. Her respiratory rate is 35 per minute*

a the most likely diagnosis is an innocent murmur
b she has no evidence of cardiac failure
c radiation to the back is suggestive of a ventricular septal defect
d a chest X-ray may be useful in her management
e these findings would be compatible with pulmonary stenosis

Knowledge — answers

Neonatology is an interesting subject for the student as it combines some physiology with a range of dramatic diseases that are almost all exclusive to the subspeciality. Questions will be asked on the changes at birth, respiratory distress syndrome, infection, prematurity, statistics, resuscitation, jaundice, and rashes. However, there are many other conditions that may also come up.

1 *Respiratory distress syndrome*
    a affects only infants born under 34 weeks
    b typically causes lobar collapse on chest X-ray
    c is prevented by surfactant therapy
    d usually presents before 5 days of age
    e maternal steroid therapy improves outcome

a **False**. Although increasingly more common with more extreme prematurity, exactly which infant will develop respiratory distress syndrome (RDS) is difficult to predict. In infants whose mothers receive no antenatal steroids, 40% will develop RDS at 30 weeks, 20% at 32 weeks, and under 1% at term. Factors associated with increased incidence include prematurity, Caesarean delivery, birth asphyxia, sepsis, and maternal diabetes. Its incidence is decreased by antenatal steroid administration and in growth-retarded infants.

b **False**. The typical radiographic appearance of RDS is of poor aeration or expansion, air bronchograms, and the ground glass appearance. Lobar collapse is a common consequence of intubation, mucus plugging, or infection. RDS appearances may be indistinguishable from congenital pneumonia.

c **False**. Surfactant therapy has been shown to reduce severity of lung disease in infants, reduces mortality, but has had no impact on disability. It is given via the endotracheal tube.

d **True**. It tends to worsen over the first 3 days and then improves. Transient tachypnoea of the newborn (TTN) is usually worst at birth and then improves over the next day or two.

e **True**. Maternal steroids have had a dramatic impact on the incidence of RDS and its complications. Dexamethasone is given intramuscularly to the mother, but then delivery must be delayed for 48 h for the full effect. It is thought to cause maturation of the surfactant synthesis and water transport systems in the fetal lung, preparing the lung for air breathing.

2   *Infants born prematurely are more likely to*
    a   die from sudden infant death syndrome
    b   have a spastic diplegia
    c   develop laryngomalacia
    d   have fractures
    e   develop right heart failure

a   **True.** The mortality is greatly increased in this group, particularly if the infant goes on to develop chronic lung disease. Sudden infant death syndrome (SIDS) and bronchiolitis are the commonest causes of death after the infant has gone home.

b   **True.** Spastic diplegia is the 'characteristic' type of cerebral palsy (CP) in graduates of the neonatal unit. Following cerebral hypoxia or intraventricular haemorrhage (IVH), both common cerebral events in infants < 32/40, there may be periventricular damage. This is the area where there are fibres running from the cortex to muscles of the lower limb.

c   **True.** Intubation, especially if prolonged, causes mucosal oedema and damage to the cartilage of the trachea. This is one reason why children are intubated with uncuffed endotracheal tubes, to reduce pressure on the trachea mucosa.

d   **True.** Metabolic bone disease is common in premature infants and predisposes to fractures. It is difficult to include enough calcium and phosphate in their intake for their needs at this time of rapid mineralization. Fractures occur most commonly at the wrist during venepuncture.

e   **True.** Right heart failure may occur as a complication of chronic lung disease. Low pulmonary vascular oxygen levels causes pulmonary vasoconstriction. Pulmonary fibrosis also increases the load on the right heart, causing hypertrophy.

3   *These features increase the suspicion of sepsis in a neonate*
    a   maternal fever (> 38.5) during labour
    b   frequent short apnoeas
    c   temperature instability
    d   vomiting
    e   antenatal membrane rupture for 21 h

a   **True.** Infection in the neonate usually presents subtly. Infection is often acquired intrapartum from the mother. Features making this more likely include maternal fever, prolonged rupture of membranes, and an offensive vaginal discharge.

b   **True**. The suggestive signs of sepsis include apnoeas, increasing oxygen requirement, feed intolerance, temperature instability, acidosis, or pallor. Each of these, when considered in their clinical context, may require further investigation.

c   **True**. As for (b).

d   **True**. As for (b).

e   **False**. Short times of membrane rupture are not considered to increase the risk of sepsis. Over 24 h in a preterm infant and over 48 h in a term infant are thought to increase this risk, although there is dispute about this. Most neonatal units perform a septic screen on such infants (FBC, blood cultures, urine culture ± LP, and give intravenous antibiotics for at least 48 h.

> *4   The following definitions are correct*
> > a   the neonatal period is from birth to 1 month of age
> > b   the perinatal period is from 28 weeks gestation to 1 month after birth
> > c   the infant mortality rate is the number of deaths in the first year per 1000 live births
> > d   preterm refers to infants born before their due date
> > e   intrauterine growth retardation means the weight of the newborn infant is below the 3rd percentile for gestational age

a   **True**. This is further split into the early neonatal period (up to 1 week) and late neonatal period (1–4 weeks).

b   **False**. This is from 28 weeks to 1 week after birth.

c   **True**. All the mortality rates are expressed per 1000 live births except perinatal and stillbirth rate, which are expressed per 1000 total deliveries.

d   **False**. This is defined as birth before 37 weeks gestation. Gestation is calculated from the mother's last menstrual period. If an early scan differs by more than 1 week from the mother's dates, the ultrasound dates are used to date the pregnancy and to give an estimated date of delivery.

e   **False**. This is an obstetric definition, based on the age of the intrauterine fetus, and its ultrasound measurements. These are plotted on a fetal growth chart and if under the 10th percentile, the term IUGR (intrauterine growth rate) is used. This is further divided into asymmetrical, where the abdominal circumference is particularly small, and symmetrical, where the whole fetus is proportionally small. The other term used is small for gestational age (SGA), which requires the newborn infants weight and its gestational age, from dates or clinical assessment.

> *5   The following statements are correct*
> > a   infant mortality rate is a marker of socio-economic deprivation
> > b   cerebral palsy is mainly caused by perinatal events
> > c   gestational age at delivery is a better predictor of outcome than birth weight

d   home births have been shown to be statistically more hazardous for the infant than hospital births

e   an infant born at 28 weeks has about a 50% chance of survival

a   **True**. The infant mortality rate (IMR) is used as a measure of social deprivation when comparing different countries. The main causes of death are SIDS, congenital abnormalities, birth asphyxia and infection. This is also discussed in Community paediatrics and development question 1.

b   **False**. About 10% of CP is caused by perinatal events, with a further 10% being caused by prematurity, 40% by postnatal illness (e.g. meningitis, trauma), and 40% by antenatal problems. This last group is least well understood.

c   **False**. Birth weight is the best single indicator.

d   **False**. Although many doctors are reluctant to encourage home deliveries, their scepticism has no statistical support. Maternal and infant mortality did not significantly decrease when there was a major change to hospital births, and now there is a move towards home deliveries where again there has been no significant rise in mortality. However, the deliveries planned for home are usually low risk and numbers are too small to observe a minor change in outcome.

e   **False**. Survival at 28 weeks is above 85% in most units at this gestation. At 26 weeks it is about 50%.

6   *In the first 10 min following birth in a healthy term neonate*
   a   pulmonary vasodilation occurs
   b   surfactant synthesis begins
   c   the ductus arteriosus closes
   d   arterial blood pressure rises
   e   right to left shunts are reduced

a   **True**. At birth the infant takes a breath and expands its lungs. Pulmonary vasodilation occurs as a result of the mechanical stretch of the lungs, the increase in pO_2 and the fall in pCO_2. This allows most of the venous blood to pass through the lungs and the pressures of the right side of the heart to fall. At the same time clamping of the umbilical arteries increases systemic resistance and hence blood pressure. These two pressure changes cause a change in the shunt at the level of the heart to stop the right to left shunt at ductus and foramen ovale.

b   **False**. This has begun before 34 weeks gestation. The presence of surfactant at birth stops the lungs collapsing after each breath and the formation of a functional residual capacity (FRC).

c   **False**. Although little right to left shunting occurs following the changes described in (a), the lumen does not close for several hours. It closes in response to rising oxygen levels and falling prostaglandin levels in the duct. Failure to close is common in preterm infants and is associated with acidosis and hypoxia. Prostaglandin synthetase inhibitors, such as indomethacin, reduce prostaglandin levels and help its closure if the duct is still patent some weeks after birth.

d   **True.** See (a).

e   **True.** See (a).

7   *During neonatal resuscitation*
  a   sodium bicarbonate can be given by an endotracheal tube
  b   atropine is used as the first measure to treat a bradycardia
  c   wrapping the infant is vital to the resuscitation
  d   any meconium should be sucked out of the trachea
  e   a heart rate of 90 is abnormally low

a   **False.** Sodium bicarbonate should only be given intravenously or intra-osseously. Adrenaline can be given in resuscitation via an endotracheal tube (ETT) or intravenously. The dose used in the ETT (0.1 ml/kg of 1 : 1000) is 10 times that used intravenously. Other routes that could be used in neonatal resuscitation include the umbilical vein and the intraosseous route.

b   **False.** The cause of almost all bradycardias in children is hypoxia. The priority in any resuscitation is the airway and breathing, so a bradycardia should be treated with clearing the airway (posture, intubation) and ventilation with a bag and 100% oxygen via mask or ETT.

c   **True.** In postnatal resuscitation the wet infant looses heat at about 0.5 °C/min. This rapidly worsens the chance of a successful resuscitation. The first step when attending any delivery is to dry and wrap the infant and place it under an overhead heater.

d   **True.** Meconium aspiration causes a pneumonitis and physically obstructs gas exchange. Meconium-stained amniotic liquor may occur in the post-term infant, but may also be a sign of fetal hypoxia. This may also cause the fetus to gasp *in utero*, aspirating the meconium. At birth, the meconium should be aspirated from the nose, mouth, and pharynx when the head is on the perineum. The vocal cords should be inspected as soon as the infant is born and if any meconium present, intubation should follow. The trachea may then be aspirated to remove any further meconium.

e   **True.** A normal rate is >100. Under 60 is treated as asystolic and cardiac massage started.

8   *Common indications that an infant has suffered intrapartum hypoxia include*
  a   hypotonia with absent reflexes
  b   poor feeding
  c   seizures
  d   excessive crying
  e   oliguria

a   **True**. Intrapartum hypoxia can cause an encephalopathy, graded 1–3. Hypotonia, no response, absent reflexes, and seizures that are difficult to control are all features of grade 3 (severe) hypoxic encephalopathy.

b   **True**. This is a feature of grade 1 (mild) encephalopathy. Others include jitteriness and being 'hyperalert'. Prognosis is very good. Poor feeding may also be due to poor positioning or maternal problems, such as engorgement, mastitis, or stress.

c   **True**. Grade 2 (moderate) encephalopathy is associated with seizures that are relatively easy to control, as opposed to the intractable seizures of grade 3. Other features include poor suck, lethargy, and mild hypotonia. Prognosis is fairly good, with only 25% having disability with this grade.

d   **True**. Excessive crying is a feature of grade 1 encephalopathy.

e   **True**. Asphyxia can affect other organs, although the brain is particularly sensitive. Acute tubular necrosis (oliguria, haematuria, then polyuria) and myocardial ischaemia with ECG changes are associated with grade 3 asphyxia and complicate the care of these infants.

9   *During intrauterine life the healthy fetus normally*
   a   makes urine
   b   swallows and sucks
   c   has regular breathing movements
   d   can move its limbs by 20 weeks gestation
   e   opens its bowels

a   **True**. Fetal urine is the main component of the amniotic liquor. Urinary tract anomalies that prevent urine production (renal agenesis, obstruction) lead to oligo- or anhydramnios. This, if long-standing causes Potter's syndrome—oligohydramnios, pulmonary hypoplasia, flat face, limb abnormalities due to compression.

b   **True**. The fetus swallows the liquor and absorbs the fluid in its small intestine. This eventually passes across the placenta to be excreted by the mother. This allows further urine to be made without causing polyhydramnios. Conversely, if there is an oesophageal or upper gastrointestinal obstruction (e.g. oesophageal atresia, duodenal atresia), polyhydramnios results.

c   **False**. The fetus 'breathes', that is it makes respiratory movements, but as its lung liquid is much more viscous than air, little fluid is moved. The movements are intermittent, increasing with gestation.

d   **True**. It has to move its limbs to ensure development of the muscles and prevent the formation of contractures and maintain joint mobility. Movements start by 16 weeks gestation.

e   **False**. Bowels are only opened and meconium passed when there is hypoxia, *in-utero* infection (especially *Listeria*) and is the post-term fetus.

10   *The following findings can be regarded as normal when found as part of a newborn examination on day 3*

    a   respiratory rate 35 breaths/min when settled
    b   marked jaundice
    c   milky discharge from the nipple
    d   asymmetric tonic neck reflex
    e   a well demarcated bluish discoloration over the buttocks

a   **True.** The neonate may normally have a respiratory rate up to 40 breaths/min, a 5 year old 25, and a 10 year old 20 breaths/min.

b   **False.** Jaundice affects 50% of infants, and is most commonly physiological. It still requires investigation, as other causes (haemolysis, infection, liver disease, etc.) may require treatment and phototherapy may be needed. Physiological jaundice is caused by the liver having a low rate of bilirubin conjugation after birth and it takes some days for this to develop. The rate is slow because the fetus can only excrete unconjugated bilirubin across the placenta, and so conjugation, although vital after birth, is not needed.

c   **True.** The fetus responds to maternal hormones and small breasts develop, even in boys. Occasionally milk can be expressed from the nipple, inappropriately called 'witch's milk'.

d   **True.** This is one of the primitive reflexes. The head is turned to one side and the arm on that side extends, while the other arm flexes at the elbow. The other reflexes are Moro, stepping, walking, sucking, rooting and truncal incurvation. There is also an upgoing plantar response. Primitive reflexes are listed in Box 5.2.

e   **True.** This is the description of a Mongolian blue spot. Other rashes commonly identified in the neonatal period include erythema toxicum (heat rash), capillary haemangiomas (stork marks), milaria, and milia. Cavernous haemangiomas (strawberry naevi) may be present at birth, but often appear later.

11   *When initiating feeding in a newborn infant*

    a   formula milk should be used before the mother's milk 'comes in'
    b   feeding more often than every 4 h should be discouraged
    c   colostrum provides little IgA for the infant
    d   the sucking reflex is not present in infants born at 37 weeks
    e   fluid requirements on the first day are about 200 ml for a 3.5 kg baby

a   **False.** Although the infant often is not satisfied by colostrum, it should provide for its fluid requirements for the first 3 days, as well as providing growth factors for the gut and some immunological protection. Formula milk alters the gut mucosa and the infant may have more difficulty in suckling from the breast once it has had several feeds from a bottle.

b **False**. Every baby is different in its feeding habit, and 'demand' feeding is now recommended.

c **False**. Colostrum is high in protein as well as IgA.

d **False**. This reflex develops at about 34 weeks gestation. Babies born before 36 weeks usually need nasogastric tube feeding as their sucking is insufficient to provide enough nutrients to grow.

e **True**. This is the day 1 requirement of 60 ml/kg but at 4 days it will need 150 ml/kg per day. An adult will only need about 40 ml/kg per day. The neonate has a high intake to compensate for its poor renal concentrating ability, and to allow a high calorie intake in liquid form. On day 1 it has high antidiuretic hormone (ADH) levels, causing an oliguria. This allows it to tolerate a low intake in the first few days as it gets used to feeding and while its mother's milk supply increases.

12 *These congenital infections commonly cause the associated feature in the newborn*
   a toxoplasmosis—microcephaly
   b rubella—cataracts
   c cytomegalovirus—hydrocephalus
   d chicken pox—scarring
   e chlamydia—pneumonitis

a **True**. Congenital infections share many features, and each has more characteristic manifestations as well. Shared features include hepatosplenomegaly, chorioretinitis, and intrauterine growth retardation. Some also have a rash (not toxoplasma), cataract (especially rubella and varicella), and haematological abnormalities [rubella, cytomegalovirus (CMV), syphilis]. Toxoplasma also causes intracranial calcification and hydrocephalus or microcephaly.

b **True**. Rubella causes micropthalmia, cataracts, patent ductus arteriosus (PDA), and deafness as well as the features listed in (a).

c **False**. CMV causes microcephaly and periventricular calcification.

d **True**. Congenital infection has a high mortality for the fetus, particularly with varicella, which is also a very serious infection for a pregnant woman. This virus causes micropthalmia and cataracts as well as cutaneous scarring.

e **True**. The fetus acquires this sexually transmitted disease at birth. Neonatal manifestations of chlamydia are conjunctivitis and pneumonitis. Treatment is with oral erythromycin and tetracycline eye drops, and appropriate management of the mother and her partner.

13 *These are features commonly found in newborn term infants with uncomplicated Down's syndrome*
   a hypertonia

     b poor feeding
     c asymmetrical growth retardation
     d brachycephaly
     e downslanting palpebral fissures

a   **False**. Down's syndrome in the neonate is not always obvious. Hypotonia is a sensitive but not specific sign.

b   **True**. Almost all Down's babies suck poorly, perhaps due to their hypotonia. Nasogastric feeding is usually needed.

c   **False**. These babies are almost always small, but show symmetrical growth retardation. Asymmetrical growth retardation is usually due to placental insufficiency. The lack of nutrients in the fetus causes the diversion of blood to the head at the expense of the trunk, to preserve brain growth. This reduces trunk growth and increases the incidence of necrotizing enterocolitis (NEC). Energy stores are reduced making the infant more susceptible to hypoglycaemia.

d   **True**. The brain is smaller and this makes the head grow less. Other cranial manifestations include a low hairline, a third fontanelle, a depressed nasal bridge and a protuberant tongue.

e   **False**. They are upslanting in trisomy 21 (going up away from the nose). Noonan's syndrome has downslanting fissures, and fetal alcohol syndrome short fissures.

14 *A infant born at 26 weeks*
     a has less little fat per kilogram than a term neonate
     b requires less fluid per kilogram than a more mature infant
     c should not be given milk until it reaches a corrected age of 34 weeks
     d is at high risk of necrotizing enterocolitis
     e is at high risk of subdural haemorrhage

a   **True**. Fat is one of the many substances including iron and IgG acquired by the fetus during late gestation. Premature delivery leaves the fetus less able to cope without energy intake than a term infant, prone to anaemia and immunologically compromised.

b   **False**. These infants tend to need more fluid than a term infant on a per kilogram basis. Fluid leaks across their permeable skins and they are unable to concentrate urine. Monitoring of the serum sodium is helpful in managing their water balance.

c   **False**. The gut is able to absorb nutrients from much earlier than this. Expressed breast milk feeding via nasogastric or orogastric tube is strongly recommended in premature infants as it decreases the incidence of NEC.

d   **True**. This disease has a high mortality and morbidity and has an incidence related mainly to birth weight. It is thought to be due to gut ischaemia, but tends to only occur after feeding.

e   **False.** The most common intracranial events are intraventricular haemorrhage (bleeding from the choroid plexus) and periventricular leucomalacia, caused by ischaemia.

15   *A baby born at 26 weeks*
   a   is more likely to die from sudden infant death syndrome
   b   is more likely to die from bronchiolitis
   c   has a mortality over 80% in England
   d   is more likely to have parents in low socio-economic groups
   e   has a 70% chance of developing cerebral palsy

a   **True.** Other factors associated with SIDS are cerebral palsy, a smoking mother, not breast feeding, twins, and sleeping prone.

b   **True.** Particularly if the infant has chronic lung disease.

c   **False.** Mortality is about 50% at present.

d   **True.** Premature delivery is strongly associated with social disadvantage.

e   **False.** About 25% will have some neurological deficit, although this may be mild.

16   *These injuries are common following an assisted delivery*
   a   fracture of the clavicle
   b   dislocation of the hip
   c   pulmonary contusion
   d   subconjunctival haemorrhage
   e   seventh cranial nerve palsy

a   **True.** This is often unrecognized by staff and parents and later found on a chest X-ray taken for another reason.

b   **False.** The trunk and legs are rarely damaged during a cephalic delivery. Congenital dislocation of the hip is screened for at the neonatal check with Barlow's and Ortolini's test. This is discussed in Rheumatology and orthopaedics question 2.

c   **False.** This injury requires a severe crushing injury to the chest. Pneumothorax affects 1% of deliveries and is due to the exertion of the first breath.

d   **True.** This is the result of venous congestion of the head and neck, which also causes petechiae.

e   **True.** This may occur as a complication of forceps delivery due to pressure on the nerve. It usually resolves rapidly.

Data interpretation and reasoning — answers

17 *A male infant is born after an uneventful pregnancy at 41 weeks gestation by
emergency Caesarean section. The indication for this was a prolonged fetal
bradycardia. The mother had previously had one Caesarean for breech presentation.
There was thick meconium present in the liquor and a fresh bleed per vaginum. The
infant was noted to have a heart rate of 40 beats/min, was pale, apnoeic, floppy, and
unresponsive.*

a   this infant has an Apgar score of 4
b   external cardiac compressions should be started
c   intravenous atropine would be useful
d   an arterial blood gas will help in the immediate management of the child
e   adrenaline can be given via the umbilical artery

a **False** b **True** c **False** d **False** e **False**

In any case history, there is likely to be irrelevant information, and some that
is vital to answering correctly. Understanding, knowledge, and interpretation of
the features in their context is being tested by these questions, which makes
them much more useful than 'knowledge' questions alone. Having said that, this
question is about neonatal resuscitation, which is fairly standard irrespective of
the preceding events.

The first measure is always drying of the baby, then clearing of the airways. If
the infant is fairly vigorous, nasal and oral suction may suffice, but in the above
situation, the infant needs its airways opened by correct head positioning and then
bag and mask ventilation to attend to its lack of breathing. An alternative approach
would be to intubate and ventilate the baby straight away. It would then be worth
reassessing the circulation. If bradycardic with rate <60, cardiac massage should
start.

If there is no response to intubation, the tube position should be rechecked.
Other strategies at this stage include adrenaline via the ETT or intravenously,
blood or plasma if the infant is shocked, and bicarbonate, although this is controversial. Adrenaline or any other sympathomimetic should never be given into an
artery, as they will cause vasospasm.

Agar scores are of some use in managing resuscitation, but more useful in
predicting long-term outcome when scored at 15 or 20 min. Given the details, this
baby has a score of 1. Atropine is of no use in managing bradycardias caused by
hypoxia (i.e. virtually all paediatric bradycardias).

Arterial blood gases are no help in neonatal resuscitation, and intervention is
based on the response to stimulation, heart rate, and colour of the infant. Blood
gases may be used later to manage ventilation.

18 *An infant age 2 h, born at 32 weeks gestation is in 50% oxygen. He has moderate chest
recession and a respiratory rate of 60 per minute. He has had several apnoeas and
bradycardias in the last hour*

This is his arterial blood gas
pH 7.19
pCO$_2$ 7.5 kPa
pO$_2$ 8.1 kPa
BE — 5.1 mmol/l

  a he has a partially compensated metabolic acidosis
  b intubation and ventilation is indicated
  c following stabilization the first intervention should be surfactant administration
  d antibiotics should be given
  e his recurrent apnoeas can be treated with caffeine or a theophylline

a **False** b **True** c **False** d **True** e **False**

In this scenario, the infant clearly has respiratory distress. The main differential diagnosis is between RDS, TTN, and infection. He is also showing signs of de-compensation—apnoeas and bradycardias. Although these are common before a postconceptual age of 34 weeks, treated with caffeine or theophylline, they may also be a sign of infection, acidosis, gastro-oesophageal reflux, and convulsions. His blood gas shows a high CO$_2$ a negative BE (i.e. excess body acid) and conse-quently he has a mixed metabolic and respiratory acidosis. The first priority is im-provement of his ventilation, either by intubation and ventilation or perhaps trying nasal CPAP (continuous positive airway pressure). Once this is established he may merit surfactant or colloid, but stabilization and reassessment on the ventilator would occur first. Surfactant is usually given via the ETT, although nebulized delivery has been tried. Antibiotics (penicillin and gentamicin) would be given after blood cultures are taken as infection could be the cause of this presentation.

Blood gas interpretation is a frequent cause of stress for the student. Simply, the first step is to identify acidosis or alkalosis from the pH. Then the BE and pCO$_2$ should be examined to see which one is responsible for the change in pH. One can now describe the situation as a respiratory or metabolic acidosis or alkalosis. To look for compensation, the other parameter (that is not causing the pH change) is examined. For instance, in a respiratory acidosis (low pH, high CO$_2$), the BE is now examined. Or in a metabolic alkalosis (high pH, +ve BE), the CO$_2$ is looked at. If there is no compensation, this other parameter is in the normal range. If there is compensation, this parameter is outside the normal range in a direction that reverses the pH change.

Using these principles, one can see there is an acidosis caused by both a high CO$_2$ and a negative BE, and no compensation.

19 *A full-term female infant is mechanically ventilated in 50% oxygen following a surgical procedure for duodenal atresia. Before operation she was self-ventilating in air. An arterial blood gas now shows the following*
    pH 7.51
    pCO$_2$ 2.4 kPa
    pO$_2$ 18.0 kPa
    BE —1.4 mmol/l

a   she is at risk of retinopathy
b   her minute volume is too high
c   she has a respiratory alkalosis
d   she should now be extubated
e   her inspired oxygen should be reduced

a **False** b **True** c **True** d **False** e **True**
This is another blood gas question. There is a high pH, a low CO_2, and an unchanged BE. The pO_2 is high. This is therefore a respiratory alkalosis, also commonly seen in asthma, but here due to overventilation in normal lungs.

In addition to lung disease, CO_2 removal is governed by the amount of gas that moves in and out of the alveoli per minute, related to the minute volume, whereas oxygenation is determined by the pulmonary blood flow, inspired oxygen concentration, and mean airway pressure.

High oxygen levels can cause retinopathy of prematurity in the period before vascularization of the retina (< 32 weeks), and oxygen toxicity particularly in the lungs may occur in any patient given > 85% oxygen for over a day, causing oedema. In this situation, the current oxygen level should be reduced, although it is not particularly harmful to the infant.

Although clearly improving, the infant would not necessarily ready for extubation at this stage

20(i)   *An infant is seen on day 3 for a routine postnatal check. The mother says he has not been breastfeeding well. The SHO examines him and finds he is centrally pink, with a good heart rate, but that he is sleepy, floppy, peripherally cold, and cyanosed. His fontanelle is slightly sunken. His temperature is 36.6°C and respiratory rate 65 per minute with no recession*

a   infection is unlikely with a normal temperature
b   respiratory illness can be ruled out clinically
c   cardiac disease is a likely cause of his signs
d   meningitis can be ruled out
e   acidosis may explain the respiratory rate

a **False** b **False** c **False** d **False** e **True**
The differential diagnosis includes sepsis, metabolic disease, and hypoglycaemia. The high respiratory rate without mention of other signs of respiratory distress suggests a metabolic acidosis. The peripheral cyanosis suggests poor perfusion and perhaps shock.

Infection is difficult to diagnose at this age. Temperature may well be absent, but if present > 38°C is strongly suggestive of infection. Other signs include apnoeas, bradycardias, feed intolerance, poor colour, and increased oxygen needs. A septic screen including a lumbar puncture is then required and appropriate antibiotics should be started.

Respiratory disease does not always present with recession. If a blood gas shows there is no metabolic acidosis, a chest X-ray would be of help to rule out a respiratory problem.

Cardiac disease is possible, with poor perfusion, and pulmonary oedema presenting with tachypnoea. It is rare that it should present at 3 days, and unusual that there is no recession as the oedema increases the work of breathing.

20(ii) *In the above scenario the following test results rapidly become available*
  blood glucose 0.3 mmol/l
  arterial blood gas:
  pH 7.12
  pCO$_2$ 3.1 kPa
  pO$_2$ 10.2 kPa
  BE −17.5 mmol/l
  a he has a metabolic acidosis
  b ventilation is not needed at this stage based on these results
  c ornithine transcarbamylase deficiency may be responsible
  d a bolus of feed is required
  e glucagon is a recognized treatment of resistant hypoglycaemia

a **True** b **True** c **True** d **False** e **True**
These results show hypoglycaemia and a partially compensated metabolic acidosis. This rules out a respiratory problem and makes a metabolic cause more likely but does not rule out sepsis. As his respiratory system is currently compensating well, ventilation will not particularly help at present, but if his condition worsens he may decompensate.

Urgent treatment for his hypoglycaemia is required as it is 'symptomatic', as shown by his floppiness. Other symptoms of hypoglycaemia include fits, jitteriness, and apnoea. Asymptomatic hypoglycaemia (usually defined as below 2.6 mmol/l) requires confirmation with a formal blood glucose if detected on a Dextrostix, and then a bolus of feed. The glucose should be rechecked after 1 h, and if still low a glucose infusion started. If symptomatic, a glucose infusion is needed (10% dextrose) and in the presence of convulsions a bolus of intravenous glucose. This baby sounds too ill to effectively absorb feed from its gut. Hypoglycaemia resistant to this infusion should first be treated by increasing the volume of glucose infusion, then increasing concentration to 15% glucose. Glucagon is useful if there is difficulty with intravenous access and in infants of diabetic mothers (low glucagon levels).

In this scenario, a metabolic defect is the likely cause of the hypoglycaemia, and urea cycle defects (e.g. ornithine transcarbamoylase deficiency) are the commonest.

21 *A woman has delivered at 23 weeks gestation following premature labour and rupture of membranes, which occurred 13 days previously*
  a if the baby is born dead, it is a stillbirth
  b no resuscitation should be offered unless the infant is vigorous
  c if the baby is born dead, the parents should not see it
  d survival in this group is above 25%
  e adrenaline should be the given in the resuscitation

a **False** b **True** c **False** d **False** e **False**

Birth at 23 weeks gestation has a mortality over 95%, with disability levels about 25% in the survivors. Resuscitation is therefore not always appropriate at the very extreme of neonatal survival at present. Most units recommend that an infant should be intubated and ventilated if it is born in good condition with a heart rate and vigorous at 23 weeks, but that adrenaline and other interventions should not be used as they do not improve survival without major disability. Technically, it is a miscarriage or abortion if born showing no signs of life before 28 weeks and a stillbirth thereafter. It is now recommended that parents have time with their stillborn infants, and where appropriate late miscarriage babies, and that they are named, buried, or whatever is culturally appropriate, as this may help recovery from the event.

22   *A term female infant is found by a midwife on day 2 to be feeding poorly, have a temperature of 37.3°C and is floppy and difficult to wake. The infant is admitted to the neonatal unit and some investigations performed*
   CSF RBC 200/mm³   Hb 17.1 g/dl
   WCC 5/mm³   WCC 2.3 × 10³/mm³
   no organisms seen   platelets 15 × 10³/mm³
   a   this result rules out meningitis
   b   the temperature is diagnostic of infection
   c   the platelet count suggest platelet consumption
   d   the white cell count suggests severe infection
   e   antibiotics should be started as soon as culture results are available

a **False** b **False** c **True** d **True** e **False**

This is another sepsis data interpretation question. Neonatal values are different to those of older children, but knowledge of the precise numbers should not be needed at undergraduate level. The CSF obviously shows a high RBC count and a normal WCC. This is against meningitis but does not rule it out. In an adult this would suggest a subdural haemorrhage, but is more likely to be due to the trauma of birth.

Temperature is within the normal range for a neonate, as they are not able to regulate their temperature well. If over 38°C or frequently over 37.5°C, infection is more likely. The FBC shows a normal Hb, which is always high in neonates to compensate for their intrauterine hypoxia. The Hb then falls to 10–11 g/dl by 6 months, then slowly rises until puberty, when it attains its adult value. Both the WCC and platelet count are abnormally low. The platelet count is low in children either because of consumption (DIC—disseminated intravascular coagulation, or immunological, as in immune thrombocytopenic purpura). The low WCC is due to septicaemia, but may also be due to chemotherapy, drugs, or maturational problems.

With a seriously ill patient, there is no time to wait for culture results, so antibiotics (e.g. penicillin and gentamicin) should be started straight away. The main causes of early neonatal infection for all infants are group B streptococcus,

Listeria and Gram-negative organisms. Later on, particularly for preterm babies, staphylococcus and *Candida* become important.

23 **A baby of 36 h age, having been born at 27 weeks has the following results**
    Na^+ *127 mmol/l*
    K^+ *3.2 mmol/l*
    urea 1.2 mmol/l

    a   these could be explained by a low urine water output
    b   fluid restriction will help to correct the problem
    c   these results can be explained by a high evaporative loss from the skin
    d   inadequate sodium in the fluids is a likely cause
    e   these results may simply reflect the mothers blood electrolytes

a **True** b **True** c **False** d **False** e **False**

The same normal range for electrolytes applies to neonates. However, the urea and creatinine levels tend to be much lower (<7.5 mmol/l and <50 μmol/l, respectively). The result above shows a low sodium and potassium. This may be due to a sampling error, but in this context is also likely to be due to water overload. Water overload may be due to excess intravenous fluid or inappropriate ADH secretion. These may be distinguished by examining urine volume and concentration. Newborn infants very commonly secrete excess ADH, and so are prone to water overload. The best treatment is moderate fluid restriction and rechecking the electrolytes after 12 h.

The normal ADH surge at birth may have developed to allow time for feeding to be established, and certainly infants need much less feed in the first few days. (60 ml/kg on the first day, rising to 150 ml/kg by the fourth). After the first week, lack of sodium in the intake is a more likely cause of hyponatraemia, as the kidneys are poor at reabsorbing sodium at this age. Normal requirements are 2–3 mmol/kg per day, falling to 1–2 mmol/kg per day by 1 year. The requirements of potassium are almost identical.

The permeability of the skin causes water to evaporate, leading to hypernatraemia, and this can be countered with the use of humidity in incubators.

Maternal and fetal values of most ions and small molecules are similar, and following birth there is some relation for the first 24 h. Glucose diffuses freely across the placenta, allowing maternal diabetes to cause a high insulin level in the fetus (consequently macrosomia and neonatal hypoglycaemia). IgG and iron are actively transported across the placenta in the last trimester.

24 **A term male is vomiting on day 2. The pregnancy and delivery have been entirely
    normal. On direct questioning, he has yet to pass meconium**

    a   the presence of abdominal distension is suggestive of bowel obstruction
    b   a small amount of milky vomiting soon after the feed over his face is normal, in
        the absence of any other findings
    c   a family history of coeliac disease is relevant to this case
    d   bilious vomiting rules out Hirschsprung's disease
    e   a PR examination is would be indicated

a **True** b **True** c **False** d **False** e **True**

Vomiting in the neonatal period is usually possetting or due to gastro-oesophageal reflux, but may be a manifestation of sepsis or obstruction. Obstruction at this age is due to atresia (e.g. duodenal), meconium ileus, Hirschsprung's disease, or mal-rotation/volvulus. Pyloric stenosis presents later (3–6 weeks), intussusception at 6–9 months and coeliac disease at 6 months and beyond.

Differentiation in the neonatal period requires a careful history and examination. Of particular note is the nature of the vomiting (possetting is described in part b), the timing of the vomiting (more significant if some time after a feed), whether it is bile stained and if there is any distension. Distension does not always occur, particularly with upper gastrointestinal obstruction. Most babies pass meconium (and urine) on the first day. If there are other features of note it may be significant that they have not passed meconium. A PR examination to feel for anal tone and to help empty a loaded rectum may be useful.

If there is concern about obstruction, a plain abdominal X-ray may be helpful (e.g. the double bubble of duodenal stenosis, dilated loops, abnormal gas pattern). A contrast meal and follow through will identify malrotation.

25 *A female infant is seen for a discharge examination on day 4. She is said to be feeding well and there is no relevant antenatal, family or birth history. The doctor examining her finds an ejection systolic murmur loudest at the lower left sternal edge, grade III. She has a liver palpable at 1.5 cm below the costal margin, and is not cyanosed. Her respiratory rate is 35 per minute*

   a the most likely diagnosis is an innocent murmur
   b she has no evidence of cardiac failure
   c radiation to the back is suggestive of a ventricular septal defect
   d a chest X-ray may be useful in her management
   e these findings would be compatible with pulmonary stenosis

a **False** b **True** c **False** d **True** e **True**

The most common causes of murmurs found in the neonatal period are innocent murmurs, ventricular septal defects (VSDs), PDAs, and pulmonary stenosis. Innocent murmurs are always soft, grade II or less, precordial, without radiation, and not associated with any other sign.

Cardiac failure in childhood presents as tachypnoea, hepatomegaly with tachycardia, sweatiness, and pallor. A liver edge palpable at 3 cm would be normal in a neonate. The spleen tip is also often palpable and the kidneys can be felt before feeding is established in some normal infants.

The individual conditions all have characteristic features, although distinguishing them in practise is more difficult. VSDs are pansystolic and precordial, radiating to the epigastrium. PDAs are best heard in the left subclavicular region, radiating to the back. Coarctation of the aorta is best heard in the upper sternum and radiates to the back. Pulmonary stenosis is best heard in the upper right sternum and radiates to the lungs.

2 Heart disease

Knowledge—questions

1 *The ductus arteriosus*
   a closes soon after the first breath
   b allows right to left shunting in the fetus
   c is closed by the action of a prostaglandin
   d is associated with a murmur audible in diastole
   e usually requires surgical closure

2 *Complications of a ventricular septal defect include*
   a cardiorespiratory failure
   b hepatomegaly
   c systemic hypertension
   d cerebral abscess
   e endocarditis

3 *The following investigations will identify the associated problems*
   a chest X-ray—pulmonary plethora
   b ECG—Wolff–Parkinson–White syndrome
   c nitrogen washout test—left to right shunt
   d four limb blood pressure—aortic stenosis
   e echocardiograph—pulmonary hypertension

4 *A 4-year-old child with congenital cyanotic heart disease is likely to*
   a be tachypnoeic
   b have hepatomegaly
   c be peripherally cyanosed
   d be dependent on ductal flow
   e have right ventricular hypertrophy

5 *An infant of 6 weeks with early congestive cardiac failure*
   a respiratory difficulty may be seen on examination
   b may have Fallot's tetralogy
   c may have excessive weight gain
   d often presents with failure to thrive
   e may have oligaemic lung fields

6   *In children with uncorrected Fallot's tetralogy*
   a   the ECG commonly shows right axis deviation
   b   Eisenmenger's syndrome may develop
   c   palliation requires creation of a left to right shunt
   d   a right to left shunt occurs at the ventricular level
   e   pulmonary artery blood flow is reduced

7   *When examining the cardiovascular system of a newborn term infant*
   a   peripheral cyanosis is common in the first hours and should be ignored
   b   a low blood pressure may be caused by sepsis
   c   heart murmurs are usually innocent at this age and should be ignored
   d   the carotid arteries should be felt to determine pulse character
   e   a liver palpable 1.5 cm below the costal margin may indicate heart failure

8   *Asystole*
   a   is the commonest ECG finding in paediatric cardiac arrests
   b   adenosine may be useful in its treatment
   c   a precordial thump should be performed
   d   often occurs following a respiratory arrest
   e   adrenaline is useful in its treatment

9   *These features are compatible with the following diagnoses in a child
     with a heart murmur*
   a   hyperdynamic precordium with a ventricular septal defect
   b   narrow pulse pressure and pulmonary stenosis
   c   a murmur radiating to the right carotid in coarctation of the aorta
   d   bounding pulses with a patent ductus arteriosus
   e   loud second sound in a ventricular septal defect

Data interpretation and reasoning—questions

10(i)   *A 3-week-old infant is seen by his family doctor as he is feeding
         poorly. The doctor finds that he has a heart rate of 260 beats/min,
         a respiratory rate of 60 breaths/min, a capillary filling time of
         3–4 s and a blood pressure of 40/25 mmHg*
   a   the prolonged filling time is likely to be due to dehydration
   b   the respiratory rate is probably raised because of cardiac failure
   c   the blood pressure is within the normal range
   d   a severe respiratory infection might be the cause
   e   poor feeding is a rare presentation for cardiac disease at this age

10(ii)   *He is referred to the local hospital for further assessment and treatment by the paediatricians. They find that, although the heart rate is 250, the capillary filling time is 2 s, and blood pressure 65/45 mmHg. Given these findings*

    a   ventricular tachycardia is the most likely diagnosis
    b   adenosine is a useful diagnostic and therapeutic agent
    c   carotid massage would be helpful
    d   maternal systemic lupus erythematosus may be the cause for the baby's arrhythmia
    e   head submersion in cold water can be used as the first approach to therapy

11   *At a hospital clinic appointment arranged because a 10-week-old child was failing to thrive, the doctor detects a heart murmur. The following features suggest a cardiac rather than another cause for his failure to thrive*

    a   murmur grade II, loudest over the precordium
    b   poor peripheral perfusion
    c   vomiting
    d   tachypnoea
    e   splenomegaly

12   *A 3-year-old girl is seen because she is unwell with a high temperature. She is known to have a ventricular septal defect. The casualty officer sees her and finds that she has a temperature of 39.1°C and a heart murmur. Infective endocarditis is made a more likely diagnosis because she*

    a   has microscopic haematuria
    b   has bounding pulses
    c   has sickle cell anaemia
    d   has a murmur loudest at the lower left sternal edge
    e   has splenomegaly

13(i)   *During a clinic visit a 6-week-old girl is found to have an ejection systolic murmur. Her heart rate is 145 beats/min, and her pulse character is normal. She has been following the 10th percentile and is breastfeeding well. Significant cardiac disease is made more likely if she also has*

    a   radiation of the murmur to the back
    b   a liver edge at 1.5 cm below the costal margin

   c a thrill
   d webbing of the neck
   e a respiratory rate of 30

13(ii) *She is referred to the hospital for further evaluation. Some*
investigations are performed
chest X-ray—increased cardiothoracic ratio, normal lung fields
ECG normal axis, no evidence of strain or conduction disturbance
four limb blood pressures: right arm 90/65; left arm 88/66; right
    leg 45/30; left leg 47/35
Based on these results and the above history and examination
   a she is not in cardiac failure
   b she probably has coarctation of the aorta
   c her normal ECG has excluded any cardiac disease
   d she is hypertensive
   e her presentation has been precipitated by closure of the ductus

14(i) *A term female infant is seen at the request of the midwife at 72 h*
of age. She has noticed that the baby has a blue tinge to her lips and
nailbeds. The colour deepens during feeding. The doctor finds that the
baby is alert but centrally cyanosed with a heart rate of 135 beats/
min and a respiratory rate of 35 breaths/min. There is minimal
respiratory distress. Auscultation reveals no heart murmur but a
single second sound. The breath sounds are equal and there are no
added sounds
   a the cyanosis may be caused by a high haemoglobin concentration
   b the single second sound may be due to similar pressures in the aorta and
      pulmonary artery
   c she is likely to be septic
   d the mother's use of phenytoin during pregnancy for her epilepsy may be
      linked to this presentation
   e the absence of a murmur makes a non-cardiac cause more likely than a
      cardiac cause for her illness

14(ii) *The infant is admitted to the neonatal unit for further evaluation.*
The following tests are performed
arterial blood gas (right radial):
pH 7.38
pCO$_2$ 3.9 kPa

pO₂ 3.7 kPa

BE − 4.2 mmol/l

chest X-ray normal

*four limb blood pressures: right arm 43/25; left arm 45/23; right
    leg 41/17; left leg 42/19*

    a she may have coarctation of the aorta

    b a significant left-to-right shunt may be responsible

    c she may have persistent pulmonary hypertension of the newborn

    d a hyperoxic (nitrogen washout) test would now be of value

    e the blood gas result confirms she has respiratory disease

Knowledge — answers

Paediatric heart disease is a particularly common topic for examiners to focus on. It is common (about 1/50 individuals will have an identifiable lesion at some point in their childhood) and it is important in terms of morbidity, mortality, hospital attendances, and resources. Fortunately, it is also easy to understand at a simple level once the anatomy and a few bits of physiology are assimilated.

Almost all of paediatric cardiology is to do with *congenital* lesions, and there are only two rare *acquired* conditions that need any mention—Kawasaki's disease and rheumatic fever/heart disease. The congenital lesions are conveniently split into acyanotic and cyanotic.

Questions can be asked about the conditions themselves, or questions can relate to presentation or management issues. In cardiology this will be with a child in heart failure, with a murmur that needs evaluation and with a cyanotic child.

    1 The ductus arteriosus

        a closes soon after the first breath

        b allows right to left shunting in the fetus

        c is closed by the action of a prostaglandin

        d is associated with a murmur audible in diastole

        e usually requires surgical closure

a   **False.** One of the bits of physiology that you need to know about is the cardio-vascular changes at birth. The fetal circulation is designed to minimize blood going to the lungs to a level that enables growth. Only about 10% of fetal cardiac output goes there. Pulmonary vasoconstriction restricts pulmonary blood flow and there are two mechanisms that shunt blood from the right side of the heart to the left—the foramen ovale and the ductus arteriosus. The fetus also sends about

40% of cardiac output to the placenta via the twin umbilical arteries so there is a relatively low systemic resistance.

At birth there is a large increase in pulmonary blood flow. Pulmonary vasodilation occurs as a result of the mechanical action of lung inflation as well as the changes in pO_2 and pCO_2. This lowers pulmonary artery pressure. It also raises left atrial pressure as more blood is returning to the left atrium. Also umbilical flow ceases so systemic vascular resistance increases, raising the systemic pressure. The combined action of these changes is to stop shunting at the atrial and ductal levels, although it is some time before the ductus fully closes.

Ductal closure is caused by a rise in pO_2 and mediated by falling levels of prostaglandins and occurs in the hours after delivery. Its closure may not happen if there is hypoxia, acidosis, or the infant is premature.

b   **True.** The ductus allows right to left shunting in the fetus because the pulmonary artery pressure is slightly higher than the aortic pressure in the fetus. After birth, pulmonary pressure falls and aortic pressure rises. So if the ductus remains patent after birth, the flow is left to right and there is excessive pulmonary blood flow and leading to congestive cardiac failure (see question 5). This explains the nature of the murmur, which is classically heard below the left clavicle and radiates through to the back. This is because the aorta overlies the pulmonary artery at the position of the ductus, which points towards the left scapula. The murmur is loudest in systole but can be heard in diastole, and is thus called 'machinery' in character. This is because there is a pressure gradient across the ductus throughout the cardiac cycle, greatest during systole.

c   **False.** Prostaglandin E_2 maintains the ductus in its open state, and a fall in its level assists ductal closure. This piece of physiology is exploited in two ways. First, in 'duct-dependent' cardiac lesions the ductus is required to keep the child alive. Here the ductus is allowing some deoxygenated blood to reach the lungs (as in pulmonary atresia, transposition of the great arteries) or blood to reach the systemic circulation (hypoplastic left heart). A prostaglandin infusion can be used to maintain ductal patency as a temporary measure before some surgical palliation is possible. In the situation where there is a patent ductus arteriosus (PDA), prostaglandin levels can be reduced by using a prostaglandin synthetase inhibitor such as indomethacin in an effort to medically close the ductus.

d   **True.** A diastolic murmur is unusual in children. Other causes include aortic or pulmonary incompetence and tricuspid or mitral stenosis. These are all uncommon. Much more common is a venous hum, caused by turbulence in the great veins.

e   **False.** Most PDAs close spontaneously during the first day of life. Of those that do not, most close in the first week, especially if any other conditions are treated. If the ductus is still patent, fluid restriction reduces the flow across the duct and its effects and thus aids closure. Indomethacin can be used if there is still a significant PDA, and if this fails the ductus would then be clipped surgically.

2   *Complications of a ventricular septal defect include*
   a cardiorespiratory failure
   b hepatomegaly
   c systemic hypertension
   d cerebral abscess
   e endocarditis

a   **True.** Congenital cardiac lesions in children can be understood fairly easily at a basic level. They can be split into acyanotic and cyanotic lesions. Essentially a cyanotic lesion is one in which insufficient blood is getting from the lungs to the systemic circulation. There might therefore be a problem with the tubes going from the body to the lungs as in pulmonary atresia (PA) or stenosis (PS), transposition of the great arteries (TGA), Fallot's tetralogy, or tricuspid atresia (TA). This leads to a right to left shunt. Alternatively, there might be a problem with the tubes connecting lungs to body as in totally anomalous pulmonary venous drainage (TAPVD).

Acyanotic lesions include every other type of cardiac lesion, and their common feature is that there is enough blood going to the lungs and returning to the body to keep the child pink. There is usually a problem with the left side of the heart and may be blockage to outflow as in aortic stenosis (AS) or coarctation of the aorta; alternatively, there may be a hole that connects the left and right side of the heart. As the left-sided pressure is higher than the right, this will produce a left to right shunt. This gives rise to a murmur, and increases right-sided pressure and ultimately causes right heart failure. The increase in flow through the lungs leads to pulmonary oedema and overloads the left side of the heart leading to left heart failure. Conditions in which all this occurs include ventricular septal defect (VSD), PDA, truncus arteriosus, and to a lesser extent an atrial septal defect (ASD).

b   **True.** Left to right shunts lead to raised systemic venous pressure. This manifests as hepatomegaly, oedema, and ascites. The liver of children is much more able to expand than that of an adult, and enlargement is easily felt, so the size of the liver is a good sign of right heart overload (heart failure or excess fluid). Dependent oedema in an infant is usually found in the sacral area, not in the ankles as in an adult.

c   **False.** A VSD will cause pulmonary hypertension but not systemic hypertension. Coarctation is the only *cardiac* condition that will. An acyanotic lesion may produce hypotension if the shunt is sufficiently large and the left heart is failing, or may cause a wide pulse pressure as in a PDA.

Pulmonary hypertension is the most serious long-term consequence of left to right shunts. In response to the raised pressure, the pulmonary arterial wall hypertrophies in an effort to restrict flow. This process becomes irreversible and leads to a progressive rise in pulmonary arterial pressure. Eventually, the pressure on the right side of the shunt is the same as that on the left. At that stage the shunt reverses and starts going right to left, and the patient becomes progressively more cyanosed, eventually dying from right heart failure. This scenario is termed Eisenmenger's syndrome. The speed at which it develops is related to the volume of the shunt and other factors (Down's children develop pulmonary hypertension more quickly).

d **True.** A cerebral abscess may either occur as a result of local infection (meningitis, otitis media, sinusitis) or be haematogenous. Haematogenous spread tends to go as far as the next vascular bed, so an abscess on the finger might cause a pulmonary abscess, or a pulmonary abscess might lead to a systemic abscess. *Staphylococcus aureus* is a common causative organism. If there is a right to left shunt (as in Fallot's or when Eisenmenger's syndrome has complicated a VSD), blood from the body may go directly to the brain, and therefore haematogenous spread may occur there. Also VSDs may be complicated by endocarditis and this may cause emboli.

e **True.** Endocarditis will unusually occur in normal undamaged hearts, caused by *Staph. aureus*. More commonly, the turbulent flow around an abnormal valve or a septal defect or a PDA causes damage to the endocardium and this allows organisms to enter and replicate. Children with congenital heart disease should receive penicillin prophylaxis if they have dental treatment or invasive procedures. *Streptococcus viridans*, *Staph. aureus*, *Strep. pneumoniae*, and other streptococci are the commonest causative organisms.

Endocarditis is suspected when there is a changing murmur, unexplained and persistent fever, embolic phenomena such as multiple abscesses and evidence of immunological activity, such as haematuria and splenomegaly.

3 The following investigations will identify the associated problems
    a   chest X-ray—pulmonary plethora
    b   ECG—Wolff–Parkinson–White syndrome
    c   nitrogen washout test—left to right shunt
    d   four limb blood pressure—aortic stenosis
    e   echocardiograph—pulmonary hypertension

a **True.** When investigating the heart of a child with a suspected problem, the doctor has only a few tools. The chest X-ray will show how much or how little blood is going to the lungs. On the film, the lungs can be divided up into the third nearest the heart, the middle third, and the peripheral third. Blood vessels should be seen in the first two-thirds but not the peripheral third. If there is too much blood in the lungs, it is termed pulmonary plethora (like upper lobe blood diversion, but in a supine infant). This is a sign of left heart failure. There may be associated pulmonary oedema. If there is a cyanotic condition in which there is too little blood going to the lungs, this may be seen as pulmonary oligaemia.

The size and shape of the heart can also be seen on the chest X-ray. Because an infant's chest is much smaller than an adult's, size can be estimated on an antero-posterior (AP) film as well as a posterior–anterior (PA) film. The cardiothoracic ratio should be under 50% (55% under 1 year), as in an adult. If it is greater than this, it is likely that there is a higher filling pressure or an outflow obstruction (AS or coarctation).

The shape of the cardiac outline can provide diagnostic information. Right ventricular hypertrophy causes the apex to look uptilted on the X-ray, and a small pulmonary artery may make the upper part of the heart look narrow. Together this produces the boot-shaped heart found in Fallot's tetralogy. Transposition of the great arteries produces the egg-on-side-shaped mediastinum. Pericardial effusions cause a water-bottle (globular) shaped heart.

However, this investigation is usually normal unless the child is symptomatic.

b   **True.** The ECG will inform about rhythm and conduction disturbances quite well, but is usually normal in VSDs, PDAs, and most common lesions. However, ASDs often are associated with a conduction defect. In Wolff–Parkinson–White (WPW), the ECG in sinus rhythm shows a d-wave, that is a slurred upstroke of the QRS complex which widens the QRS complex. It represents ventricular pre-excitation caused by conduction to the ventricles through the fast conducting bundle of Kent. This condition can lead to supraventricular tachycardia.

c   **False.** The nitrogen washout or hyperoxic test distinguishes between systemic hypoxia caused by inadequate pulmonary blood flow (e.g. pulmonary atresia) and that caused by pulmonary disease. The patient is placed in 100% oxygen and the arterial pO_2 monitored. If the child has inadequate pulmonary blood flow, the blood leaving the lungs will be fully saturated and raising inspired oxygen will do little to increase oxygen delivery to the body and hence pO_2. If there is respiratory disease, there is enough blood leaving the lungs, but it is just not containing enough oxygen. By increasing the alveolar pO_2, more diffuses into the blood and hence there is a rise in systemic pO_2 is seen of at least 15 kPa (113 mmHg) in the pre-ductal blood. Therefore, this test will distinguish between a right to left shunt and a respiratory problem. The only exception is persistent pulmonary hypertension of the newborn (see question 5 of the Data interpretation and reasoning section).

d   **False.** The four limb blood pressure is a useful test for diagnosis of coarctation of the aorta. Here the blood pressure in the arms (especially the right) is higher than that in the legs because of the obstruction in the aorta. AS has a narrow pulse pressure.

e   **True.** The echocardiograph is a very good tool for looking at the structure and dynamic function of the heart and will diagnose any structural defect in the heart. Also by doing calculations based on the rate of flow at a particular part of the heart and the size of the lumen, a pressure difference can be established.

4   A 4-year-old child with congenital cyanotic heart disease is likely to
  a   be tachypnoeic
  b   have hepatomegaly
  c   be peripherally cyanosed
  d   be dependent on ductal flow
  e   have right ventricular hypertrophy

a   **False.** A child with cyanotic heart disease is blue because of poor blood flow from the lungs to the systemic circulation. There is nothing wrong with the lungs themselves. Tachypnoea may be a sign of lung disease with normal blood gases (asthma, pulmonary oedema) or of abnormal blood chemistry (acidosis, high pCO_2). The pO_2 does not affect the respiratory centre until it is very low.

These facts are useful clinically as cyanosed children with few respiratory signs usually have a cardiac problem whereas those with marked signs usually have respiratory or metabolic disease.

b   **False.** Hepatomegaly is the result either of liver enlargement caused by liver disease (hepatitis, storage disorders) or systemic venous congestion. The liver may also be palpable because of lung hyperexpansion.

In children with cyanotic heart disease there is rarely a problem with systemic venous congestion until there is end-stage disease. There is a right to left shunt, but there is usually no obstruction. On the other hand acyanotic heart disease with a left to right shunt often causes hepatomegaly, due to right ventricular failure.

c   **True.** Of course the child will be peripherally cyanosed. There are no conditions which have central cyanosis but not peripheral cyanosis. However, there may be peripheral cyanosis without central cyanosis in situations where there is poor peripheral perfusion (dehydration, hypovolaemia, cold).

Cyanosis needs about 5 g/dl of deoxyhaemoglobin, which can happen at a saturation of 75% in a neonate (Hb concentration about 20 g/dl) and at about 50% in an older child (Hb concentration more like 10 g/dl).

d   **False.** Cyanotic heart disease may be 'duct dependent', but it is extremely unlikely at the age of 4. Duct dependent lesions are discussed in question 1

e   **True.** Ventricular hypertrophy will occur if there is prolonged excessive work for the muscle to do. In cyanotic heart disease the right ventricle has to pump blood at systemic pressure across a right to left shunt and so the hypertrophy develops. It will also develop if there is outflow obstruction (pulmonary stenosis). Left ventricular hypertrophy develops with aortic stenosis, coarctation, or hypertension.

Right atrial hypertrophy is a common complication of right ventricular hypertrophy and lung disease.

   5   *An infant of 6 weeks with early congestive cardiac failure*
   a   respiratory difficulty may be seen on examination
   b   may have Fallot's tetralogy
   c   may have excessive weight gain
   d   often presents with failure to thrive
   e   may have oligaemic lung fields

a   **True.** Congestive cardiac failure occurs in an infant when there is left heart failure and right heart failure, caused most often by acyanotic heart lesion with a left to right shunt (VSD, PDA, truncus arteriosus, and coarctation with a septal defect). The excessive pulmonary blood flow overloads the left heart and leads to a raised pulmonary venous pressure. This produces interstitial and ultimately alveolar oedema. This makes the lungs stiff so that recession will be noted on respiratory examination, and raises the respiratory rate.

b **False.** Fallot's tetralogy (pulmonary stenosis, overriding aorta, VSD, and right ventricular hypertrophy) results from unequal division of the embryological truncus arteriosus and malalignment with the developing ventricular septum. It is a cyanotic condition as the right ventricular outflow is shunted to the systemic circulation. Neither ventricle is acutely overloaded so no congestive cardiac failure can develop.

c **True.** The weight may increase because of oedema, the result of systemic venous congestion. Being dependent oedema, it is typically sacral.

d **True.** Even though there may be oedema and weight gain, a more common presentation is with failure to thrive. There are plenty of reasons why as congestive cardiac failure increases energy expenditure (increased cardiac and respiratory work due to the shunt and pulmonary oedema, respectively) and reduces energy intake (poor feeding).

e **False.** He will have plethoric lung fields because of the increased pulmonary blood flow. Oligaemic fields are found with cyanotic heart lesions.

6 *In children with uncorrected Fallot's tetralogy*
    a the ECG commonly shows right axis deviation
    b Eisenmenger's syndrome may develop
    c palliation requires creation of a left to right shunt
    d a right to left shunt occurs at the ventricular level
    e pulmonary artery blood flow is reduced

a **True.** Axis deviation is one of the important things to look for on a paediatric ECG. Where the axis is depends on the relative size of the muscle mass in the left and right ventricles, so a hypertrophied right ventricle (part of the tetralogy) will cause right axis deviation. Left ventricular outflow obstruction will similarly cause a left axis deviation.

The axis is calculated from the relative sizes of lead I and AVF. You can work it out exactly using vectors or you can look for an isoelectric lead and say the axis is about 90° away from this. In newborns the mean axis is +135° with a wide normal range, but by 6 weeks is +80°. By 4 years it is in the adult range. This reflects the right ventricle becoming relatively smaller as it no longer needs to pump at systemic pressure, as it does in the fetus.

A more basic approach is to see if leads I and AVF show a positive deflection. In a neonate, AVF should be positive. If negative in its deflection, this is always abnormal, and implies major structural or conductive abnormalities. In older children, both I and AVF should be positive.

b **False.** As discussed above, Eisenmenger's syndrome is the consequence of a reversal of a left to right shunt as a result of progressive pulmonary hypertension.

Fallot's never has a left to right shunt, but children with VSDs, PDAs, and even ASDs may go on to develop Eisenmenger's.

c   **True.** The immediate problem with Fallot's children is that there is insufficient blood reaching the lungs. This tends to present as cyanosis in the first few months of life as the duct finally closes (closure is delayed if there is hypoxia). Corrective surgery is technically difficult at this stage, and so a left to right shunt is created to take systemic blood and divert it into the pulmonary vascular tree. The best known shunt is the Blalock–Taussig shunt, which takes a subclavian artery and connects it to a pulmonary artery. It leaves a thoracotomy scar and a continuous shunt murmur under the clavicle. It can be done on either side. This allows the infant to grow (albeit a bit cyanosed) until big enough for corrective surgery.

d   **True.** There is an obstruction to right ventricle outflow via the pulmonary artery and a VSD, so the right ventricle pumps blood straight into the left ventricle and aorta, in a right to left shunt.

e   **True.** As discussed above flow is reduced. Children with Fallot's also suffer 'spelling' in which there is pulmonary infundibular spasm. This acutely reduces the blood flow to the lungs and the child becomes more hypoxic. It is relieved either by raising systemic resistance (squatting or other manoeuvres that flex the hips) or by relieving the infundibular spasm (propranolol, morphine, correcting acidosis).

7   *When examining the cardiovascular system of a newborn term infant*
    a   peripheral cyanosis is common in the first hours and should be ignored
    b   a low blood pressure may be caused by sepsis
    c   heart murmurs are usually innocent at this age and should be ignored
    d   the carotid arteries should be felt to determine pulse character
    e   a liver palpable 1.5 cm below the costal margin may indicate heart failure

a   **True.** A useful system for the routine examination of the cardiovascular system (CVS) is shown in Box 2.1. The presence of centrally cyanosis is determined by looking at the lips and tongue, peripheral cyanosis from the nailbeds. If the patient is blue, there is either a cardiovascular or a respiratory problem, and these can be distinguished by the presence or absence of other respiratory signs. If the newborn is blue because of heart disease, a precordial heave, single second sound, and a murmur may be found. In older children it is always worth looking for the thoracotomy scar used to make a shunt.

On the other hand peripheral cyanosis affecting hands and feet is normal for the first day and simple reflects poor peripheral circulation.

b   **True.** Neonatal sepsis can lead to a death in a very short time. The neonate has limited immunity and septicaemia with group B streptococcus, *Listeria* and Gram negatives is relatively common. The blood pressure falls because there may be vasodilation, poor cardiac output, and a capillary leak of plasma. Acidosis develops which further reduces cardiac output. Septic neonates need volume

Box 2.1   Scheme for the examination of the cardiovascular system

Is the child blue or pink?
Are there scars (thoracotomy or sternotomy)?
Heart rate, fast, slow, or normal?
Tachycardic or with respiratory distress?
Visible cardiac impulse?
Thrills or heave?
Murmur present?
Grade and timing of the murmur
Heart sounds I and II character
Other added sounds?
Hepatomegaly or peripheral oedema?
Femoral arteries—palpable?
Pulse character
Blood pressure

expansion to boost preload for the heart and ionotropes to increase contractility as well as other supportive measures. Deciding which is needed at a particular time is not always easy, especially as most newborns do not have a central venous line to determine preload! They do have the liver, so that if the liver is not enlarged and the blood pressure low with poor perfusion, volume is needed, whereas if the liver is enlarged ionotropes are probably needed.

Other causes for a low blood pressure (a rough guide is that the mean pressure in mmHg should be above the gestation in weeks) include prematurity and haemorrhage.

c   **False**. Distinguishing innocent and pathological murmurs is a very common topic in examinations. An innocent murmur is one associated with no cardiac disease and usually represents turbulent blood in the great veins or blood flow across aortic or pulmonary valves. The characteristics of innocent murmurs are that they are short, systolic, precordial and do not radiate, and are not associated with a thrill or any other signs of cardiac disease. They often alter with posture.

In the neonatal period there are often heart murmurs particularly caused by the closing duct. Even if a murmur in the newborn period is 'innocent' in character, there should still be some investigations as the murmur may be the start of a congenital heart disease presentation in a rapidly changing neonatal circulation. An ECG and chest X-ray can be done initially and if abnormal or if the baby symptomatic, an echocardiogram performed.

If a murmur is discovered in an older child that is innocent in character, it is not always necessary to investigate, because the CVS is more stable and the murmur is not likely to be the presentation of a more serious illness.

d   **False**. It is very difficult to feel the carotids in a neonate as their necks are short and fat! Pulse character is best felt in the femorals or brachial arteries. Pulse character is useful to help diagnose PDAs aortic stenosis and coarctation.

e   **False**. This is normal. Over 3 cm would be considered abnormal and evidence of possibly cardiac failure.

8   *Asystole*
   a   is the commonest ECG finding in paediatric cardiac arrests
   b   adenosine may be useful in its treatment
   c   a precordial thump should be performed
   d   often occurs following a respiratory arrest
   e   adrenaline is useful in its treatment

a   **True**. The commonest adult arrhythmia causing circulatory arrest is ventricular fibrillation (VF). This is generated by diseased myocardium. In children myocardial disease is uncommon and the commonest arrest arrhythmia is asystole, usually secondary to hypoxia. Electromechanical dissociation, secondary to hypovolaemia or pneumothorax is less common but commoner than VF. The commonest arrhythmia caused by cardiac disease is a supraventricular tachycardia.

A 'sinus arrhythmia' is the name given to the rise and fall in heart rate during the respiratory cycle. Heart beats are closer together during expiration. The loss of sinus arrythmia is seen with autonomic nervous system dysfunction.

b   **False**. Adenosine is a blocker of the A/V node and has a very short half-life. Its only function is in the evaluation and treatment of 'narrow complex tachycardias' in which the child is cardiovascularly stable. As the narrow complex reflects synchronous depolarization of the ventricles, the impulse must be carried normally across the myocardium. This means these tachycardias are usually atrial in origin but are occasionally ventricular. If atrial, they involve a wave of depolarization cycling through the A/V node. Administration of adenosine temporarily blocks the conduction and slows the tachycardia if the tachycardia is supraventricular.

If the child is cardiovascularly compromised, synchronous d.c. cardioversion is required.

c   **False**. The only role of a precordial thump is at the onset of VF. It is reasonable to try a thump if there is no cardiac output following a witnessed collapse in the community *in an adult* as VF is by far the most likely cause. The only children who have VF are those who have had cardiac surgery.

d   **True**. Epiglottitis, severe asthma, bronchiolitis, and inhaled foreign bodies are common precursors to cardiac arrest.

e   **True**. Adrenaline increases the electrical excitability of the myocardium. After its administration, a rhythm may be seen that is either functional or treatable (e.g. VF). Adrenaline and electricity are not the main priorities in a paediatric cardiac arrest. The most important step is securing the airway and oxygenating the child.

Only then should cardiac massage be started and only then further measures (drugs etc.) be given. These steps are outline in Box 2.2.

Box 2.2   Treatment of asystole in children

Secure airway, ventilate with 100% oxygen
Start compressions
Adrenaline 0.1 ml/kg of 1 : 10000 i.v.
Consider fluids 10 ml/kg or bicarbonate, wait 3 min
Adrenaline 0.1 ml/kg of 1 : 1000 i.v.
Continue repeating this dose every 3 min
Consider calcium
Stop at 30 min from start of arrest

---

9   *These features are compatible with the following diagnoses in a child with a heart murmur*

   a   hyperdynamic precordium with a ventricular septal defect
   b   narrow pulse pressure and pulmonary stenosis
   c   a murmur radiating to the right carotid in coarctation of the aorta
   d   bounding pulses with a patent ductus arteriosus
   e   loud second sound in a ventricular septal defect

a   **True**. A hyperdynamic precordium is the physical sign that results from increased cardiac work or cardiomegaly. This may be because a ventricle is pumping against a resistance (PS, AS, coarctation) or is having to pump an excessive amount of blood (VSD, PDA, or in high output cardiac failure). This sign may accompany heart failure, but may just be the heart compensating.

b   **False**. PS cannot affect the pulse—it is on the wrong side of the heart. AS will cause a narrow pulse pressure (little difference between the systolic and diastolic pressures).

The signs of pulmonary stenosis do not need to be memorized—they can all be worked out. As there is an obstruction to right ventricular outflow there may be a precordial heave and cardiomegaly, an a murmur corresponding to the timing of the flow (systole). This will be loudest nearest the site of the obstruction (pulmonary area) and radiate to where the blood is going (the lungs). As there is an obstruction, less blood may reach the lungs, producing cyanosis. This sort of approach can be used to predict correctly most of the physical signs related to cardiac defects.

c   **False**. A coarctation murmur is systolic, is heard in the upper left sternum and radiates through to the back (like a PDA murmur), in the direction in which the blood is going. The obstruction is usually below the left subclavian artery, but occasionally is at the origin of this artery. In an infant, radiofemoral delay cannot be felt, so low volume or impalpable femoral arteries should alert the doctor to the possibility of a coarctation. In older children delay may be observed. At all ages, the blood pressure is higher in upper limbs. There may also be evidence of heart failure, particularly if there is a septal defect.

The only murmur radiating to the carotid is the AS murmur.

d   **True**. They bound like the pulse in aortic regurgitation. This is because the systemic blood drains rapidly into the low resistance pulmonary bed, causing a collapsing pulse. An easily palpable dorsalis pedis in an infant is probably a bounding pulse and there should be a wide pulse pressure. Other causes include CO_2 retention and septicaemia (peripheral vasodilation).

e   **False**. VSDs have a pansystolic murmur as the pressure difference across the hole exists before the mitral and tricuspid valves close and after the outflow valves shut again. The second sound is often then obliterated by the murmur.

A loud second sound is heard when there is an excessive outflow tract pressure (systemic or pulmonary hypertension) that causes forceful shutting of the aortic or pulmonary valves.

Reasoning and data interpretation — answers

10(i)   *A 3-week-old infant is seen by his family doctor as he is feeding poorly. The doctor finds that he has a heart rate of 260 beats/min, a respiratory rate of 60 breaths/min, a capillary filling time of 3–4 s and a blood pressure of 40/25*

a   the prolonged filling time is likely to be due to dehydration
b   the respiratory rate is probably raised because of cardiac failure
c   the blood pressure is within the normal range
d   a severe respiratory infection might be the cause
e   poor feeding is a rare presentation for cardiac disease at this age

a   **False**   b   **True**   c   **False**   d   **False**   e   **False**

A cardiac scenario will most probably involve the presentation and management of either heart failure, cyanotic heart disease or an asymptomatic murmur. All of these are illustrated here. As ever with scenarios there will be relevant and irrelevant information and perhaps normal data. Always one is looking for a bit of specific or diagnostic information. Here it is the heart rate of 260. In branch (a), while it is true that dehydration may increase capillary filling time (CFT) and tachypnoea (due to acidosis) and even a tachycardia, it is certainly not likely to cause a heart rate of 260 beats/min, which is only in practice caused by a cardiac problem. Similarly, a respiratory infection will not be the cause. This may be indicated by fever and chest signs. Tachypnoea is not a very reliable indicator of a chest infection, as it is mostly caused by the raised temperature.

Any heart rate over 180 in an infant is defined as a tachycardia. By far the commonest rhythm is a supraventricular tachycardia (SVT). Some of these of the patients will have Wolff–Parkinson–White syndrome. The bundle of Kent between the atria and ventricles allows premature ventricular depolarisation when in sinus rhythm, seen as a δ-wave on the ECG (slurred upstroke to the QRS complex). Other causes of a heart rate of 260 include conducted atrial flutter or fibrillation and fast ventricular tachycardia.

Normal capillary filling is less than 2 s. The prolonged filling time simply reflects poor peripheral perfusion, but other information is needed to distinguish between cold, hypovolaemia, low cardiac output, or vasoconstriction as its cause. Here we are told the child is tachypnoeic (normal < 40 at this age), has a low blood pressure and a prolonged CFT and tachycardia. Tachycardia can reduce the heart's efficiency as there is too little time for the ventricles to fill adequately. This reduces cardiac output and leads to pulmonary venous congestion and oedema (a cause for the tachypnoea). Also in an attempt to maintain blood pressure, peripheral vasoconstriction occurs, hence there is a prolonged filling time. Catecholamines are released, which causes the infant to be sweaty and pale. All of these factors, especially the raised respiratory rate reduce the appetite of the infant and make feeding difficult. Furthermore, aspiration of the feed is much more common in an infant with a rate above 60 breaths/min.

> 10(ii) He is referred to the local hospital for further assessment and treatment by the paediatricians. They find that although the heart rate is 250, the capillary filling time is 2 s, and blood pressure 65/45 mmHg. Given these findings
>
> a ventricular tachycardia is the most likely diagnosis
> b adenosine is a useful diagnostic and therapeutic agent
> c carotid massage would be helpful
> d maternal systemic lupus erythematosus may be the cause for the baby's arrhythmia
> e head submersion in cold water can be used as the first approach to therapy

a **False** b **True** c **False** d **False** e **True**

The baby seems to have improved, with a faster CFT and better blood pressure. An ECG performed now will show if the child has a narrow complex tachycardia (probably an SVT) or a broad complex tachycardia (probably VT, but very unusual in an otherwise healthy heart). If the child were cardiovascularly compromised, d.c. synchronous shocks should be used to return the heart to sinus rhythm. As he is cardiovascularly uncompromised, vagal manoeuvres can be used. These include facial ice, eyeball pressure, and head submersion (the diving reflex). You should warn the parents about what you are going to do first! Valsalver manoeuvres and carotid massage can work, but are not suitable for a child of 3 weeks. Adenosine (see above) will be helpful in this situation.

Maternal systemic lupus erythematosus is associated with congenital complete heart block that is permanent, as well as rash, anaemia, thrombocytopenia, and neutropenia in the neonatal period.

> 11 At a hospital clinic appointment arranged because a 10-week-old child was failing to thrive, the doctor detects a heart murmur. The following features suggest a cardiac rather than another cause for his failure to thrive
>
> a murmur grade II, loudest over the precordium
> b poor peripheral perfusion

c vomiting
d tachypnoea
e splenomegaly

a **False** b **True** c **False** d **True** e **False**

Failure to thrive is a common presentation of acyanotic cardiac disease in infancy. Other causes are discussed in Growth and nutrition question 5. Cyanotic heart disease is not commonly associated with failure to thrive as there is usually no associated heart failure. However, acyanotic conditions (VSD most commonly) reduce nutrient intake (poor feeding) and increase energy expenditure (tachypnoea, non-compliant lungs, increased cardiac work). This causes failure to thrive.

This question is looking for features of significant cardiac disease. A grade II murmur loudest over the precordium is typical of an innocent murmur and so would not make a cardiac cause more likely. Heart lesions that cause heart failure are either associated with no murmur where the defect is so big there is little turbulence or a loud murmur (grade III+, where there is a large flow through a modest defect). Poor peripheral perfusion may indicate that there is not enough blood entering the systemic circulation, probably because of a large left to right shunt. Tachypnoea, tachycardia, an active precordium, and oedema would be expected in an infant with a cardiac cause for failure to thrive, as heart failure would be present.

Vomiting is a non-specific sign of illness in children and can be brought on by a wide range of problems, as discussed in Gastroenterology question 3. It is not a particular feature of cardiac disease. Splenomegaly may occur in cardiac disease, but in this scenario, it is much more likely that it is a sign of infection. Otherwise it may be caused by infiltration or storage disorders.

12 *A 3-year-old girl is seen because she is unwell with a high temperature. She is known to have a ventricular septal defect. The casualty officer sees her and finds that she has a temperature of 39.1°C and a heart murmur. Infective endocarditis is made a more likely diagnosis because she*

a has microscopic haematuria
b has bounding pulses
c has sickle cell anaemia
d has a murmur loudest at the lower left sternal edge
e has splenomegaly

a **True** b **False** c **False** d **False** e **True**

Endocarditis should be considered in any child who has a fever and a heart murmur, and is part of the differential diagnosis in a patient with a prolonged fever or positive blood cultures. On the other hand heart murmurs are often found in children with fevers. The hyperdynamic circulation of a febrile child makes any murmur easier to hear, be it innocent, a pulmonary or aortic flow murmur or a venous hum.

Infective endocarditis has signs that are attributable to the mechanical problem directly (a murmur that is changing or associated with worsening cardiac function). There are also features related to the infective process (metastatic infection, persistent swinging fever) and immunological phenomena (microscopic haematuria, splenomegaly, splinter haemorrhages). The organisms most commonly responsible are *Strep. viridans*, *Strep. pneumoniae*, *Staph. aureus*, and other streptococci.

Bounding pulses are found in children who are septic or with carbon dioxide retention (peripheral vasodilation), or have PDAs. Sickle cell anaemia is often accompanied by a pulmonary flow murmur (ejection systolic murmur loudest at the right upper sternal edge) as the anaemia leads to a high cardiac output. Murmurs loudest at the left sternal edge are much more likely to be innocent than anything else, and so this finding does not support the diagnosis of endocarditis, as she is already known to have a VSD.

> *13(i)   During a clinic visit a 6-week-old girl is found to have an ejection systolic murmur. Her heart rate is 145 beats/min, and her pulse character is normal. She has been following the 10th percentile and is breastfeeding well. Significant cardiac disease is made more likely if she also has*
>
> a   radiation of the murmur to the back
> b   a liver edge at 1.5 cm below the costal margin
> c   a thrill
> d   webbing of the neck
> e   a respiratory rate of 30

a **True**   b **False**   c **True**   d **True**   e **False**

This question is about identifying an innocent murmur. Innocent murmurs are typically short, systolic, precordial, do not radiate, and are not associated with a thrill or any other signs of cardiac disease. They can also alter with posture. Children with these murmurs probably do not have significant cardiac disease. In this scenario, there is no indication from the history that there is any cardiac disease. On the other hand, cyanotic spells, poor feeding, laboured or fast breathing (not 30/min), sweatiness, and pallor are symptoms of cardiac disease. A weight following the 10th percentile is also normal.

Radiation of the murmur to the back is a sign of either a PDA or coarctation, and a thrill implies the murmur is at least grade IV (Box 2.3). Webbing of the neck is a dysmorphic feature associated with Turner's or Noonan's syndromes. These are reviewed in Growth and nutrition question 4. Dysmorphic features in a child with a murmur makes it more likely that there is an associated cardiac lesion. Other common associations include Down's syndrome, and the CHARGE and VATER associations. CHARGE stands for Coloboma, Heart, Atresia choanae, Retarded growth and development, Genital problems, and Ear anomalies. VATER stands for Vertebral anomalies, Anal anomalies, Tracheo-Esophageal fistulae, Renal, and Radial. The message is simple—the formation of the heart is very complex and many genetic anomalies will cause a heart defect.

The liver edge can be up to 3 cm below the costal margin in a neonate and still be normal. This is because the chest is relatively small and the lungs therefore push

---

Box 2.3 Grades of murmur

Grade I Audible only by cardiologist
Grade II Soft
Grade III Loud, but no thrill
Grade IV Loud, associated with a thrill
Grade V Can be heard without the stethoscope
Grade VI Can be heard at the end of the bed

---

the liver into the abdomen. Furthermore, the pelvis cannot fully accommodate the bladder and so this is an abdominal organ during the first months. All this makes the infant's abdomen fairly distended.

13(ii)   *She is referred to the hospital for further evaluation. Some investigations are performed*
chest X-ray—increased cardiothoracic ratio, normal lung fields
ECG normal axis, no evidence of strain, or conduction disturbance
four limb blood pressures: right arm 90/65; left arm 88/66; right leg 45/30; left leg 47/35

Based on these results and the above history and examination

a   she is not is cardiac failure
b   she probably has coarctation of the aorta
c   her normal ECG has excluded any cardiac disease
d   she is hypertensive
e   her presentation has been precipitated by closure of the ductus

a **True** b **True** c **False** d **True** e **False**
These are the standard investigations for use in a child with an asymptomatic murmur. The normal ECG makes a major cardiac lesion less likely, but has not excluded a smaller lesion. Its main function is to determine the axis of the heart and any conduction or rhythm disturbances, as discussed in questions 3 and 6 of the knowledge section. The chest X-ray shows an increased cardiothoracic ratio, meaning that the cardiac shadow is too big for the size of the child. Dilatation of the ventricles and atria is the most common cause of this, but there might be pericardial fluid or thickened muscle to account for the large heart.

The atria and ventricles dilate when the ventricles are unable to fully eject the blood put into them, and this will occur if there is too much blood going into them (left to right shunt, high output cardiac failure, fluid overload) or resistance to ejection of blood (AS, coarctation). This corresponds with excessive preload and afterload. Pericardial fluid may accumulate with infective processes (*Staph. aureus*, *Haemophilus influenzae* type B, *Strep. pneumoniae*, *Coxsackie* virus), juvenile rheumatoid arthritis and rheumatic fever. The muscle may be thickened with cardiomyopathy and storage disorders.

In this child, there is no evidence of increased vascular markings in the lungs, but there is an increased cardiothoracic ratio. This suggests that there is an increased resistance to the outflow of blood. Support for this is gained from the high blood pressure in the arms, and the difference between arm and leg blood pressures. This is good evidence of coarctation of the aorta.

Coarctation can present in many different ways. It may be identified in a newborn examination, where the femorals may be weak or absent. It may be identified as a heart murmur with associated hypertension. It may be diagnosed incidentally as a raised blood pressure when it is measured for screening. As one of the treatable causes for hypertension, its diagnosis is important to reduce long-term complications.

This presentation has nothing to do with the ductus, as this will have closed long before the clinic visit.

14(i)   A term female infant is seen at the request of the midwife at 72 h of age. She has noticed that the baby has a blue tinge to her lips and nailbeds. The colour deepens during feeding. The doctor finds that the baby is alert but centrally cyanosed with a heart rate of 135 beats/min and a respiratory rate of 35 breaths/min. There is minimal respiratory distress. Auscultation reveals no heart murmur but a single second sound. The breath sounds are equal and there are no added sounds

a   the cyanosis may be caused by a high haemoglobin concentration
b   the single second sound may due to similar pressures in aorta and pulmonary artery
c   she is likely to be septic
d   the mother's use of phenytoin during pregnancy for her epilepsy may be linked to this presentation
e   the absence of a murmur makes a non-cardiac cause more likely than a cardiac cause for her illness

a **False** b **True** c **False** d **True** e **False**

Cyanosis is either due to a respiratory problem or a right to left shunt. The absence of any other respiratory signs is suggestive of a cardiac problem, and this age is typical for the presentation of lesions such as transposition of the great arteries (TGA), and pulmonary atresia (PA). These are all duct-dependent lesions, in which the ductus is allowing blood to mix between pulmonary and systemic circulations in TGA, and some systemic blood to reach the lungs in PA. The single second sound is due to the pulmonary component of the second sound being very quiet (as the outflow tract is small) or because the left and right sides of the heart are working at similar pressures. Even in the absence of a murmur, a cardiac cause is much more likely given the history and examination. Other possibilities might include respiratory distress syndrome (RDS), chest infection, aspiration, and sepsis. All of these should be, but not always will be accompanied by some chest signs.

At birth the haemoglobin concentration will be high, but even then the saturation will be at least as low as 75% to cause cyanosis. As the fetal haemoglobin has a higher oxygen affinity than adult haemoglobin, this means that a newborn with a saturation of 75% has a much lower pO_2 than an adult with the same saturation. Hence central cyanosis is a serious sign.

Phenytoin is one of the few drugs that may cause cardiac malformations if taken by the mother in pregnancy. Fetal alcohol syndrome includes VSDs and ASDs as part of its spectrum. Patients with epilepsy who become pregnant must be counselled as carbamazepine, valproate, and phenytoin are all associated with neural tube defects and neonatal haemorrhage. Folate supplements during the pregnancy and vitamin K prophylaxis for the newborn is strongly recommended. Other anticonvulsants are not recommended.

14(ii)   The infant is admitted to the neonatal unit for further evaluation. The following tests are performed
arterial blood gas (right radial):
pH 7.38
pCO$_2$ 3.9 kPa
pO$_2$ 3.7 kPa
base excess − 4.2 mmol/l
chest X-ray normal
four limb blood pressures: right arm 43/25; left arm 45/23; right leg 41/17; left leg 42/19

a   she may have coarctation of the aorta
b   a significant left-to-right shunt may be responsible
c   she may have persistent pulmonary hypertension of the newborn
d   a hyperoxic (nitrogen washout) test would now be of value
e   the blood gas result confirms she has respiratory disease

a **False**   b **False**   c **True**   d **True**   e **False**
All of these test results are normal, except perhaps there is a slightly wide pulse pressure. The most valuable test for use in a cyanosed child who may have cardiac disease is the hyperoxic or nitrogen washout test. This helps distinguish a respiratory problem from a shunt as the cause of the cyanosis. This test is discussed in question 3.

A left to right shunt can only cause cyanosis if there is pulmonary oedema, but there is no clinical evidence to support this or changes on the chest X-ray. Coarctation is not possible either based on the scenario or the four limb blood pressure readings.

Persistent pulmonary hypertension of the newborn (PPHN), also termed persistent fetal circulation (PFC) is the term given when there is continued pulmonary vasoconstriction after birth. In the fetus, this vasoconstriction is vital to reduce blood flow to the lungs, but after birth the pulmonary vessels should dilate to allow gas exchange. PPHN is occasionally primary, but more often secondary to sepsis, RDS, meconium aspiration, and other conditions. There are usually some respiratory signs and changes on chest X-ray relating to a primary respiratory problem. A hyperoxic test may show little rise in pO$_2$, but there may be vasodilation occurring in response to the higher oxygen levels and there may be a large component of respiratory disease in the pathology that leads to a larger rise in pO$_2$.

The blood gas result shows a low pO$_2$, but is otherwise normal. Respiratory diseases typically have either a low or high pCO$_2$.

3 Respiratory disease

Knowledge — questions

1 *Pulse oximetry*

   a is useful in the triage of acute asthma
   b cannot be used in African patients
   c shows blood pressure
   d measures oxygen content of the blood
   e is useful in triage of children following smoke inhalation

2 *Bronchiolitis*

   a usually presents with poor feeding
   b is responsible for the admission of 2% of infants each year
   c has a peak incidence in the autumn
   d commonly results in hypernatraemia
   e is unlikely if parainfluenza virus is isolated from a nasopharyngeal aspirate

3(i) *A 4-year-old boy has been diagnosed as having asthma. When considering how to treat the child*

   a a spacing device will probably provide the best drug delivery for maintenance treatment
   b dry powder delivery devices will be poorly tolerated at this age
   c his parents should be encouraged to stop smoking as this will reduce the severity of his disease
   d a peak flow meter will not be of help in his management
   e a home nebulizer would be appropriate at this stage

3(ii) *His mother asks what is involved in the treatment of asthma. It would be correct to say that*

   a his growth will probably be reduced
   b inhaled sodium methotrexate will stabilize mast cells
   c he should be started on salbutamol as his first medication
   d oral prednisolone might be given for acute attacks
   e a chest X-ray will be needed in each acute attack to rule out infection or pneumothorax

4   **Stridor in children**

   a   is usually associated with drooling
   b   may be congenital
   c   requires urgent intubation
   d   is associated with *Haemophilus influenzae* infection
   e   is also known as 'croup'

5   **When examining the respiratory system of a boy of 4 months**

   a   recession is characteristic of a lower airways problem
   b   flaring of the ali nasi implies there is respiratory distress
   c   a respiratory rate of 35 is abnormal
   d   hyperexpansion is a sign of an expiratory obstruction
   e   expiratory crackles would be a sign typical of bronchiolitis

6   **The following chest X-ray appearances are consistent with the associated conditions**

   a   hyperexpansion—bronchiolitis
   b   lobar collapse—asthma
   c   normal lung fields—foreign body inhalation
   d   lobar consolidation—streptococcal pneumonia
   e   indistinct right hemidiaphragm—right middle lobe pneumonia

7   **Otitis media**

   a   is almost always viral
   b   may be diagnosed after visualizing a dull and injected tympanic membrane in a febrile child
   c   is more common in children with Down's syndrome
   d   is best treated with oral penicillin
   e   is a common cause of speech delay

8   **Upper respiratory tract infections in infants**

   a   are viral in over 90% of cases
   b   often cause loose motions
   c   commonly cause vomiting
   d   occur over six times a year for most children
   e   may be the cause of wheeze

9   **The diagnosis of cystic fibrosis**

   a   may be made antenatally
   b   is likely if there is a high immunoreactive trypsin level
   c   is made by finding a high faecal fat content
   d   cannot be made using a sweat test in small infants
   e   is made in all of infants with meconium ileus

10   Sleep apnoea
    a   is best diagnosed by admitting the child for nocturnal pulse oximetry
    b   may lead to pulmonary hypertension
    c   requires tonsillectomy
    d   may impair school performance
    e   is often due to allergy

Data interpretation and reasoning — questions

11   A boy of 18 months is brought to the emergency department by his
    mother. The triage nurse notices that he has an inspiratory stridor, is
    holding his neck extended, and is drooling. His pulse is recorded as
    175 beats/min, respiratory rate 40, and temperature 38.5°C. He also
    has a blue tinge to his tongue and seems agitated. To manage him
    correctly
    a   an urgent lateral neck X-ray should be obtained
    b   arterial blood gases will be needed to determine the need for intubation
    c   broad-spectrum antibiotics should be given before anything else is done
    d   high flow oxygen may reduce his agitation
    e   his siblings will need prophylaxis

12   A 2-month-old inpatient has a respiratory rate of 50 and chest
    recession. An arterial blood gas is taken
    pH 7.36 (7.35–7.45)
    pCO_2 7.2 kPa (4.5–6.0)
    pO_2 11.2 kPa (10.0–14.0)
    BE +11.3 mmol/l (+5.0 to − 5.0)
Now it can be said that
    a   he has a respiratory acidosis
    b   chronic respiratory disease is probably the cause of his high pCO_2
    c   the cause of these results may be vomiting
    d   hypoventilation is the cause for the high pCO_2
    e   the positive BE has compensated for a respiratory problem

13   A 13-month-old boy presents with difficulty in breathing. In the past
    he has been admitted with bronchiolitis and is being seen in the
    asthma clinic. The following features increase the possibility of an
    inhaled foreign body

a   lobar collapse on chest X-ray
b   temperature 38.2°C
c   bilateral crackles
d   bilateral hyperexpansion
e   cyanosis in air

14(i)   *A girl of 7 months is seen with a cough by her family doctor. She has*
already been ill for 1 week with a cough, poor feeding, and a
temperature. She has had similar symptoms twice in the last
3 months and each time was prescribed amoxycillin. On the first of
these occasions she had a normal chest X-ray taken. The doctor
examines her and finds that she is alert and interested in her
surroundings. She has a respiratory rate of 50 with mild recession. On
auscultation wheeze was audible on both sides of her chest. She is pink
in air and cardiovascular examination is unremarkable. Her mother
is worried that she will develop asthma. She is more likely to be
correct because

a   her temperature is 37.7°C
b   there is a family history of urticaria
c   both the child's parents smoke cigarettes
d   she had bronchiolitis 3 months ago
e   she improves after a salbutamol nebulizer

14(ii)   *The doctor would have good reason to*

a   start inhaled steroids
b   prescribe a course of a different antibiotic
c   repeat the chest X-ray
d   perform a sweat test
e   arrange for a home nebulizer

15(i)   *A 4-year-old girl who is a known asthmatic presents to the*
emergency department at 23.00 with her father. She is managed in
conjunction with the asthma clinic at the hospital and is currently on
beclomethasone 200 µg twice a day and salbutamol 200 µg after
she takes the beclomethasone or when she needs it. She takes both with
a spacer. Today she has been taking the salbutamol every hour all day
but is no better. In the past she has been admitted with her asthma five
times and once went to the paediatric intensive care unit. Last week
she saw her family doctor with oral candidiasis

a   the candidiasis is probably iatrogenic

b   she is taking her medicines correctly
c   the beclomethasone can be increased during attacks
d   she will get better drug delivery from a dry powder delivery device
e   she should have been brought earlier in the day

15(ii)   She is given a salbutamol nebulizer immediately by the nurse. The nurse also records that her pulse is 160 beats/min, respiratory rate 65 breaths/min, and her saturation 83% in air. She is no better after the nebulizer and so the doctor is called urgently. He listens to her chest and finds poor breath sounds and no wheeze. To manage her well he could now

a   give a loading dose of aminophylline
b   give her oral prednisolone
c   take an arterial blood gas
d   site an intravenous line and give hydrocortisone
e   repeat the salbutamol nebulizer

16   A 9 year old is admitted to the intensive care unit as he has failed to improve with half-hourly salbutamol nebulizers, intravenous hydrocortisone, and an aminophylline infusion. He is now looking tired. An arterial blood gas is taken while he is breathing oxygen via a face mask

pH 7.18 (7.35–7.45)
pCO_2 7.5 kPa (4.5–6.0)
pO_2 13.1 kPa (10.0 14.0)
BE −1.2 mmol/l (+5.0 to −5.0)

From this it can be said that

a   his oxygen should be turned down
b   a salbutamol infusion could be of benefit
c   mechanical ventilation should now be started
d   a low minute volume is responsible for his high pCO_2
e   his negative BE implies there is a metabolic acidosis

17   A 4 year old is brought to his family doctor with a sore throat. The doctor is worried that he has glandular fever (infectious mononucleosis). The following features make this diagnosis more likely than another cause of a sore throat

a   he has a palpable liver 3 cm below the costal margin
b   his temperature is 38.9°C
c   a fine maculopapular rash on the trunk

d pustules on the tonsils
e slightly enlarged cervical lymph nodes

Knowledge — answers

1 Pulse oximetry
  a is useful in the triage of acute asthma
  b cannot be used in African patients
  c shows blood pressure
  d measures oxygen content of the blood
  e is useful in triage of children following smoke inhalation

a **True.** The most widely used instrument for monitoring the progress of children with a wide variety of problems is the pulse oximeter. It works by measuring the absorbence of light at different frequencies, exploiting the fact that oxyhaemoglobin and deoxyhaemoglobin have different absorbence spectra. It measures the differences in absorbence occurring during a pulse and so eliminates the effect of absorbence by the tissues. Hence the machine gives an output of percentage saturation and pulse rate. Both of these measurements are useful in the triage of acute asthma (shown in Box 3.1) and for any respiratory problem. It can be used in the continued monitoring of patients with other diseases.

Box 3.1   Features identifying severity in acute asthma, adapted from National Asthma Campaign guidelines

	Mild	Moderate	Severe
Cyanosis	No	In air	In oxygen
Exhaustion	No	—	Present
Sentences	>8 words	5–8 words	<5 words
Consciousness	Quiet	Restless	Agitated/depressed
Sternal retraction	Absent	Moderate	Marked
Wheeze	Minimal	Marked	Silent chest
Peak expiratory flow rate	>50% of normal	33–50% of normal	<33% of normal

b **False.** There are not many situations where the device will not work. Differences in skin colour are allowed for by the machine. Poor peripheral perfusion, found in very sick children may lead to unreliable readings.

c **False.** It does not show blood pressure.

d   **False.** It only measures the percentage of haemoglobin that is oxyhaemoglobin and pulse rate. Also it offers no measure of pO_2. Oxygen delivery is related to the product of saturation and haemoglobin concentration. Therefore the pulse oximeter will falsely reassure in an anaemic patient, who will be well saturated even if oxygen delivery is low. Children with sickle cell disease or newborns can have a high levels of HbF (high affinity) may be well saturated but with a low pO_2.

e   **False.** Carboxyhaemoglobin (being cherry red in colour) fools the machine. It counts this as oxyhaemoglobin, so giving a much higher saturation than is actually present. Carbon monoxide combines with haemoglobin to make carboxyhaemoglobin. This is much more stable than oxyhaemoglobin and so in effect reduces the amount of haemoglobin available for oxygen transport. Reversion to haemoglobin is slow and aided by a high pO_2, so hyperbaric oxygen is used if the carboxyhaemoglobin percentage is high.

2   *Bronchiolitis*
   a   usually presents with poor feeding
   b   is responsible for the admission of 2% of infants each year
   c   has a peak incidence in the autumn
   d   commonly results in hypernatraemia
   e   is unlikely if parainfluenza virus is isolated from a nasopharyngeal aspirate

a   **True.** Carers are always able to give a feeding history and tell you about the contents of the nappy! Poor feeding is a common presentation of a wide variety of paediatric conditions—infections and respiratory problems being the most common. Other features in the history consistent with bronchiolitis include—mild fever, runny nose, wet or bubbly cough, vomiting with the cough, and loose stools, or more seriously cyanosis and apnoea. Signs consistent with bronchiolitis include respiratory distress (flaring of the ali nasi, tracheal tug, supra clavicular, intercostal, sternal and subcostal recession, and tachypnoea), crackles, and wheeze. As it is a small airways problem, these are louder on expiration. A low grade fever may be found and there may be evidence of dehydration.

Investigations are often not required, except for a nasopharyngeal aspirate (NPA) to identify a causative agent by immunofluorescence. A chest X-ray is useful to rule out a pneumonia that may be secondary to the bronchiolitis or collapse, but hyperexpansion is the most usual finding. Electrolytes should be measured if there is concern about the feeding.

Treatment is supportive—tube feeding or an intravenous infusion may be needed, and oxygen is given by headbox or nasal cannulae. Occasionally, deterioration may lead to mechanical ventilation. The role of the antiviral agent ribavirin is controversial. Its enthusiasts only recommend it where the disease is likely to have a poor outcome. This is most likely in infants who have chronic lung or cardiac disease. Most of the deaths from bronchiolitis occur in ex-premature infants.

b   **True**. It is the commonest cause of admission in the winter and the commonest cause for infants. Asthma is the commonest cause of admission in 1–14 year olds, with 10–20% of patients having this diagnosis.

c   **False**. For poorly understood reasons, the peak is always in the winter. Infants under 12 months are most affected.

d   **False**. Commonly, there is a mild hyponatraemia, the result of inappropriate antidiuretic hormone secretion. This is discussed in more detail in the Nephrology questions 7 and 12. Bronchiolitis can occasionally result in a high sodium. Hypernatraemia will occur when there is a loss of water in excess of sodium, the result of hyperventilation and poor fluid intake.

e   **False**. Bronchiolitis is most commonly caused by respiratory syncytial virus. A host of other viruses may be responsible, such as parainfluenza, adenovirus, and rhinovirus. Bronchiolitis is primarily a clinical diagnosis and isolation of a virus only supports this—isolation of the virus may be an incidental finding, or the virus may be causing another disease. For instance respiratory syncytial virus (RSV) can also cause pneumonia and upper respiratory tract infections (URTIs). Parainfluenza is the commonest cause of croup.

Isolating a virus is useful as it enables infection control procedures to be rational (you would not want a RSV+ve infant nursed near a parainfluenza +ve infant even if they both have bronchiolitis.

3(i)   A 4-year-old boy has been diagnosed as having asthma. When considering how to treat the child

   a   a spacing device will probably provide the best drug delivery for maintenance treatment
   b   dry powder delivery devices will be poorly tolerated at this age
   c   his parents should be encouraged to stop smoking as this will reduce the severity of his disease
   d   a peak flow meter will not be of help in his management
   e   a home nebulizer would be appropriate at this stage

a   **True**. Asthma is something that must be understood well by undergraduates. There is much that can be asked about its presentation, treatment, and epidemiology. Furthermore, the drugs used and administration is different in children to adults and alters as the child ages. Lastly, the prevalence of asthma is increasing and its cause is not known.

The first branch deals with the treatment devices. There are three ways a drug can be carried into the lungs via the respiratory tract to give 'topical' treatment—as an aerosol, as a powder, and via a nebulizer. The nebulizer delivers large doses with relatively large amounts actually reaching the lung. This is used in the treatment of moderate to severe attacks. Any age can use this as it requires no cooperation for drug delivery (an infant crying has a good inspiration). Dry powder devices require a child to inhale a powder. This requires cooperation and the doses given are small, so it is only used for mild attacks and maintenance treatment. Children

under 5 are less likely to tolerate this device. Aerosol devices are the most used for
adult—particularly the metered dose inhaler (MDI). This requires more technique—inhalation at the same time as the can is pressed—and so is not suitable
for most children under 10 years. Even then it has a high delivery to the pharynx.
To get around the co-ordination problem the 'autohaler' has been developed, which
is a breath-activated MDI. More practically for children, spacing devices can be
used. A MDI is used to put the drug into a plastic spacer and the child breaths the
agent from the spacer using a mouthpiece and valve. Some 2 year olds can even
master this, and by putting a mask on to the mouthpiece, it can be used at any
age. Larger doses can be put into the spacer and there is a relatively high rate of
delivery to the lung . It can be used in mild attacks as well as maintenance treatment. The delivery devices are summarized in Box 3.2.

Box 3.2   Drug delivery devices for asthma

	Type	Ages	Drugs delivered
Metered dose inhaler (MDI)	Aerosol	10+	Salbutamol, ipratropium, beclomethasone, salmeterol, terbutaline, budesonide, chromoglycate
MDI with spacer	Aerosol	3+	As above
MDI with spacer and mask	Aerosol	Any	As above
Autohaler	Aerosol	7+	Salbutamol, beclomethasone
Turbohaler	Dry powder	4+	Terbutaline, budesonide
Diskhaler	Dry powder	4+	Salbutamol, salmeterol, beclomethasone
Rotacaps, via Rotahaler	Dry powder	5+	Salbutamol, beclomethasone
Spinhaler	Dry powder	4+	Chromoglycate
Accuhaler	Dry powder	4+	Salbutamol, salmeterol
Nebulizer	Nebulized	Any	Salbutamol, terbutaline, beclomethasone, budesonide
Oral		Any	Salbutamol, prednisolone, aminophylline
Intravenous		Any	Salbutamol, terbutaline, hydrocortisone, aminophylline

Even if the correct device is used, ongoing advice on technique will be needed.
Drugs may also be given orally. The obvious disadvantage is that side-effects are
more common, so the oral route is only used in three situations: oral salbutamol
in infants with mild symptoms where a spacer is not wanted, to give oral prednisolone in an acute attack, and when aminophylline is given for nocturnal cough.

b **False.** Some 4 year olds will manage a dry powder device. It is much more convenient than the only alternative at this age—the MDI with a spacer.

c **True.** There are many external factors implicated in the aetiology of asthma including cigarette smoking and the house dust mite. Pollution has been shown not to be an important factor.

d **False.** Children with established asthma will have differing needs for their medicine at different times. Parents should be advised to how and when to increase treatment and when to seek further help. One indicator would be a fall in the peak expiratory flow rate (PEFR). In response to this the parents could increase the dose of inhaled steroids or bronchodilator. The PEFR is also used in the definition of severity of attacks. Under 33% indicates a life-threatening attack and under 50% a severe attack. Some children at 4 years can be taught how to use the device.

e **False.** Home nebulizers are best used for children with established severe asthma to reduce admissions and reduce the need for oral steroids. They can be dangerous as the child can be managed at home by parents even when fairly severe. Children may then present very late.

> *3b   His mother asks what is involved in the treatment of asthma. It would be correct to say that*
> a   his growth will probably be reduced
> b   inhaled sodium methotrexate will stabilize mast cells
> c   he should be started on salbutamol as his first medication
> d   oral prednisolone might be given for acute attacks
> e   a chest X-ray will be needed in each acute attack to rule out infection or pneumothorax

a **False.** Long-term *systemic* steroids can cause Cushing's syndrome. They also cause premature fusion of the epiphyseal plate, arresting growth early. Cushing's is most commonly associated with nephrotic syndrome, malignancies, juvenile rheumatoid arthritis, and bronchopulmonary dysplasia. There will be no growth suppression associated with inhaled steroids and or the 3-day courses of oral steroids used in acute asthmatic attacks. Undertreated asthma does reduce growth as the child will have increased respiratory work and a reduced appetite.

b **False.** Methotrexate is a folic acid antagonist used in chemotherapy. Sodium chromoglycate is used as the second step in asthma treatment, once it is established the child needs more than occasional salbutamol to keep his disease at bay. It does not work in every child, but as it is free of side-effects it is worth trying. The next step is inhaled steroids. Both chromoglycate and inhaled steroids are called 'preventers' and should be used so that 'relievers' such as salbutamol or terbutaline need only be used occasionally.

c **True.** Chronic symptoms should always be sought when asthmatics are seen. Cough at nights, during exercise, and on cold exposure gives an idea of the level of control between attacks. Inhaled salbutamol is the first step in asthma management. Terbutaline via a dry powder device could also be used in an older child. See Box 3.3 for stepwise treatment details.

Box 3.3   Stepwise treatment for asthma

Step 1   Intermittent inhaled B$_2$ agonists, maximum once a day

Step 2   β$_2$ agonists PRN plus inhaled sodium chromoglycate (if effective) or low-dose inhaled steroids

Step 3   β$_2$ agonists PRN plus regular high dose inhaled steroids consider long acting B$_2$ agonists or short course oral steroids

Step 4   β$_2$ agonists PRN plus very high dose steroids via spacer consider oral theophylline or steroids

Step down when improved

---

d   **True.** Very mild attacks can be managed at home by increasing (or starting) inhaled steroids. Here it is particularly important to use the bronchodilator *before* the steroid. Attacks not responding to inhaled bronchodilators will need nebulizer treatment and oral steroids. Prednisolone is used at a dose of 2 mg/kg for 3 days. Hydrocortisone is used intravenously for more severe attacks, if the child is too ill to drink the prednisolone or is vomiting . The time it takes for the drug to work is the same (about 8 h) whichever route is chosen. Acute asthma treatment is outline in Box 3.4.

Box 3.4   Treatment for acute asthma

Oxygen if desaturated

Nebulized salbutamol 2.5–5 mg

Nebulized salbutamol 2.5–5 mg

Oral prednisolone 2 mg/kg

Half-hourly or continuous nebulized salbutamol 2.5 mg

Nebulized ipratropium bromide 125 μg

Aminophylline loading dose 5 mg/kg (if not already on aminophylline)

Aminophylline infusion 1 mg/kg per h

Hydrocortisone 4 mg/kg

Salbutamol infusion 1–5 μg/kg per min

---

e   **False.** Chest X-rays carry a very small risk of malignancy. This is increased if there are many repeated exposures or the individual is young. Therefore, X-rays are avoided in acute asthma. Even if taken they usually only show hyperexpansion (flattened diaphragms, horizontal ribs, over 5½ anterior ribs ends). The indications for an X-ray are asymmetrical signs (there might be collapse, pneumothorax, or infection), life-threatening asthma, and the first episode, as there may be a congenital anomaly masquerading as asthma.

4 Stridor in children

  a is usually associated with drooling
  b may be congenital
  c requires urgent intubation
  d is associated with *Haemophilus influenzae* infection
  e is also known as 'croup'

a **False**. Stridor is a harsh inspiratory noise. There may also be an audible expiratory noise, but it is always quieter than the inspiratory noise. This is a characteristic feature of an upper airways obstruction (nose to major bronchi) as opposed to lower airways obstructions that always make louder expiratory noises than inspiratory noises (e.g. asthma, bronchiolitis). Stridor is associated with a number of conditions, but not all are serious.

Drooling implies the child cannot swallow its saliva—a feature of laryngeal, pharyngeal, or oesophageal pathology, and common in epiglottitis.

b **True**. Stridor may also be caused by congenital lesions such as laryngo- or tracheomalacia, in which there is a local defect in the airway cartilage, or by mediastinal vascular anomalies. Stridor may also be caused by infections [laryngo-tracheobronchitis (LTB), epiglottitis, tracheitis], pharyngeal problems (e.g. sleep apnoea) or by an aspirated foreign body.

c **False**. Most children with croup do not need intubation at all. These children should have nebulized steroids as these have been shown to speed recovery.

Intubation is needed to maintain the airways of a child or allow ventilation when there is respiratory failure. The airways will not be protected if there is a reduced conscious level (a Glasgow Coma Score less than 8). Intubation may also be needed if there is airways pathology—most commonly causes by LTB, but more dramatically with epiglottitis. Children with tracheitis commonly need intubation. Indications for intubation are cyanosis, severe recession, or bradycardia. A 'croup call' is made and senior anaesthetist, ENT surgeon, and paediatrician attend for the intubation. Nebulized adrenaline can be given by as a temporary measure.

d **True**. *Haemophilus influenzae* type B (HIB) is the cause of epiglottitis. Parainfluenza, measles, RSV and other viruses can all cause LTB. Tracheitis is usually caused by *Staphylococcus aureus*. Children with epiglottitis tend to have a short history (<24 h) and are classically toxic, with a high fever, drooling, and sit in the tripod position with an extended neck. They may not have been immunized against HIB or be one of the vaccination failures (<5%). Those with LTB have a barking cough, tend to be under 18 months, have a fever under 38.5 °C, do not drool or have such a severe airways problem. The history is often at least 2 days, and the symptoms worse at night. However, the decision to intubate should be based not on the presumed diagnosis but on the condition of the child.

e   **False**. Stridor is a sign of croup, but not the disease itself.

>   5   *When examining the respiratory system of a boy of 4 months*
>   a   recession is characteristic of a lower airways problem
>   b   flaring of the ali nasi implies there is respiratory distress
>   c   a respiratory rate of 35 is abnormal
>   d   hyperexpansion is a sign of an expiratory obstruction
>   e   expiratory crackles would be a sign typical of bronchiolitis

a   **False**. Recession occurs when there is an increased work of inspiration. This may be because there is an inspiratory obstruction (e.g. croup), or because the lungs are difficult to inflate (e.g. pulmonary oedema) or if the child is trying to inspire quickly because of some other problem, such as expiratory obstruction (e.g. asthma). The only signs that distinguish upper and lower airways problems are stridor and wheeze.

b   **True**. Respiratory distress incorporates tachypnoea, flaring of the ali nasi, tracheal tug, supra clavicular, intercostal, sternal and subcostal recession. It is the body's adaption to a perceived need to increase alveolar ventilation. The nostrils offer most airways resistance so the ali nasi flare during inspiration in small children.

c   **False**. The upper limit of normal under 1 year is 40 breaths/min. From 1 to 10 years the upper limit is 30 and over 10 years is 20 breaths/min.

d   **True**. Difficulty expiring will lead to hyperexpansion, or air trapping. This is because the small airways narrow and obstruct in expiration. Signs of hyper-expansion are an increased anteroposterior diameter of the chest, a liver edge over 3 cm below the costal margin, and a hyper-resonant chest. Hyperexpansion is most commonly found in asthma and bronchiolitis.

e   **True**. Expiratory crackles and wheeze are typical signs of bronchiolitis.
     Auscultation in children is frequently difficult because they may not always be cooperative! Plenty can still be gained because, even when crying, the inspira-tory phase can be heard, and the breath sounds noted. These can be described as bronchial or vesicular. The younger the child, the more bronchial are the breath sounds, as the bronchi are closer to the stethoscope. If they are louder or harsher on one side there may be consolidation on that side or a pneumothorax on the other. In the inspiratory phase crackles may also be heard. Coarse inspiratory sounds are large airways sounds and frequently bilateral, and may be found in diseases such as LTB or even a runny nose. Fine, late inspiratory sounds usually come from the bronchioles as they open, and are associated with pulmonary

oedema and pneumonia. Expiratory sounds are typical of small airways disease, with expiratory crackles in bronchiolitis and wheeze in asthma.

Percussion is a useful adjunct to auscultation, but may be poorly tolerated by the child.

6   *The following chest X-ray appearances are consistent with the associated conditions*
   a   hyperexpansion—bronchiolitis
   b   lobar collapse—asthma
   c   normal lung fields—foreign body inhalation
   d   lobar consolidation—streptococcal pneumonia
   e   indistinct right hemidiaphragm—right middle lobe pneumonia

a   **True**. The radiographic features of hyperexpansion are discussed in question 3(ii), and are most often associated with bronchiolitis or asthma.

Poor expansion on a chest X-ray is probably seen because film has been exposed when the child was not taking a large inspiration. The heart seems large, lung fields bilaterally streaky or hazy, and fewer than $4\frac{1}{2}$ anterior rib ends are showing. Poor expansion is also seen in respiratory distress syndrome with air bronchograms and a ground glass appearance. Poor expansion may be unilateral or localized if there is collapse due to bronchial obstruction. This may occur as a result of mucus (asthma or bronchiolitis) or a foreign body inhalation. Here there will be an abnormally high diaphragm, mediastinal shift, rib crowding and movement of lung markings (e.g. lateral fissure) as well as increased opacity in the affected area.

b   **True**. Asthma most commonly causes hyperexpansion. Other appearances seen include collapse or consolidation, as these children are more prone to have chest infections. Pneumothorax may also be found.

c   **True**. The X-ray is frequently normal in foreign body inhalation. On the other hand, there may be unilateral hyperexpansion (caused by the foreign body obstructing expiration more than inspiration) or collapse (if the obstruction is complete). Just occasionally the foreign body is visible. Peanuts, which are involved in the majority of foreign body inhalations are not radiodense.

Children with symptoms and signs suggestive of foreign body inhalation should be bronchoscoped. Sudden onset of cough, lobar pneumonia with a poor response to antibiotics or localized chest signs should prompt consideration of a bronchoscopy. Children from 6 to 24 months are most affected.

d   **True**. *Strep. pneumoniae* is the commonest cause of lobar pneumonia. Other organisms including *Mycoplasma*, *Haemophilus* (not type B), and viruses tend to cause a more diffuse bronchopneumonia. *Staph. aureus* is an uncommon cause of pneumonia and associated with a severe pneumonia, which may have fluid levels visible on the X-ray.

e   **False**. The edge between lung and surrounding tissue becomes indistinct when the density of the lung increases in that piece of lung. This may be because there is consolidation, collapse, fluid, or a mass. The lung bordering the right diaphragm is the right lower lobe and the right middle consolidation is seen as an indistinct right heart border. The interpretation of other lung field changes is outlined in Box 3.5.

Box 3.5   Interpretation of common chest X-ray appearances

Pattern	Cause	Appearance	Aetiology
Symmetrical	Effusion	At bases, fluid level	Hypoproteinaemia, heart failure, pneumonia
	Pulmonary oedema	Opacity spreading from hilum	Hypoproteinaemia, heart failure
		Kerley B lines, fluid in horizontal fissure	
	Bronchopneumonia	Patchy opacities especially along bronchi	*Mycoplasma*, cystic fibrosis
	Poor expansion	Diffuse haziness, under $4\frac{1}{2}$ anterior rib ends	
Asymmetrical	Effusion	At base, usually R, fluid level	Subphrenic abscess, abdominal disease
	Tumour	Solid mass, round	Neuroblastoma
Lobar pattern	Consolidation	No volume loss, air bronchograms	*Strep. pneumoniae*
	Collapse	Volume loss, no air bronchograms	Mucus plugging, Foreign body
Indistinct R mediastinum		Right Upper Lobe	
Indistinct R heart border		Right Middle Lobe	
Indistinct R hemidiaphragm		Right Lower Lobe	
Indistinct L mediastinum		Left Upper Lobe	
Indistinct L hemidiaphragm		Left Lower Lobe	

---

7   *Otitis media*

a   is almost always viral
b   may be diagnosed after visualizing a dull and injected tympanic membrane in a febrile child
c   is more common in children with Down's syndrome
d   is best treated with oral penicillin
e   is a common cause of speech delay

a   **False.** The majority of otitis media episodes are caused by bacteria, of which *Haemophilus influenzae* (not type B) and *Strep. pneumoniae* are the commonest causes. Bacterial otitis media may be distinguished from its viral counterpart as it is more likely to be unilateral and the child more likely to be toxic. However, a viral URTI may be complicated by a bacterial otitis media as the inflammation may obstruct the Eustachian tube and this predisposes to bacterial infection.

b **True**. These are the signs of otitis media. The normal tympanic membrane should be pearly-white and reflective of the light of the otoscope. It may appear as pale and thickened if there is scarring or a perforation may be seen. A blue-grey indrawn tympanic membrane is found with serous otitis media.

c **True**. As with most things, otitis media is more common in children with Down's syndrome. This is one of several treatable causes of delayed intellectual development in Down's children, along with hypothyroidism and myopia.

d **False**. If bacterial otitis media is diagnosed, antibiotics should be given. Amoxycillin or erythromycin are the most commonly used as they are active against the commonest organisms. Penicillin is used in only a few situations in paediatrics where activity against streptococcus only is needed. It is therefore used as prophylaxis in children with nephrotic syndrome and sickle cell anaemia and for treatment of a suspected bacterial pharyngitis and neonatal septicaemia (group B streptococcus). For pharyngitis, group A *Strep.* (*pyogenes*) is the most serious causative organism, but infectious mononucleosis is also likely. Other antibiotics (e.g. ampicillin) often cause a rash when there is infectious mononucleosis.

e **True**. Speech delay results from chronic otitis media or glue ear. Other causes of speech delay include other causes of hearing loss, environmental deprivation, and global developmental delay. This topic is covered in more detail in Community paediatrics and development question 17.

Otitis media may also be complicated by local extension of the infection to cause mastoiditis, cerebral abscess or meningitis.

8 *Upper respiratory tract infections in infants*
   a   are viral in over 90% of cases
   b   often cause loose motions
   c   commonly cause vomiting
   d   occur over six times a year for most children
   e   may be the cause of wheeze

a **True**. Most URTIs are viral, notably caused by the rhinovirus. Sinusitis is frequently bacterial, but is uncommon in infancy as the frontal and maxillary sinuses only develop during childhood as the mid-face grows.

b **True**. URTIs typically present with poor feeding, a low grade temperature, a runny nose, and a cough. There is often vomiting associated with the cough and the vomitus is usually mucusy. Loose stools are often found and may be greenish if the baby has not been eating. This frequently alarms parents but this is simply a starvation stool—the colour of bile.

c **True**. Many illnesses in infancy result in vomiting. Overfeeding and gastro-oesophageal reflux are the commonest causes of chronic vomiting in infancy. Febrile illnesses can all cause vomiting and URTIs and lower respiratory tract infections both cause reflex vomiting with coughing. The commonest surgical presentations in the first year are pyloric stenosis, intussusception, and mal-rotation.

d   **True**. It is true!

e   **True**. Wheeze is a result of small airways narrowing. Asthma is difficult to diagnose under the age of 1, as the definition of asthma incorporates repeated bronchospasm, and it is difficult to exclude other causes. Infants who have had bronchiolitis frequently go on to wheeze with each URTI for up to 1 year after the initial episode. Reactive bronchoconstriction may also occur in infants who have an URTI even without antecedent bronchiolitis. It has been suggested that this may be related to 'fetal smoking'. Recurrent reflux also can cause wheeze as the only symptom.

> **9   *The diagnosis of cystic fibrosis***
> a   may be made antenatally
> b   is likely if there is a high immunoreactive trypsin level
> c   is made by finding a high faecal fat content
> d   cannot be made using a sweat test in small infants
> e   is made in all of infants with meconium ileus

a   **True**. There are many ways to approach the diagnosis of cystic fibrosis (CF). The disease is caused by a defect in the gene that encodes the cystic fibrosis transport regulator (CFTR), a transmembrane protein that regulates chloride and also sodium channels in epithelia. The main organs affected are lungs, liver, pancreas, and the gut. In these organs the epithelium is unable to secrete enough salt and water, so the mucus is too thick. In the lungs this leads to poor mucus clearance and infection. In the liver, cirrhosis and in the pancreas chronic pancreatitis causing malabsorption.

To make the diagnosis genetic techniques can be used, even antenatally using chorion villus sampling. There over 200 mutations so far identified, and these account for over 85% of affected individuals, so genetic techniques will usually be helpful, but not always. Even then it will only give a genotype, and will not give a prognosis. The commonest mutation is known as $\Delta F508$.

b   **True**. The gold standard method for making phenotypic diagnosis is a sweat test. However, collection of an adequate volume of sweat is difficult in infants, so other tests can be used. Immunoreactive trypsin is measured from the serum and is high in children with CF.

c   **False**. Malabsorption is almost universal in children with CF, and so CF is part of the differential diagnosis in a child who is failing to thrive. Malabsorption occurs as a result of the pancreatic dysfunction. A high faecal fat content will be present. Unfortunately, this is not diagnostic. Other common causes include cow's milk protein intolerance and gluten enteropathy. This is further discussed in Gastroenterology question 7.

d   **False.** Sweat tests measure sweat sodium content, which will be high in CF patients. This is because these individuals are unable to reabsorb the salt from the sweat ducts. The method can be used in infants but it is a more difficult than in older children as a small volume of sweat gives unreliable results. The technique used is called pilocarpine iontophoresis.

e   **False.** Many infants with meconium ileus have CF. It presents as bilious vomiting after birth with delayed passage of meconium and is caused by an unusually sticky meconium.

10   *Sleep apnoea*
    a   is best diagnosed be admitting the child for nocturnal pulse oximetry
    b   may lead to pulmonary hypertension
    c   requires tonsillectomy
    d   may impair school performance
    e   is often due to allergy

a   **True.** Sleep apnoea is caused by upper airways obstruction. During sleep and when supine the tissues of the nasopharynx relax and fall posteriorly into the airways and lead to snoring and apnoea. Parents of affected children often complain the noise is so bad even they can't sleep. During the daytime the children may be sleepy. The best way to make the diagnosis is to admit the child for nocturnal pulse oximetry. This allows objective assessment of the problem. There will be apnoea and desaturation in badly affected children.

b   **True.** The hypoxia that occurs as a result of the apnoea can lead to pulmonary hypertension. Failure to thrive and developmental delay may also result.

c   **False.** Large tonsils and adenoids are the usual cause. Most children with sleep apnoea will benefit for removal of these glands, but it is not always needed. The other indication for removal of tonsils and adenoids is recurrent tonsillitis that causes the child to miss a significant amount of school, quinsy, and chronic otitis media.

d   **True.** Other common causes include poor vision, poor hearing, and behavioural problems.

e   **False.** Sleep apnoea is a mechanical problem.

Data interpretation and reasoning—answers

11   *A boy of 18 months is brought to the emergency department by his mother. The triage nurse notices that he has an inspiratory stridor, is holding his neck extended and is drooling. His pulse is recorded as 175 beats/min, respiratory rate 40 and temperature 38.5°C. He also has a blue tinge to his tongue and seems agitated. To manage him correctly*

a   an urgent lateral neck X-ray should be obtained
b   arterial blood gases will be needed to determine the need for intubation
c   broad-spectrum antibiotics should be given before anything else is done
d   high flow oxygen may reduce his agitation
e   his siblings will need prophylaxis

a **False**   b **False**   c **False**   d **True**   e **True**

Reasoning and data interpretation questions are designed to test if the candidate can decide the appropriate management for a given situation, which is more difficult than simply knowing whether something is right or wrong. In this scenario there is a child with a stridor. This sign is often not associated with serious disease, but on the other hand the child may be about to die from airway obstruction. Here we are given additional information to help decide how best to treat him.

Every disease causes local effects and may also cause systemic effects. In terms of local effects of the problem, he has an extended neck, which children adopt to open the airways, as an anaesthetist will to ventilate by mask. He is also drooling, which implies he is not able to swallow saliva. Babies from about the age of 6 to 14 months drool even when well as they are upright and do not attempt to swallow all their saliva out of their mouths. Drooling may also be caused by a neuro-muscular problem (IXth or Xth cranial nerve palsy, cerebral palsy) or local inflammation (pharyngitis, tonsillitis, quinsy, or epiglottitis).

The degree of recession also gives some information about the amount of obstruction, but is influenced by other factors such as agitation and tiredness.

In terms of systemic signs of illness in the child, he is cyanosed in air and agitated. Cyanosis implies there is either cyanotic congenital heart disease or a respiratory emergency, and he must be evaluated (airway and breathing) and treated urgently. The first measure will be face mask oxygen. Agitation is one of the cerebral effects of hypoxia, and may progress to coma, fits and eventually death. Hypercarbia, on the other hand causes vasodilation, manifest as headache and eventually coma. This boy also has a tachycardia, and all these reasons indicate that he is severely ill with an airway problem.

High flow oxygen may reduce his agitation, but on the other hand may increase it as he may become even more distressed by a face mask. In children with stridor, care should be taken to minimize their anxiety—they should be kept with their parent in a calm atmosphere, but they also need to be closely observed, as they may collapse at any time.

In this question a number of investigations are suggested, but only investigations that provide useful information to alter management without significant risk to the patient should ever be used. A lateral neck X-ray may show the swollen epiglottis, but provides little information useful for management—he will need intubation based on clinical information (degree of recession, severity of stridor, oxygen requirement, pulse, conscious level) rather than radiographic appearances. An arterial blood gas will probably be abnormal, but will certainly distress the child and make his airway problem worse. Even siting an intravenous line should not be done until the airway are secured by intubation, and then antibiotics given (a third-generation cephalosporin such as cefotaxime) that will be active against HIB, as this is the only organism responsible for epiglottitis.

Prophylaxis is indicated for all HIB infections for close contacts with oral rifampicin. This agent is also used in the prophylaxis of meningococcal disease. Prophylaxis is further discussed in Immunology/infectious diseases question 1.

12　*A 2-month-old inpatient has a respiratory rate of 50 and chest recession. An arterial blood gas is taken*
　　pH 7.36 (7.35–7.45)
　　pCO_2 7.2 kPa (4.5–6.0)
　　pO_2 11.2 kPa (10.0–14.0)
　　BE +11.3 mmol/l (+5.0 to − 5.0)

Now it can be said that
　　a　he has a respiratory acidosis
　　b　chronic respiratory disease is probably the cause of his high pCO_2
　　c　the cause of these results may be vomiting
　　d　hypoventilation is the cause for the high pCO_2
　　e　the positive BE has compensated for a respiratory problem

a **False**　b **True**　c **False**　d **False**　e **True**

Blood gas interpretation is outlined in question 18 of the neonatal section. It can be seen that there is a high pCO_2 and BE, but there is neither acidosis nor alkalosis. There is a fully compensated respiratory acidosis or a metabolic alkalosis. The scenario states that there is respiratory distress and tachypnoea, implying that there is a primary respiratory problem. If the hypercarbia is long-standing, the acidosis is corrected by the excretion of an acid urine.

The most likely cause of this infant's disease is bronchopulmonary dysplasia, a form of chronic lung disease following respiratory distress syndrome. Hypoventilation can cause a high pCO_2, but this is not the case in this scenario. Hypoventilation is rare in paediatric populations—most commonly it is caused by opiates or a central nervous problem. A high pCO_2 may also be caused by respiratory disease, acute or chronic.

Vomiting can alter the blood chemistry if severe enough because it leads to the loss of acid, water, chloride, and sodium ions. The best known situation is with pyloric stenosis, where there is a hypokalaemic metabolic alkalosis. The reasons for this are outlined in Nephrology question 11. This would not explain the high CO_2.

13　*A 13-month-old boy presents with difficulty in breathing. In the past he has been admitted with bronchiolitis and is being seen in the asthma clinic. The following features increase the possibility of an inhaled foreign body*
　　a　lobar collapse on chest X-ray
　　b　temperature 38.2°C
　　c　bilateral crackles
　　d　bilateral hyperexpansion
　　e　cyanosis in air

a **True** b **True** c **False** d **False** e **True**

This child is statistically the right sex and age (6–24 months) to inhale a foreign body. His respiratory distress may be also due to a bronchiolitis exacerbation or asthma. Features in the history of an inhaled foreign body are a sudden onset of cough, with or without a history of choking. Signs vary depending on the size of object inhaled, where it is lodged, and how long it has been there. If a large airway is obstructed, there may be cyanosis or even death. Breath sounds are reduced unilaterally or in the area to which air entry is obstructed. If there is partial blockage, unilateral hyperexpansion results. If the blockage is more complete collapse results. Infection commonly develops after several days, and may give rise to a high fever.

14(i)   *A girl of 7 months is seen with a cough by her family doctor. She has already been ill for 1 week with a cough, poor feeding, and a temperature. She has had similar symptoms twice in the last 3 months and each time was prescribed amoxycillin. On the first of these occasions she had a normal chest X-ray taken. The doctor examines her and finds that she is alert and interested in her surroundings. She has a respiratory rate of 50 with mild recession. On auscultation wheeze was audible on both sides of her chest. She is pink in air and cardiovascular examination is unremarkable. Her mother is worried that she will develop asthma. She is more likely to be correct because*

a   her temperature is 37.7°C
b   there is a family history of urticaria
c   both the child's parents smoke cigarettes
d   she had bronchiolitis 3 months ago
e   she improves after a salbutamol nebulizer

a **False** b **True** c **True** d **False** e **True**

Recurrent cough is a common problem in childhood. The differential diagnosis is listed in Box 3.6 with distinguishing features for each condition. Here this girl presents with a cough and respiratory difficulty. She also has a wheeze which makes bronchiolitis and asthma more likely, although she may have reactive bronchospasm secondary to a URTI. Foreign body inhalation and pneumonia are unlikely as the signs are bilateral, and upper airway problems unlikely (e.g. postnasal drip) because no nocturnal symptoms are mentioned and there are signs suggestive of small airways disease. The history of repeated chest infections raises the possibility of CF or an immunodeficiency, such as IgA or IgG subclass deficiency both of which can cause chest infections.

This question is asking for features that make asthma more likely. A family history of atopy (asthma, eczema, allergic rhinitis, urticaria, and migraine) is one of these. Cigarette smoking by the parents will also increase the chance of the child having asthma as well as other respiratory infections. There has been much debate about the effect of pollution on the incidence of asthma, but it is certain that it is not a major factor. The contribution that pets make triggering and in the continuation of a child's asthma is very variable. For some individuals removal of a pet does improve symptoms markedly, but may be traumatic for the child. The house dust

Box 3.6 Causes of recurrent cough

Asthma	Atopic, worse at night
Cystic fibrosis, bronchiectasis	Failure to thrive, recurrent infections
Chronic sinusitis with a postnasal drip	Atopic, worse at night
Gastro-oesophageal reflux with aspiration	Worse on lying down, recurrent infections
Pertussis	Initially coryzal with paroxysmal cough
Foreign body	Abrupt start of symptoms
H-type tracheoesophageal fistula	Recurrent infections

mite is more important is asthma, but removal of this agent from a house is impossible. Dust reducing measures can improve symptoms.

A raised temperature does not increase the chance of asthma but makes it more likely that there is an URTI. Response to salbutamol is not characteristic of asthma, as it merely indicates that there is bronchospasm and $\beta2$ receptors present on bronchial smooth muscle. This muscle is not often present before the child is 1 year old, except in infants with bronchopulmonary dysplasia. However, response to salbutamol is much more likely if the infant has asthma. In the first year, ipratropium bromide is more likely to work as a bronchodilator, as it acts as an acetylcholine antagonist.

Bronchiolitis has not been shown to increase the chance of a child developing asthma, although both present similarly, and as both are common, asthma may carry on from bronchiolitis.

14(ii)   The doctor would have good reason to
   a   start inhaled steroids
   b   prescribe a course of a different antibiotic
   c   repeat the chest X-ray
   d   perform a sweat test
   e   arrange for a home nebulizer

a   **False**   b   **False**   c   **False**   d   **False**   e   **False**

Given the information above, bronchiolitis, asthma, or perhaps a viral pneumonia are the most likely causes for the baby's problems. It would be appropriate to start a bronchodilator via a spacer and mask to see if it had any effect. A nebulizer would be inappropriate at this stage (see question 3i). At a later stage inhaled steroids could be added in. There are no indications to start antibiotics, as the child is not unwell with signs to suggest a chest infection. The sweat test would certainly cause alarm and be inappropriate unless the child was having well documented chest infections or not growing well. A repeat chest X-ray would not be indicated unless there were localizing signs or a high fever suggestive of bacterial pneumonia.

15(i)   *A 4-year-old girl who is a known asthmatic presents to the emergency department at 23.00 with her father. She is managed in conjunction with the asthma clinic at the hospital and is currently on beclomethasone 200 μg twice a day and salbutamol 200 μg after she takes the beclomethasone or when she needs it. She takes both with a spacer. Today she has been taking the salbutamol every hour all day but is no better. In the past she has been admitted with her asthma five times and once went to the paediatric intensive care unit. Last week she saw her family doctor with oral candidiasis*

a   the candidiasis is probably iatrogenic
b   she is taking her medicines correctly
c   the beclomethasone can be increased during attacks
d   she will get better drug delivery from a dry powder delivery device
e   she should have been brought earlier in the day

a **True** b **False** c **True** d **False** e **True**

This girl has both bad chronic asthma (she uses regular doses of inhaled steroids and attends the asthma clinic) and is prone to severe attacks (previous visit to intensive care). Now she has been using the salbutamol hourly. Patients should see a doctor if they are not getting relief from bronchodilators every 4 h. Delay in presentation means that the attack is well advanced before systemic steroids are given and is more likely to result in death.

This question is about maintenance treatment and advice. Here she is *not* taking the steroid after the bronchodilator and so less steroid can reach the bronchi. She is, however, using a spacing device which gives excellent drug delivery at any age. She and her parents should be told to put the puffs (typically two to four) from the MDI into the spacer and then for her to breathe in and out through the mouthpiece at least 20 times, moving the valve. She will get no better delivery from a dry powder device, and it is likely not to be as well tolerated.

With topical steroids, systemic effects are reported, but rare and usually mild, whereas local effects are common. Oral candidiasis is one of these, but it is less likely to occur if the mouth is washed out after inhalation.

When an attack is coming on or likely (the child has an URTI), the parents can be instructed to increase the dose of bronchodilator or steroid. This, as long as well supervised with clear limits as to when to seek further medical attention, reduces hospital attendance and helps avoid systemic steroids.

15(ii)   *She is given a salbutamol nebulizer immediately by the nurse. The nurse also records that her pulse is 160 beats/min, respiratory rate 65 breaths/min and her saturation 83% in air. She is no better after the nebulizer and so the doctor is called urgently. He listens to her chest and finds poor breath sounds and no wheeze. To manage her well he could now*

a   give a loading dose of aminophylline
b   give her oral prednisolone
c   take an arterial blood gas
d   site an intravenous line and give hydrocortisone
e   repeat the salbutamol nebulizer

a **False** b **True** c **False** d **False** e **True**

She has a severe attack, as manifest be the tachypnoea, tachycardia, desaturation, and reduced breath sounds. There is no wheeze because she is not moving enough air in and out to wheeze. Box 3.1 shows features that distinguish attacks of different severity.

In this situation, when there is no response to this first nebulizer, a second salbutamol nebulizer should be given and the patient loaded with oral prednisolone. The indications for intravenous hydrocortisone are life-threatening attacks, inability to swallow and vomiting, where prednisolone will not be absorbed. Aminophylline can be given if she is still 'severe' after the nebulizers and steroids. A loading dose should be given if the child is not already on aminophylline, and then an infusion continued. A salbutamol infusion is also effective, and is used when the child is still severe despite aminophylline, although recent research has shown that its use at admission reduces hospital stay. Both of these agents cause hypokalaemia, tachycardia, and vomiting. Ipratropium bromide can be given as a nebulized inhalation as it is sometimes of benefit.

If there is still no response to these agents or the child is deteriorating, arterial blood gases can be used to determine the need for ventilation. Deranged gases are tolerated up to a point as ventilation of asthmatics is difficult and hazardous.

16 *A 9 year old is admitted to the intensive care unit as he has failed to improve with half-hourly salbutamol nebulizers, intravenous hydrocortisone, and an aminophylline infusion. He is now looking tired. An arterial blood gas is taken while he is breathing oxygen via face mask*
   pH 7.18 (7.35–7.45)
   pCO_2 7.5 kPa (4.5–6.0)
   pO_2 13.1 kPa (10.0–14.0)
   BE −1.2 mmol/l (+5.0 to −5.0)

From this it can be said that

   a his oxygen should be turned down
   b a salbutamol infusion could be of benefit
   c mechanical ventilation should now be started
   d a low minute volume is responsible for his high pCO_2
   e his negative BE implies there is a metabolic acidosis

a **False** b **True** c **True** d **True** e **False**

If patients with severe asthma attacks do not improve, their respiratory muscles become tired and then they are unable to overcome their airways resistance. They may then deteriorate rapidly. This may be seen as worsening conscious level and deteriorating blood gases.

Here the boy has a respiratory acidosis that, being acute, is not compensated. The BE is within the normal range. Carbon dioxide levels rise if the minute volume is low—that is the volume of gas breathed in (or out) in a minute. This is the product of the respiratory rate and tidal volume. Here his tidal volume is probably reduced as he has airways obstruction.

In this situation, his treatment should be reviewed to see if anything else that can be done or if there are any treatable complications. His nebulizer frequency could be increased to give continuous nebulized salbutamol and he could have a salbutamol infusion. Also a chest X-ray would be a good idea to rule out a pneumothorax. If pneumothoraces are bilateral clinical diagnosis can be difficult.

17   A 4 year old is brought to his family doctor with a sore throat. The doctor is worried that he has glandular fever (infectious mononucleosis). The following features make this diagnosis more likely than another cause of a sore throat

   a   he has a palpable liver 3 cm below the costal margin
   b   his temperature is 38.9°C
   c   a fine maculopapular rash on the trunk
   d   pustules on the tonsils
   e   slightly enlarged cervical lymph nodes

a **True** b **False** c **True** d **False** e **False**

Sore throats are a very common cause of visits to the family doctor. Most are viral and if bacterial *Strep. pyogenes* is the most likely organism. There is no way to be sure of the type of organism form the appearance of the throat, but it is likely to be redder with pustules in bacterial pharyngitis. Also viral infections tend to cause milder illnesses with a lower temperature, less systemic upset, and tend to have less effect on appetite and swallowing than streptococcal pharyngitis. Children with suspected viral pharyngitis should have a throat swab and paracetamol but no antibiotics.

Glandular fever, also called infectious mononucleosis (IM) is usually accompanied by a pharyngitis that is sometimes pustular, and there is often marked systemic upset. Local lymph nodes are usually enlarged in URTIs, but in children with IM enlarged nodes will be found in other areas. Other distinguishing features include a maculopapular rash, and hepato- or splenomegaly. Again no specific treatment is indicated, but a throat swab will rule out bacterial infection. A Monospot test may be positive and a full blood count may show atypical lymphocytes.

Streptococcal pharyngitis can also cause a number of distant effects, including erythematous rash (scarlet fever), erythema nodosum, nephritis, and arthritis.

If a bacterial sore throat is suspected again a throat swab should be taken and the child started on penicillin, which will be active against streptococci, but is not so likely to bring out a rash as other antibiotics, notably ampicillin.

4 Nephrology

Knowledge — questions

1 A 9-year-old boy is taken to his family doctor because it was noticed that his urine was pink. There is no relevant past medical history. The following pieces of additional information would provide an explanation for his pink urine

   a he has just finished a 2 day prophylaxis course of rifampicin
   b his father has long-standing kidney disease
   c his blood pressure is 90/65
   d he is deaf
   e he is currently ill with a sore throat

2 A 4-year-old boy is found to have a blood pressure of 125/95 at a clinic visit for an unrelated problem

   a unilateral kidney disease cannot be the cause
   b essential hypertension cannot be the cause at this age
   c vesico-ureteric reflux is a likely aetiological factor
   d the femoral pulse must be examined
   e he should be started on antihypertensives while awaiting further investigation results

3 When managing a child who has had an urinary tract infection

   a an intravenous urogram is a useful first-line investigation
   b an ultrasound is useful in the acute phase to demonstrate obstruction
   c to identify renal scarring children under 1 year should have a DMSA scan
   d constipation may predispose to further infections
   e a high blood pressure indicates renal damage has probably occurred

4 A 3-year-old girl presents with periorbital oedema

   a the blood albumin level will be low
   b probably has low complement factors
   c proteinuria, haematuria, and hypertension indicates she has the nephrotic syndrome
   d frusemide treatment should be used to reduce the oedema
   e may be at increased risk of pneumococcal peritonitis

5   *Concerning glomerulonephritis*
   a   streptococcal infection may precipitate glomerulonephritis and lead to nephritic syndrome
   b   features of minimal change nephropathy may be seen by light microscopy in some areas of a renal biopsy
   c   children with nephrotic syndrome are best treated after a renal biopsy
   d   minimal change nephropathy is characteristically associated with a highly selective proteinuria
   e   massive proteinuria is a common feature of children with nephritic syndrome

6   *Acute renal failure in children*
   a   may lead to convulsions
   b   often leads to hyperkalaemia
   c   is often precipitated by intravascular volume depletion
   d   should be treated initially using dialysis
   e   often includes a polyuric phase

7   *Urine tests*
   a   will show a low specific gravity if the child has inappropriate antidiuretic hormone levels
   b   will be positive for ketones in a child who has not eaten for 36 h
   c   usually demonstrates nitrites in bacterial urine infections
   d   will demonstrate microscopic haematuria in a proportion of normal individuals after exercise
   e   often show a raised white cell count with a systemic leucocytosis

8   *Urine organisms*
   a   treatment of *Proteus* infections is aided by the acidification of the urine
   b   pseudomonal urine infection is frequently resistant to amoxycillin
   c   *Escherichia coli* is the commonest organism responsible for urine infections in girls
   d   *Mycobacterium tuberculosis* is a cause of 'sterile pyuria'
   e   *Streptococcus faecalis* is not sensitive to trimethoprim

Data interpretation and reasoning — questions

9(i)   *A child of 5 is seen because his parents have noticed swelling around his eyes. The diagnosis of nephrotic syndrome is made more likely than another cause for his illness because he is also found to have*

a   macroscopic haematuria
b   liver edge palpable at 3 cm below the costal margin
c   temperature 38°C
d   maculopapular rash
e   a distended abdomen

9(ii)   *In this child the following results become available*
urinary protein dipstix ++++
urine microscopy: RBC, 20 mm³; WCC, <5 mm³
albumin 18 g/dl
Na⁺ 135 mmol/l
K⁺ 3.9 mmol/l
urea 3.4 mmol/l
antistreptolysin O titre negative
complement levels normal

a   he is in renal failure
b   albumin should be given
c   these results are compatible with nephritic syndrome
d   he does not have pyuria
e   oral steroids should form part of his treatment

10(i)   *A female infant of 6 months age presents with five loose stools in
the past 24 h and a temperature of 38.5°C, but is not clinically
dehydrated or cardiovascularly compromised. She is feeding well, is
alert, and interested in her surroundings. A partial septic screen is
performed*
Hb 12.7 g/dl
WCC 14.5 × 10³/mm³
PL 453 × 10³/mm³
Na⁺ 143 mmol/l
K⁺ 3.8 mmol/l
U 3.7 mmol/l
clean catch urine
    cloudy appearance
    RBC 25/mm³
    WBC 75/mm³
    no organisms seen
blood cultures pending

a   a diagnosis of a urinary tract infection can now be made
b   a suprapubic aspirate should now be performed

    c she has microscopic haematuria
    d she should be started on aspirin
    e antibiotics should be withheld until culture results are available

10(ii)   *This girl's urine culture grows* **Escherichia coli** *$>10^5$ colony forming units/ml. She is discharged on a 1 week course of trimethoprim and seen in the outpatient clinic at the end of this course. She has made a good recovery and is now virtually back to normal*

    a a DMSA scan will be needed to identify vesico-ureteric reflux
    b a renal ultrasound may identify scarring
    c organisms may still be present in the urine even if the infection has been successfully treated
    d antibiotics should be stopped until all the investigations are completed
    e a micturating cysto-urethrogram must be delayed for 6 weeks to prevent false positive results

11   *A male infant is admitted at the age of 7 weeks. He has been vomiting all his feeds for 3 days and now has a reduced urine output. He still seems hungry. He has no temperature. Some results are now available*

    Na^+ 132 mmol/l
    K^+ 2.8 mmol/l
    urea 8.2 mmol/l
    creatinine 90 μmol/l
    urine clear
    urine pH 6.2

    a his vomiting has left him sodium depleted
    b urine and creatinine levels are normal
    c the potassium is high because renal tubular function is poor
    d systemic acidosis has made his urine pH acidotic
    e fluid replacement should occur before any surgical intervention

12   *A 5-month-old boy is admitted to the ward with a 3-day history of cough and runny nose. He has not taken any solids for 2 days. He has had four 90 ml bottles of formula milk and has wet two nappies in the last 24 h. Examining him, his temperature is 37.3°C, his heart rate is 135 beats/min, his respiratory rate is 55/min, and he has moderate chest recession. He is not clinically dehydrated. Some investigations are performed, mainly because of his poor urine output*

Hb 9.7 g/dl
WCC 5.7 × 10³/mm³
platelets 296 × 10³/mm³
Na⁺ 128 mmol/l
K⁺ 3.3 mmol/l
urea 1.9 mmol/l
osmolality 272 mmol/l

   a he should be cross-matched for a blood transfusion
   b his urine is likely to be inappropriately concentrated
   c urine sodium concentration is probably high
   d his fluid intake is reduced
   e the most likely diagnosis is an upper respiratory tract infection

13   *These results are obtained from a 2-year-old boy who has presented*
     with a convulsion. He is well known to the casualty department, who
     have seen him on several occasions with various injuries. Now his
     carer says he has been vomiting
     Na⁺ 165 mmol/l
     K⁺ 4.3 mmol/l
     urea 3.7 mmol/l
     creatinine 45 mmol/l

These results are explained by the fact that

   a he has been given only formula milk to drink in the last 2 days
   b his mother has inadvertently given dioralyte at 10 times the correct
      strength
   c further questioning reveals he also has profuse diarrhoea
   d he has just been resuscitated with a large bolus of 0.9% sodium chloride
      solution
   e he has been poisoned with salt

Knowledge — answers

Paediatric nephrology and urinary medicine is a complicated subject; however, at
undergraduate level it is dominated by only a few conditions that are simple to
understand and fairly common. You are almost certain to be asked about urinary
tract infections in regard to their presentation, treatment, and investigation. Adult
and paediatric urinary tract infections (UTIs) differ markedly in their significance
and implications and examiners like to check you know this. The other major
condition that is asked about is nephrotic syndrome, as it is the most common
paediatric kidney disorder in the Western world. The rest of undergraduate paedi-

atric renal/fluid questions will either be to do with interpretation of electrolyte results or other manifestations of kidney disease.

These questions mainly focus on these areas.

1 A 9-year-old boy is taken to his family doctor because it was noticed that his urine was pink. There is no relevant past medical history. The following pieces of additional information would provide an explanation for his pink urine

    a he has just finished a 2 day prophylaxis course of rifampicin

    b his father has long-standing kidney disease

    c his blood pressure is 90/65

    d he is deaf

    e he is currently ill with a sore throat

a   **True.** Urine is coloured by a variety of substances. Some colour it red, such as beetroot and rifampicin. Urine can also be coloured by poisons such as benzene and carbon tetrachloride. None of these reddening substances will test positive for blood on Dipstix testing, and a careful history should identify them in the clinical setting.

Rifampicin is given to all close contacts of an index case with meningococcal disease twice a day for 2 days to prevent secondary cases. Alternatively ciprofloxacin can be used.

b   **True.** There are several familial kidney disorders of which Alport's syndrome is the most significant and serious. This affects the ears, with sensorineural deafness, eyes with cataracts and keratoconus, and the kidneys, with progressive renal failure and haematuria. Other familial conditions causing haematuria are much more benign.

Even if you knew nothing about Alport's, this would still have been a good guess!

c   **False.** This is a normal blood pressure for a 9 year old. A raised blood pressure may indicate renal disease, particularly reflux nephropathy, and is part of the nephritic presentation.

Numbers and normal ranges are difficult to learn and even more so in paediatrics, where they are different for each age. As a rough guide, the 95th and 5th percentiles for systolic blood pressure are roughly 115 mmHg and 78 mmHg, respectively, at 12 months. They rise about 1 mmHg/year thereafter. In exams data will usually be well outside the normal range.

d   **True.** This branch is again trying to make the connection with Alport's syndrome.

e   **False.** Two conditions link sore throats with renal disease. Post-streptococcal glomerulonephritis (PSGN) typically occurs 7–21 days after a bout of streptococcal pharyngitis. Only certain strains of organism can cause the complement activation that leads to glomerulonephritis (GN). A nephritic syndrome develops (hypertension, oedema, haematuria, oliguria) and this can lead to heart failure or seizures. Treatment is entirely supportive with diuretics and antihypertensives. Prognosis is excellent, and most children are symptomatically better in 1–2 weeks. C3 levels are low, but C4 normal.

The other renal disease linked to upper respiratory illness is IgA nephropathy, also called Berger disease. This presents as bouts of haematuria 1–2 days after respiratory infections. There are no other nephritic features and the C3 is normal.

> 2   *A 4-year-old boy is found to have a blood pressure of 125/95 at a clinic visit for an unrelated problem*
>   a   unilateral kidney disease cannot be the cause
>   b   essential hypertension cannot be the cause at this age
>   c   vesico-ureteric reflux is a likely aetiological factor
>   d   the femoral pulse must be examined
>   e   he should be started on antihypertensives while awaiting further investigation results

a   **False**. It is actually the most common renal cause. Systemic hypertension is children is almost always caused by raised levels of hormones—renin, catecholamines, or steroids. Essential hypertension is relatively uncommon at this age. A kidney damaged by disease (e.g. reflux nephropathy) will have a lower glomerular filtration rate (GFR) and thus produce more renin. Coarctation and unilateral renal artery stenosis will reduce GFR and raise renin by the same mechanism.

b   **False**. Essential hypertension is a rare cause at this age, but becomes more likely as the child gets older. It is the diagnosis only after careful exclusion of all other primary causes.

c   **True**. Vesico-ureteric reflux (VUR) is an important preventable cause of adult kidney disease and is the most common pathological cause of long-standing hypertension in children. VUR is found in 20–50% of children who present with UTIs depending on age and sex. Children with UTIs may also have anatomical anomalies.

d   **True**. Coarctation of the aorta is an important preventable cause of hypertension. It may be picked up in the newborn examination, the femoral arteries may be impalpable and later on there may be radiofemoral delay. If there is any doubt, the blood pressure in each of the child's limbs (a four-limb blood pressure) can be measured. This will identify the right arm or upper body hypertension characteristic of the condition.

e   **False**. The stress of a clinical situation or mild illness is enough to raise a child's blood pressure. The size of the cuff may also be incorrect, leading to error. The blood pressure should be rechecked before further investigations unless there are other signs of renal disease.

> 3   *When managing a child who has had an urinary tract infection*
>   a   an intravenous urogram is a useful first-line investigation
>   b   an ultrasound is useful in the acute phase to demonstrate obstruction

    c to identify renal scarring children under 1 year should have a DMSA scan
    d constipation may predispose to further infections
    e a high blood pressure indicates renal damage has probably occurred

a **False**. The purpose of any investigation is to provide information that alters
management and thus reduces morbidity or mortality. In a child who has had a
UTI there are two potential adverse outcomes: further UTIs and permanent renal
damage. Permanent renal damage from UTIs occurs as a result of an infection
ascending from the bladder. Such damage probably never occurs after the age of 5.

Investigations in those under 5 are designed therefore to identify those who
have already suffered renal damage, as these children should receive prophylaxis
against further infections. A DMSA scan is the best way to do this, although ultrasound can identify small scarred kidneys.

Under 1 year the damage may not already have happened, and so investigations
in this age group are designed to look also for factors predisposing to ascending
infection. By far the most common cause is VUR, best diagnosed with a MCUG
(micturating cysto-urethrogram). A plan for investigation is shown in Box 4.1.

Box 4.1   Investigation of a proven urinary tract infection

Over 5 years	Ultrasound	Further tests if recurrent	
1–5 years	Ultrasound	DMSA	MCUG if DMSA or ultrasound abnormal
Under 1 year	Ultrasound	DMSA	MCUG

Prophylactic antibiotics for those under 5
Abdominal X-ray if *Proteus* UTI
All tests except ultrasound must wait 6 weeks
Ensure UTI has cleared

An intravenous urogram will identify an obstruction in the system. It is used if a
part of the urinary tract is dilated (as seen on ultrasound), but there is no reflux
seen on MCUG. This is unusual in children.

b **True**. It will identify obstruction if the ureters are >5 mm in diameter,
depending on who is doing the test. It is particularly useful if the child is taking
some time to respond to treatment, as a stagnant pool of obstructed urine will be
difficult to clear of organisms without drainage.

DMSA and MCUG tests on the other hand must wait until 6 weeks after the
UTI or there may be false positive results.

c **True**. As discussed in part (a). If there is scarring or evidence of reflux, the
child must continue on prophylaxis until the reflux has stopped or he or she is
too old to scar.

d **True**. Constipation leads to incomplete bladder emptying and this can cause UTIs. Constipation should always be treated with the UTI and dietary change initiated if this is needed.

On the other hand a UTI may present as diarrhoea with a fever. For this reason any child with diarrhoea should have a urine sent for culture.

e **True**. Other indications are scarred kidneys on DMSA or ultrasound. At the most extreme, poor growth, rickets, and deranged blood chemistry may occur.

   4 *A 3-year-old girl presents with periorbital oedema*
   a   the blood albumin level will be low
   b   probably has low complement factors
   c   proteinuria, haematuria, and hypertension indicates she has the nephrotic syndrome
   d   frusemide treatment should be used to reduce the oedema
   e   may be increased at risk of pneumococcal peritonitis

a **False**. Causes for periorbital oedema include nephrotic syndrome, local infection, angioneurotic oedema, acute nephritis, and heart failure. Minimal change nephropathy is associated with a highly selective proteinuria. The damage to the basement membrane makes it leaky to small negatively charged proteins. This means large amounts of albumin and lesser amounts of other proteins such as immunoglobulins are lost.

b **False**. Glomerulonephritis causes low complement by consumption, but levels are typically normal in minimal change glomerulonephropathy, the most common cause of nephrotic syndrome.

c **False**. This is the nephritic syndrome. Features of the nephrotic syndrome are oedema, hypoalbuminaemia, proteinuria, and hypercholesterolaemia. The syndrome does not give information about the pathology, although 80% of children with nephrotic syndrome have minimal change nephropathy.

d **False**. It is only used in children where there is massive scrotal or pulmonary oedema. Frusemide works by increasing the loss of salt and water from the intravascular compartment. Fluid then passes into this space from the tissues. As nephrotics are already tending towards intravascular depletion, frusemide can be dangerous.

Salt-poor albumin can be used in this situation to reduce oedema in combination with diuretics. It leads to a temporary shift of water out of the tissues into the vessels. It can then be excreted in the urine. However, this albumin will also be lost in the urine so the effect is temporary. Also the fluid shifts can lead to heart failure and pulmonary oedema, so patients receiving albumin must be closely monitored.

e **True**. Any ascitic fluid can become infected. Children with nephrotic syndrome are immunocompromised because of immunoglobulin loss. Encapsulated organisms such as *Strep. pneumoniae* are a particular problem so prophylaxis with penicillin is recommended.

5   *Concerning glomerulonephritis*

   a   streptococcal infection may precipitate glomerulonephritis and lead to nephritic syndrome

   b   features of minimal change nephropathy may be seen by light microscopy in some areas of a renal biopsy

   c   children with nephrotic syndrome are best treated after a renal biopsy

   d   minimal change nephropathy is characteristically associated with a highly selective proteinuria

   e   massive proteinuria is a common feature of children with nephritic syndrome

a   **True**. As already discussed, certain strains of β-haemolytic streptococcus can lead to a GN. Hepatitis B is also able to do this. Both are associated with types of proliferative GN, typically presenting as nephritic syndrome.

b   **False**. The only changes seen in minimal change GN are seen by electron microscopy, which identifies fusion of the podocytes.

c   **False**. A diagnosis is always a useful thing to have, but making one with a potentially hazardous investigation that is unlikely to alter management is not a good idea. As 80–90% of children with typical nephrotic syndrome will have steroid-sensitive GN, a biopsy is only done if the patient does not improve after 4 weeks of steroids or relapses as soon as doses are reduced. This identifies those children who have another type of GN that might need treatment with another drug and has a different prognosis.

d   **True**. As discussed already in question 4. Other types of GN do not tend to cause such a selective proteinuria, as the damage to the glomerulus is more severe.

e   **False**. This is typical of nephrotic syndrome and exceeds 1 g/m^2 per day of protein. Nephritic syndrome causes a moderate proteinuria of the order of 0.5 g/m^2 per day.

6   *Acute renal failure in children*

   a   may lead to convulsions

   b   often leads to hyperkalaemia

   c   is often precipitated by intravascular volume depletion

   d   should be treated initially using dialysis

   e   often includes a polyuric phase

a   **True**. Acute renal failure (ARF) is divided into pre-, intra- and post-renal causes. All share a lack of glomerular filtration, and this leads to a raised renin, and hence angiotensin level, causing hypertension. This is worsened by the volume overload that may develop. Hypertensive encephalopathy can precipitate convulsions and is treated with antihypertensives as well as fluid restriction, diuretics, and dialysis.

b   **True**. Potassium retention occurs because renal tubular function is lost in ARF. Normally, potassium is secreted in the distal tubule in exchange for sodium. Sodium retention is also a problem, but as it also leads to water retention, Na^+

levels do not rise. Sodium can also be excreted more easily as glomerular filtrate contains more sodium than potassium, so that in the absence of tubular function, it is easily lost from the body.

c   **True**. This is prerenal dehydration. A low blood volume eventually leads to a reduced GFR. This also reduces the nutrient supply to the proximal and distal tubules. These cells die, causing acute tubular necrosis. At this stage the urine is highly concentrated. When intravascular volume is restored, GFR returns, but because the tubules are still not working, the urine is copious and resembles filtered plasma in its biochemistry.

d   **False**. Dialysis is reserved for those not responding to supportive treatment (fluid and salt restriction, antihypertensives) and who are likely to develop a serious complication (encephalopathy, hyperkalaemia).

e   **True**. The polyuric phase, as discussed in (c), typically starts 7–10 days after the presentation of ARF. During this phase, fluids must be liberalized and electrolytes maintained to meet the renal losses.

7   *Urine tests*
   a   will show a low specific gravity if the child has inappropriate antidiuretic hormone levels
   b   will be positive for ketones in a child who has not eaten for 36 h
   c   usually demonstrates nitrites in bacterial urine infections
   d   will demonstrate microscopic haematuria in a proportion of normal individuals after exercise
   e   often show a raised white cell count with a systemic leucocytosis

a   **False**. Inappropriate antidiuretic hormone (ADH) inappropriately concentrates the urine when the plasma concentration (osmolality) is low. When there is inappropriate ADH the urine therefore has a high specific gravity.
   ADH is secreted by the posterior pituitary in response to a high plasma osmolality. It acts on the distal tubule and leads to an increase in the permeability of the membrane to water. This allows an increase in the reabsorption of water and a reduction in the serum osmolality. Aldosterone, on the other hand is secreted in response to hypovolaemia, and leads to sodium and hence water reabsorption. This corrects the hypovolaemia.

b   **True**. Ketone bodies are made in response to low insulin levels. As glucose levels fall during fasting, glucagon rises and insulin falls. This leads to gluconeogenesis and lipolysis producing ketones.

c   **True**. Nitrites are made from nitrates by bacteria, so the test for urinary nitrites can aid in the Dipstix identification of a child who might have a UTI.

d   **True**. Haematuria can occur after exercise in normal individuals.

e   **True**. A pyuria is also found with renal tract inflammation and renal or urinary infection.

8 *Urine organisms*
   a   treatment of *Proteus* infections is aided by the acidification of the urine
   b   pseudomonal urine infection is frequently resistant to amoxycillin
   c   *E. coli* is the commonest organism responsible for urine infections in girls
   d   *M. tuberculosis* is a cause of 'sterile pyuria'
   e   *Strep. faecalis* is not sensitive to trimethoprim

a   **False**. *Proteus* acidifies the urine. This leads to the formation of ammonium phosphate stones. Unfortunately, manipulating pH does not help eliminate any organisms.

b   **True**. *Pseudomonas* is frequently resistant to commonly prescribed antibiotics. Amoxil often eliminate streptococci, but will be less effective against *E. coli* and other common urinary organisms.

c   **True**. UTIs are primarily caused by bowel organisms, such as *E. coli*. In the first year boys are almost as likely as girls to get UTIs but later girls are more susceptible (3% of girls and 1% of boys have had a UTI by the age of 11.

d   **True**. Sterile pyuria describes the situation when there are raised white cells in the urine, but there is no growth. Causes include inflammation in the renal tract, difficult to culture infections as in renal tuberculosis, systemic leucocytosis.

e   **False**. This is the best oral antibiotic for UTIs as judged by its efficacy, side effects and cost. It is active against *E. coli*, *Strep. faecalis* and *Proteus*. spp.

Data interpretation and reasoning — answers

9(i)   *A child of 5 is seen because his parents have noticed swelling around his eyes. The diagnosis of nephrotic syndrome is made more likely than another cause for his illness because he is also found to have*

   a   macroscopic haematuria
   b   liver edge palpable at 3 cm below the costal margin
   c   temperature 38°C
   d   maculopapular rash
   e   a distended abdomen

a **False** b **False** c **False** d **False** e **True**
This is a question about the differential diagnosis and clinical evaluation of periorbital swelling in children. The most likely cause is nephrotic syndrome, but heart failure, liver disease, angioneurotic oedema, and local infection may also be considered. Each of the branches of this type of question will either contain a non-discriminating feature or a feature of another disease (false branches) or a fairly characteristic feature of the disease (true branches). A bit of technique is needed as you must carefully read the stem to see how characteristic the feature has to be to make it 'true'. Here it says 'made more likely', so a 'true' branch

will contain a feature more commonly found in association with the suggested diagnosis than anything else in the differential. If it had said '. . .the diagnosis is confirmed by. . .' a characteristic feature would be needed. A distended abdomen may be found with liver disease or right heart failure, due to ascites but is particularly associated with nephrotic syndrome, so this is true. A rash is an unusual accompaniment of nephrotic syndrome, and would make you question the diagnosis. Other systemic infections, viral or streptococcal might cause such a rash and be associated with facial swelling. Henoch−Schönlein purpura (HSP) typically causes a vasculitic petechial and purpuric rash on the legs and buttocks. Other features of this disease include renal and abdominal involvement as well as joint pain and swelling. About 90% present with haematuria and 10% go on to develop some renal impairment. A urine Dipstix test for blood is therefore a useful test in children with a rash and abdominal pain. Occasionally, HSP can be complicated by intussusception.

Macroscopic haematuria is not typical feature of nephrotic syndrome, and would suggest nephritic syndrome (other features hypertension, haematuria, and oedema). A slightly raised temperature (<37.5°C) is often found in nephrotics, but a higher temperature is more likely to be found in other conditions, such as periorbital infection. The liver edge at 3 cm is suggestive of liver disease (hepatitis, storage or metabolic disease) or right heart failure. The liver is often palpable <3 cm in young children, but slowly disappears as the child's chest grows.

9(ii)   *In this child the following results become available*
   urinary protein dipstix ++++
   urine microscopy: RBC, 20 mm³; WCC, <5 mm³
   albumin 18 g/dl
   Na⁺ 135 mmol/l
   K⁺ 3.9 mmol/l
   urea 3.4 mmol/l
   antistreptolysin O titre negative
   complement levels normal

   a he is in renal failure
   b albumin should be given
   c these results are compatible with nephritic syndrome
   d he does not have pyuria
   e oral steroids should form part of his treatment

a **False** b **False** c **False** d **True** e **True**

Not surprisingly for this chapter the patient's data are compatible with renal disease! He now has almost enough features to say he has nephrotic syndrome (see Box 4.2), but not nephritic syndrome. Red cells in the urine is not uncommon in nephrotic syndrome but typical of nephritic syndrome. Pyuria is increase of the white cells in the urine (>10/mm³), and associated with urinary infection, inflammatory conditions of the renal tract such as GN and systemic leucocytosis. Renal failure requires the failure of sodium, potassium, or water control. Proteinuria, acidosis, or rickets may accompany these features.

Box 4.2   Features of nephrotic and nephritic syndromes

Nephrotic	Nephritic
Microscopic haematuria	Haematuria
Selective, massive proteinuria	Proteinuria
hypertension unusual	Hypertension
Oedema, ascites prominent	Less oedema
Hypoalbuminaemia	Albumin normal or near normal
Hyperlipidaemia	Normal lipids
Good urine output	Oliguria

The treatment of nephrotic syndrome is supportive and immunosuppressive. Salt and fluid intake is restricted and bed rest can be of help, although keeping a child of 5 in bed is not so easy! High dose prednisolone is used until the proteinuria has reduced and then the dose tailed off slowly. A renal biopsy is considered if there is no response to steroids or repeated relapses when they are reduced. As discussed in the knowledge section, a low albumin alone is not an indication for parenteral albumin, as it does not change the course of the disease and can be dangerous.

10(i) *A female infant of 6 months age presents with five loose stools in the past 24 h and a temperature of 38.5°C, but is not clinically dehydrated or cardiovascularly compromised. She is feeding well, is alert, and interested in her surroundings.*
A partial septic screen is performed
Hb 12.7 g/dl
WCC 14.5 × 10³/mm³
PL 453 × 10³/mm³
Na⁺ 143 mmol/l
K⁺ 3.8 mmol/l
U 3.7 mmol/l
clean catch urine
    cloudy appearance
    RBC 25/mm³
    WBC 75/mm³
    no organisms seen
blood cultures pending

a   a diagnosis of a urinary tract infection can now be made
b   a suprapubic aspirate should now be performed
c   she has microscopic haematuria
d   she should be started on aspirin
e   antibiotics should be withheld until culture results are available

a **False** b **False** c **True** d **False** e **False**
This is a typical scenario for an infant with a UTI, with fever and a diarrhoea. Other common presentations include irritability, septicaemia, and in the older

child loss of urinary control. In this situation, even with a well looking child, some would advocate a lumbar puncture, but for most a thorough examination and the above investigations are all that is usually required. These results are suggestive of a UTI, as there is a pyuria, but confirmation with positive cultures is needed before the diagnosis can be made. A clean catch urine (CCU) is good enough for management in this situation. A suprapubic aspirate (SPA) is the 'gold standard' but as the child has already passed urine this approach would not be successful even if it were wanted. This technique can be used up to the age of about 9 months, when the bladder is no longer an abdominal organ. A 23G needle under suction is inserted into the mid-line angling posteriorly and inferiorly until urine is obtained. A catheter may be passed temporarily to obtain a specimen (a CSU), but this is often more difficult and distressing than an SPA. Any organisms found to grow from a CCU, CSU, or SPA are considered to represent a UTI. Bag urine specimens are frowned upon but often performed as they require less time to do. A negative culture result is believable, but growth, particularly mixed growth without pyuria is less so. Perhaps their only place is as a screening tool in children who are very unlikely to have UTIs with the understanding that a further test may need to be done.

Useful normal values for urine are < 5 RBCs/high power field and < 10 WBCs /mm^3. Any values above this represent haematuria or pyuria. There should be no bacteria, but the urine frequently contains crystals.

Treatment for a febrile child with a leucocytosis and pyuria should involve antibiotics active against typical urine infecting organisms (*E. coli*, *Proteus*, *Pseudomonas*, *Strep. faecalis*, *Klebsiella*) before culture results are known. If the child is fairly well and taking oral fluids, trimethoprim can be used, but if not a third-generation cephalosporin such as cefotaxime is needed. As soon as the child improves and culture and sensitivities are known, an oral antibiotic can be started.

Aspirin is a potentially dangerous drug in febrile children < 12 years as it can rarely lead to Reye's syndrome (hepatic encephalopathy). The only situations in which it is used is in Kawasaki disease, for its anti-inflammatory and antiplatelet actions, and in juvenile rheumatoid arthritis.

10(ii)   *This girl's urine culture grows E. coli $> 10^5$ colony forming units/ml. She is discharged on a 1 week course of trimethoprim and seen in the outpatient clinic at the end of this course. She has made a good recovery and is now virtually back to normal*

   a   a DMSA scan will be needed to identify vesico-ureteric reflux
   b   a renal ultrasound may identify scarring
   c   organisms may still be present in the urine even if the infection has been successfully treated
   d   antibiotics should be stopped until all the investigations are completed
   e   a micturating cysto-urethrogram must be delayed for 6 weeks to prevent false positive results

a   **False**   b   **True**   c   **False**   d   **False**   e   **True**
The strategy and purpose of investigating children who have had UTIs has already

been discussed in question 3 and Box 4.1. A DMSA, being a test that measures blood flow will give information about areas that are poorly perfused (scarred or recently infected) and will measure the relative perfusion of both kidneys. Unlike the MCUG, the DMSA test cannot directly identify reflux, only its effects. Both the DMSA and MCUG must be delayed 6 weeks as they may show false positive results earlier, due to oedema.

An ultrasound detects differences in absorption of the waves. Water is particularly poor at absorbing ultrasound, so a difference between a water filled space and the surrounding tissue can be seen. This makes it particularly useful in visualizing the bladder, kidneys, and ventricular system. Ultrasound passes poorly through gas filled spaces, so a gas-filled abdomen can reduce the value of the examination. Resolution is good, but a ureter <5 mm may be missed. The difference in the absorption of renal scarred tissue and neighbouring parenchyma can be seen on ultrasound, but this is less sensitive than a DMSA. The renal ultrasound is particularly useful in acute or chronic renal failure, where it will distinguish between pre-renal (normal kidneys), intra-renal (bright kidneys in ARF or small scarred kidneys in chronic renal failure) and post-renal (dilated collecting system).

A repeat urine culture should be taken after 1 week of treatment or earlier if the child is not improving to see if it has cleared. Any remaining organisms at this stage means that the organism is resistant to the antibiotic used or it is not entering the child! If a child has a UTI, a further scarring may occur. For this reason prophylactic antibiotics should be given until a predisposition to UTIs is ruled out.

11   *A male infant is admitted at the age of 7 weeks. He has been vomiting all his feeds for*
3 days and now has a reduced urine output. He still seems hungry. He has no
temperature. Some results are now available
Na$^+$ 132 mmol/l
K$^+$ 2.8 mmol/l
urea 8.2 mmol/l
creatinine 90 μmol/l
urine clear
urine pH 6.2

a   his vomiting has left him sodium depleted
b   urine and creatinine levels are normal
c   the potassium is high because renal tubular function is poor
d   systemic acidosis has made his urine pH acidic
e   fluid replacement should occur before any surgical intervention

a **True** b **False** c **False** d **False** e **True**
This scenario is included in the renal section as it concerns the renal response to systemic dehydration. Dehydration is caused by loss of body water and is measured in percentage of body mass. The different clinical pictures depend on what else is lost with the water. Diarrhoea or stoma losses are primarily small intestinal fluid and so alkali and potassium is lost in addition to the water and sodium. The result is hypokalaemia and acidosis. Loss of stomach contents is a loss of water,

acid, and sodium but less potassium. The resultant blood chemistry depends on the body's response to the situation as well as any administered fluids (such as bottled water or sodium rich cow's milk).

The overriding homeostatic response of the body is to maintain blood pressure, and it worries less about potassium levels, acidosis or osmolality. A reduced renal GFR leads to renin production, which raises angiotensin levels and blood pressure. Aldosterone levels rise, increasing sodium and water reabsorption. Also ADH secretion is stimulated, retaining water. The renal reabsorption of sodium increases in the distal tubule. As more sodium is reabsorbed hydrogen or potassium ions are excreted into the urine. So, in severe volume depletion there may be a potassium depletion as a result of a renal loss. This is also the cause for the total body hypokalaemia found in diabetic ketoacidosis. If vomiting occurs to cause the volume depletion, the body is usually alkalotic, but the urine is in-appropriately acid as a result of the H^+ loss.

Urea and creatinine levels are normally lower in children. The creatinine comes from muscle cell turnover and is almost entirely excreted by glomerular filtration. There is little reabsorption of this substance. This means that its normal level relates to muscle bulk and will rise if there is muscle injury or a reduction in GFR. Urea is made as a result of protein turnover in the liver (ingestion, muscle catabolism) and is both filtered and to some extent reabsorbed. Levels will rise if the GFR is reduced but also if there has been a period of fasting or a gastro-intestinal bleed (a large protein meal). Its levels will be low in liver failure.

12   *A 5-month-old boy is admitted to the ward with a 3-day history of cough and runny nose. He has not taken any solids for 2 days. He has had four 90 ml bottles of formula milk and has wet two nappies in the last 24 h. Examining him, his temperature is 37.3°C, his heart rate is 135 beats/min, his respiratory rate is 55/min, and he has moderate chest recession. He is not clinically dehydrated. Some investigations are performed, mainly because of his poor urine output*
Hb 9.7 g/dl
WCC $5.7 \times 10^3/mm^3$
platelets $296 \times 10^3/mm^3$
Na^+ 128 mmol/l
K^+ 3.3 mmol/l
urea 1.9 mmol/l
osmolality 272 mmol/l

   a   he should be cross-matched for a blood transfusion
   b   his urine is likely to be inappropriately concentrated
   c   urine sodium concentration is probably high
   d   his fluid intake is reduced
   e   the most likely diagnosis is an URTI

a   **False**   b   **True**   c   **True**   d   **True**   e   **False**
Here is an infant with a moderate respiratory illness, a low grade fever, and reduced feeding. (As an easy to remember rough guide, an infant normally takes the equivalent of one ounce/kg of feed = 30 ml/kg every 6 h once on solids.) The

differential diagnosis would include bronchiolitis, another viral or bacterial chest infection, heart failure, and possibly a metabolic disorder leading to acidosis. The data show a slightly low haemoglobin, electrolytes, and osmolality. This strongly suggests inappropriate ADH secretion. The other causes of hyponatraemia (hypoaldosteronism, diarrhoea with a hyponatraemic fluid replacement) really do not fit the scenario. The diagnosis would be made with a paired urine and plasma osmolalities. Inappropriate ADH is fairly common in bronchiolitis, but is rarely severe. Other causes include intracranial pathology (trauma, bleeds, infection) other pulmonary conditions (pneumonia, asthma), DDAVP (synthetic ADH) and other drugs as well as the incredibly rare ADH secreting tumours.

Inappropriate ADH leads to an inappropriate reabsorption of water in the kidneys when they really should be letting it go. The urine is therefore concentrated with a high sodium and the blood dilute.

This may account to some extent for the low Hb, but at this age it is usually low anyway. Two to 6 months is the nadir for the blood Hb. The fetus is polycythaemic and has a Hb of about 20 g/dl. This is because the uterine environment is so hypoxic it needs the extra Hb to get an adequate oxygen delivery. After birth less Hb is needed so little Hb is made for some months. Instead the iron is recycled and used in growth. Iron deficiency is very common at about 6 months as demands are high and intake may be poor. There is little iron in breast milk and solid feeds may not be well established. A transfusion should only be given if the benefits outweigh the risks. For a growing and basically healthy baby, a low Hb > 6 g/dl is unlikely to cause compromise. In sick or oxygen dependent infants, a HB > 10 g/dl is more desirable.

13   *These results are obtained from a 2-year-old boy who has presented with a convulsion.*
    He is well known to the casualty department, who have seen him on several occasions
    with various injuries. Now his carer says he has been vomiting
    Na+ 165 mmol/l
    K+ 4.3 mmol/l
    urea 3.7 mmol/l
    creatinine 45 μmol/l

These results are explained by the fact that

    a   he has been given only formula milk to drink in the last 2 days
    b   his mother has inadvertently given dioralyte at 10 times the correct strength
    c   further questioning reveals he also has profuse diarrhoea
    d   he has just been resuscitated with a large bolus of 0.9% sodium chloride solution
    e   he has been poisoned with salt

a   **False**   b   **True**   c   **False**   d   **False**   e   **True**

Hypernatraemia is a serious and fairly uncommon situation. As with all data questions, the examiner is trying not to test just knowledge, but the candidate's ability to put bits of knowledge together and reach conclusions. This can be done even if you have never read or even heard of the topic. Here is a child who has a high sodium, but the rest of the data are normal. This might be an artefact, but the scenario states that the child has had a convulsion, one of the expected consequences of hypernatraemia. Blood investigation artefacts can be divided into those whose errors originate in the body and those which occur after the sample is taken. The first group includes the 'drip arm' sample, where the sample comes from a vein distal to the site of an intravenous infusion. The result is therefore tending towards the fluid instilled. This is suggested by stem (d), but even 0.9% saline has only 150 mmol/l of sodium. It would have diluted the sodium concentration in the blood if used in this child. This makes 0.9% sodium chloride a useful fluid in the volume resuscitation of children dehydrated and shocked as a result of diarrhoea and vomiting before the sodium level is known.

Hypernatraemia may be caused by excess of sodium or a depletion of water. Salt poisoning is thought to be the commonest cause of a sodium over 165 mmol/l, and a form of Munchausen's syndrome by proxy. Depletion of water in excess of sodium can occur when there is body fluid loss (diarrhoea, insensible losses) and replacement with fluid of higher sodium concentration. This could be with incorrectly mixed Dioralyte or even cow's milk (sodium = 22 mmol/l), but not formula milk (sodium = 8–10 mmol/l).

Treatment of dehydration is further discussed in Neurology question 8d.

5 Neurology

Knowledge — questions

1 *Children with cerebral palsy*
   a are usually born prematurely
   b have physical signs that change with time
   c often fail to thrive
   d are always handicapped
   e usually walk with a wide-based gait

2 *A 6-week-old boy, who was born at term, is found to have a head circumference above the 97th centile*
   a his large circumference might be linked directly to a forceps delivery
   b his large head circumference may be familial
   c the best screening test to rule out hydrocephalus in this situation is a computed tomography scan
   d signs associated with hydrocephalus include sun-setting eyes and prominent scalp veins
   e a ventriculoperitoneal shunt can be inserted if he has hydrocephalus

3 *In the early neonatal period, convulsions*
   a are usually secondary to hypoglycaemia, hypoxia, or an abnormal electrolyte level
   b should be treated initially with sodium valproate
   c could be the first indication of idiopathic epilepsy
   d are most often tonic-clonic and generalized
   e are associated with a high (over 70%) chance of cerebral palsy

4 *Spina bifida*
   a is associated with a low maternal α-fetoprotein during pregnancy
   b can lead to chronic renal failure
   c may be assymptomatic
   d is less likely to occur if the mother is given intramuscular vitamin B_{12}
   e commonly leads to upper motorneurone signs in the legs

5 *An infant is brought to her family doctor because her mother noticed a squint. It is more likely there is identifiable disease causing this if*
   a she is 2 weeks old

b she is not fixing and following at 10 weeks
c there is a family history of strabismus
d the infant has features of a congenital infection
e it is convergent and intermittent

6   *These neurological manifestations are commonly associated with the following skin lesions*

a infantile spasms and depigmented patches
b focal seizures and maxillary capillary haemangioma
c neck stiffness and vesicular rash with pustules and crusting
d squint and eczema
e leg hypotonia and mid-line sacral hairy naevus

7   *Epilepsy in children*

a usually presents as a febrile convulsion
b may present as poor school performance
c is best treated with phenobarbitone
d causes developmental delay
e affects 0.5% of the school age population

8   *The anterior fontanelle*

a can be felt to pulse
b usually bulges when the infant has meningitis
c is used for ultrasound scans
d is depressed if there is dehydration
e closes slowly in infants deficient of vitamin D

9   *A child is seen because his mother thinks that his muscles are becoming weak*

a a high blood creatine phosphokinase level implies the child may have muscle disease
b Gower's sign (using his hands to assist standing) is a sign specific to Duchenne muscular dystrophy
c he may have myasthenia gravis
d the weakness may be related to a metabolic disorder
e progressive descending weakness over a week is typical of Guillain–Barré syndrome

10 *The following signs are typically found with these associated conditions*

a an abnormal Moro response and Erb's palsy
b scissor gait and cerebral palsy

    c unilateral loss of facial sensation and Bell's palsy
    d strabismus and tuberculous meningitis
    e fasciculation and cerebral palsy

11   *Ataxia in children*
    a is commonly found in 'clumsy' children
    b leads to a wide-based gait
    c is a common presentation of Wilson's disease
    d is occasionally associated with chicken pox
    e is usually caused by a primary cerebellar lesion

12   *An infant of 3 months with meningitis is likely to have*
    a a rash
    b a stiff neck
    c a poor outcome
    d a fever
    e a high polymorphonucleocyte count in their cerebrospinal fluid

Data interpretation and reasoning—questions

13(i)   *A 14-month-old girl is brought to the emergency department by ambulance. She was found by her mother to be 'shaking', unresponsive with her eyes deviated upwards. The shaking stopped after about 3 min but restarted just before arrival at the emergency department. On arrival she is centrally cyanosed and not breathing. She is moving her limbs at about 3 beats/s. She is unconscious and her temperature is 39.2°C. The doctor should*
    a first establish intravenous access
    b give paracetamol syrup by mouth
    c secure the airway by intubating her
    d if the seizure is prolonged give diazepam rectally or intravenously
    e give antibiotics immediately

13(ii)   *The convulsion stops. This convulsion is more likely to be a manifestation of another problem rather than a simple febrile convulsion because*
    a she is pale, with a capillary filling time of 4 s
    b she was unable to sit unsupported before she became ill
    c her blood sugar is 1.2 mmol/l

d   she has six café-au lait patches
e   her 4-year-old brother had febrile convulsions when young

14(i)   *A 5-month-old boy is brought to the emergency department. He*
was found unconscious early that morning by his father who went
to wake him up for a feed. He has previously been well. Examining
him, he is pink and well perfused. There is no respiratory distress
and he has a respiratory rate of 25. His blood pressure is 85/50 and
pulse rate 130. He has no rash. His tone is reduced but there are no
other abnormal neurological findings. Some blood results rapidly
become available
Na^+ 131 mmol/l
K^+ 3.7 mmol/l
urea 2.1 mmol/l
glucose 8.9 mmol/l
haemoglobin 9.5 g/dl
white cell count 15.3 × 10^3/mm^3
platelets 179 × 10^3/mm^3

Based on these results and his clinical condition
a   he is unconscious because he is anaemic
b   a convulsion could be the cause
c   his sodium should be corrected urgently
d   he is likely to have had an intracranial bleed
e   he must not have a lumbar puncture if his anterior fontanelle is bulging

14(ii)   *Cerebrospinal fluid is collected and analysed*
red cells 35 mm^3
white cells 450 mm^3 polymorphonucleocytes
no organisms seen
glucose 1.3 mmol/l
protein 0.8 g/l

Now
a   bacterial meningitis has been ruled out
b   the cerebrospinal fluid glucose level has made viral meningitis less
    likely
c   he should now be given intramuscular penicillin
d   the red cell count indicates there has been a subarachnoid haemorrhage
e   encephalitis is the most likely diagnosis

15   *A 10-year-old girl is seen by a paediatrician because she has been having recurrent headaches for the past 6 months. The following features make migraine a more likely cause for her problem than any other diagnosis*

  a they are worse in the morning
  b a family history of epilepsy
  c her aunt has migraines
  d the headaches are associated with abdominal pain
  e there is also photophobia

16   *A 3-year-old girl is seen in outpatients at the request of her family doctor. She has had three episodes of 'twitching' in the last 2 months each lasting several minutes and terminating spontaneously. A full neurological examination is normal. Idiopathic epilepsy is a more likely cause of her episodes because*

  a she had a febrile convulsion at the age of 13 months
  b she becomes cyanosed before each attack
  c they all have occurred during her sleep
  d her uncle has idiopathic epilepsy
  e all of the episodes were preceded by an emotional outburst

17(i)   *A 5-year-old boy is brought into the resuscitation room having fallen 3 m from a tree. He was initially unconscious but then began to speak to the ambulance officers on the way to hospital. Now he is making incomprehensible groans, has a flexor response to pain, and opens his eyes to command. He has a pulse of 130, a blood pressure of 110/70, and a capillary filling time (CFT) of 4 s. He is not cyanosed, but is having difficulty breathing. There is a large contusion on the right side of his head and he has blood coming from his right ear. There are several minor cuts and grazes to the rest of his body. The following steps would now be appropriate*

  a he should be nasally intubated
  b a hard neck collar should be applied
  c he should be given 10 ml/kg of colloid intravenously
  d once stabilized, he should have a magnetic resonance imaging of his brain
  e he should be given mannitol

17(ii)   *The CT shows a base of skull fracture and a small intracranial bleed. Concerning his further management*

a rising pulse and falling blood pressure indicate rising intracranial pressure
b unequal pupils may indicate that his intracranial pressure is rising
c a head up posture reduces his intracranial pressure
d anticonvulsants should be avoided
e he should be fluid restricted

Knowledge — answers

Neurology is one of the larger areas in paediatrics, particularly in examinations. As neurological patients often have long-standing diseases that may be disabling, they are seen in the community by a variety of professionals, and these children may require frequent hospitalization. As they are often 'stable' and have reliable signs they make up a core of children for clinical examinations in paediatrics.

As with most of the other paediatric subspecialties, there are only a few diseases that students are expected to know in detail, and these can be easily understood. The most important chronic conditions to know about are cerebral palsy and epilepsy. Other chronic conditions worth understanding are hydrocephalus, and neuromuscular and neurocutaneous disorders. Acute disorders to know are infective (meningitis and encephalitis), or involve the acute management of convulsions (and febrile convulsions) or coma. One can also be asked about the interpretation of symptoms (e.g. headache), signs, and investigations. These questions aim to cover these topics.

1 *Children with cerebral palsy*
   a are usually born prematurely
   b have physical signs that change with time
   c often fail to thrive
   d are always handicapped
   e usually walk with a wide-based gait

a **False.** Cerebral palsy (CP) is defined as a 'constant but not unchanging deficit resulting from a lesion in the motor part of the developing brain'. There may be other associated problems such as blindness, hearing loss, and epilepsy. In terms of pathology, there has been a brain lesion in the past and there is now no further active healing of the injury. This has left a constant deficit, but it changes as the child grows older and the rest of its brain continues to develop. The commonest causes are shown in Box 5.1. Premature infants are more likely to develop CP than other children, but because extreme prematurity is uncommon, premature infants only make up under 10% of the CP population.

b **True.** This is the essence of CP. Normal children also have changing neurology. At birth the brain is poorly myelinated and the cortex relatively non-functional.

Box 5.1   Causes of cerebral palsy

Antenatal	Genetic
	Cerebral malformation
	Intrauterine vascular events
	Infection
Perinatal	Birth asphyxia, infection
	Intraventricular haemorrhage
	Hypoglycaemia
	Hyperbilirubinaemia
Postnatal	Trauma
	Infection
	Hypoglycaemia
	Hydrocephalus

Many of the early responses (see Box 5.2) that a baby makes are later suppressed as the cortex becomes dominant. Fixing and following and smiling are the early indicators of cortical function.

Box 5.2   Reflexes

Period	
Moro	<5 months
Stepping	>4 months
Walking	>4 months
Grasp	>4 months
Asymmetric tonic neck	<5 months
Rooting	>4 months
Spinal incurvation	Any
Lateral parachute	6 months+
Forward parachute	6 months+
Upgoing plantar	<12 months
Downgoing plantar	>12 months
Diving	Any

Infants with CP may be hypotonic or hypertonic or neither, but this is likely to change along with their posture and reflexes as the child grows. Most often an 'upper motor neurone posture' is adopted with hypertonia and flexed elbows and wrists, with extended ankles. There is usually persistence of the primitive reflexes and persistently upgoing plantar reflexes.

CP children often undergo surgery, which may alter signs, particularly if there are releases of contractures.

c   **True**. Failure to thrive is a very common problem for CP children. Difficulty in feeding occurs as a result of poor sucking and swallowing and there may also be gastro-oesophageal reflux. Children will also be more often systemically unwell (chest infections and urine infections) so may have a reduced appetite and increased energy expenditure.

Many children with CP are identified in follow-up clinics after hospitalization (after meningitis or head injury), but they may also be identified as an children with convulsions, delayed developmental milestones, or failure to thrive.

d   **False**. Handicap is different from disability, and neither are synonymous with CP. Handicap is the inability to perform a task (e.g. getting to a shop, toileting, communicating), whereas disability is the inability of the body to work (e.g. seeing, standing, sphincter control, speaking). The goal of treatment for CP patients is to reduce disability by reducing muscle spasm and contractures and to give them ways to improve body function using the abilities they have. Then handicap can be reduced by aids, such as wheelchairs, handrails, communication aids, and the like.

e   **False**. The wide-based gait is typical of children with poor proprioception or cerebellar pathology. Children with CP are most likely to have a scissor gait with toe walking. Other gaits are shown in Box 5.3 with their associated causes.

Box 5.3	Gaits	
Scissor	Hypertonic hip adductors	Cerebral palsy
Tip toe	Hypertonic ankle extenders	Cerebral palsy
Wide based	Cerebellar dysfunction	Varicella or brain tumour, drugs
Waddling	Weak proximal muscles	Muscular dystrophy
Limp	Musculoskeletal problem	Dislocated hip, scoliosis
	hemiparesis	Cerebral palsy

2 *A 6-week-old boy, who was born at term, is found to have a head circumference above the 97th centile*

   a his large circumference might be linked directly to a forceps delivery
   b his large head circumference may be familial
   c the best screening test to rule out hydrocephalus in this situation is a CT scan
   d signs associated with hydrocephalus include sun-setting eyes and prominent scalp veins
   e a ventriculoperitoneal shunt can be inserted if he has hydrocephalus

a   **False**. Paediatric students are often worried about neurological examination technique. In some ways it is more similar to the adult technique than other systems. The main components are outlined in Box 5.4. There is a particular emphasis on the anterior fontanelle (AF), head circumference, and examination of the spine. The brain of a newborn is extremely large for the size of the body when compared with other species. In order to enable birth, the bones of the skull do not fuse before birth so that the head shape can 'mould' as the head fits through the tight birth canal. The fontanelles and sutures are gaps in between these bones. The posterior fontanelle should close by 3 months and the anterior by 18 months at the latest. In an infant with open sutures the head circumference directly reflects the volume of brain and fluid inside. This means that raised intracranial pressure will not occur.

Box 5.4   Neurological screening examination for children

Observation
        evidence of dysmorphism
        microcephalic or large head
        abnormal posture
        skin manifestation of neurological disease
        atrophy of any muscle groups
        can the child see, hear, move
Palpate anterior fontanelle
Cranial nerve examination as appropriate
Tone, power (antigravity movement can be observed during play)
Deep tendon reflexes
Primitive reflexes

The head circumference is increased if there is too much fluid (hydrocephalus) or megalencephaly, as occurs in Sotos syndrome or another space occupying lesion (tumour, haemorrhage). A small head is the result of premature fusion of the sutures (when the head may also be abnormal in shape) or a small brain.

Forceps deliveries can be traumatic, but only damage external structures— facial nerve palsies and bruising are the commonest problems. Ventouse deliveries cause local swelling (a chignon) and a cephalohaematoma.

b   **True.** This is the commonest cause of a large head. Investigations should be performed on children with head circumferences that are crossing centiles or those with developmental delay, as this may reflect a brain disease. Other indications for investigations include bony disease and an abnormal head shape.

c   **False.** A CT would work, but for a screening tool an ultrasound scan is far superior. These involve no radiation exposure and are simple, cheap and sensitive for hydrocephalus. Ultrasound is particularly good at delineating fluid/tissue boundaries, ideal for hydrocephalus. Unfortunately, once the AF is closed, the ultrasound is not useful.

d   **True.** Other signs in hydrocephalus include transillumination of the head and fullness of the AF.

e   **True.** The blockage to flow either occurs at the aqueduct of Sylvius (non-communicating hydrocephalus) or at the arachnoid granulations (communicating hydrocephalus). The common causes are congenital malformations, meningitis, intraventricular haemorrhage, and tumours.

If the hydrocephalus is steadily increasing, eventually the brain is stretched and compressed. In the short term this leads to paralysis of the upward gaze (sun setting eyes) and ataxia, but will damage the brain in the long term.

There are several treatments for hydrocephalus. Acetazolamide temporally reduces CSF production. If drainage is needed, but the problem is expected to resolve, repeated lumbar punctures or tapping the lateral ventricle via the AF can be undertaken. For the longer term, a ventriculoperitoneal or ventriculo-atrial shunt is inserted. However, these can get infected or blocked as they have to stay in for many years.

3   *In the early neonatal period, convulsions*
   a   are usually secondary to hypoglycaemia, hypoxia, or an abnormal electrolyte level
   b   should be treated initially with sodium valproate
   c   could be the first indication of idiopathic epilepsy
   d   are most often tonic-clonic and generalized
   e   are associated with a high (over 70%) chance of cerebral palsy

a   **True.** Seizure activity in children changes in its nature and aetiology with age. This is outlined in Box 5.5. In the neonatal period, convulsions are usually secondary to a metabolic derangement, hypoxic encephalopathy, meningitis, or drug withdrawal. The commonest causes at this age are a low blood sugar, sodium, calcium, or magnesium, and the convulsion may be the manifestation of a metabolic disorder (e.g. organic acidaemias and urea cycle defects). Hypoxic encephalopathy is outlined in The newborn question 8. In association with convulsions there may be irritability, abnormal tone, poor feeding, and jitteriness. Meningitis should always be suspected in a neonate with a convulsion, and CSF obtained for analysis if the baby is stable enough for a lumbar puncture.

b   **False.** Sodium valproate is a very useful anticonvulsant for older children with all forms of epilepsy. It is relatively free of side-effects compared with the other agents, although liver function must be monitored. However, it is not used for the control of ongoing seizures. After checking the airways, breathing and circulation, as with any child having a convulsion, the blood sugar should be checked immediately and intravenous dextrose given if needed. In the neonatal period the first agent used is phenobarbitone, although phenytoin is also useful. Diazepam is

Box 5.5   Age and seizures

Age	Aetiology	Treatment	Prognosis
Neonatal	Hypoxic, intraventricular haemorrhage, infection, metabolic (e.g. hypoglycaemia), cerebral malformation, idiopathic	Of cause and phenobarbitone	Variable
Infancy	Infantile spasms	Vigabatrin, ACTH	Poor in 50%
	Febrile	Antipyretics	30% recur
	Idiopathic		
Childhood	Febrile	Antipyretics	Excellent
	Idiopathic	Valproate	Good
	Absence	Valproate	Excellent

used as the first agent in older children (see question 13i) but is avoided in neonates as it is slowly metabolized and depressant to respiration.

c   **True**. It may be the beginning of idiopathic epilepsy, but this is unusual, and only considered after other causes have been eliminated and treated.

d   **False**. To have a tonic-clonic convulsion, there needs to be a myelinated brain as only this will transmit impulses fast enough for the whole body to shake at once. Neonates have more subtle manifestations including shaking of one limb progressing to others, apnoeas, myoclonic jerks, sucking, and eye deviation.

e   **False**. The overall chance of neurological sequelae following a neonatal seizure is about 30%, but depends on the aetiology. Structural lesions are most serious.

4   *Spina bifida*
    a   is associated with a low maternal α-fetoprotein during pregnancy
    b   can lead to chronic renal failure
    c   may be asymptomatic
    d   is less likely to occur if the mother is given intramuscular vitamin B_{12}
    e   commonly leads to upper motorneurone signs in the legs

a   **False**. Spina bifida (SB) is one manifestation of a neural tube defect (also anencephaly and encephalocele). SB is itself classified according to which structures are involved. SB occulta is a defect in the dorsal spinal arch, where there is often a pigmented or hairy patch overlying the defect but may be found incidentally on an X-ray. With meningoceles there is a meningeal sac protruding from the back, and with meningomyeloceles the sac is made of meninges and spinal cord.

A high α-fetoprotein (αFP) may be found when there is a leak from the fetus of αFP, caused by open SB and abdominal wall defects (gastroschisis). A low αFP is found in Down's syndrome.

SB can be diagnosed antenatally on ultrasound.

b   **True.** The consequences of SB depend on which structures are involved and at what spinal level. Those above L3 are much more disabling than those below. Upper motor neurone type lesions cause spasticity in the legs that make walking difficult and may lead to dislocation of the hips. Neuropathic bladder and bowel leads to incontinence, urinary tract infections, and constipation.

c   **True.** SB occulta can be asymptomatic. On the other hand surgery may be required to close a defect and a multidisciplinary team employed to reduce disability and handicap, with physiotherapists to reduce spasticity, orthopaedic surgeons to repair dislocated joints and release contractures, occupational therapists to maximize function, and paediatricians to manage other aspects of treatment.

d   **False.** The administration of folic acid periconceptually and for the first weeks of pregnancy has dramatically reduced the incidence of SB, particularly in those mothers who have already had a child with SB. Its mode of action is not known.

Vitamin B_{12} is one of several vitamins whose deficiency can cause neurological manifestations. B_1 (thiamine) deficiency causes polyneuropathy and opthalmoplegia, B_6 deficiency seizures, B_{12} deficiency peripheral neuropathy, and degeneration of the lateral spinal columns.

e   **True.** Other causes are CP, spinal trauma, stroke, tumours, metabolic disease, and demyelinating syndromes.

5   *An infant is brought to her family doctor because her mother noticed a squint. It is more likely there is identifiable disease causing this if*

a   she is 2 weeks old
b   she is not fixing and following at 10 weeks
c   there is a family history of strabismus
d   the infant has features of a congenital infection
e   it is convergent and intermittent

a   **False.** Strabismus is common in the neonatal period as the neural mechanisms for conjugate gaze are not fully developed. If it is intermittent and convergent up to the age of 6 weeks with a normal red reflex and normal neurology no action need be taken. Squint may be identified as an asymmetrical light reflex in an infant. In cooperative children, the cover test can be used to confirm the presence of a squint or identify a latent squint.

An examination protocol suitable for screening for neonatal neurological problems is shown in Box 5.6.

b   **True.** Strabismus may be a manifestation of either an ophthalmic disorder or a neurological problem and the first symptom of either problem may be delay in

---

Box 5.6   Neonatal neurological examination

Observation	Moving all limbs equally
	Size of head
	Any dysmorphic features
	Able to fix visually
Palpation	Anterior fontanelle
	Tone of muscles
	Neck tone in suspended prone position
Reflexes	Primitive
	Moro if asymmetrical signs

---

fixing and following. Ophthalmic causes include chorioretinitis (congenital infection), cataract (idiopathic or secondary to storage disorders), refractive errors, and later retinoblastoma.

c   **True**. Squints can run in families. If not treated early, the neural pathways that handle the visual stimuli do not develop and so the child will never be able do 'see' with that eye. This is called amblyopia.

d   **True**. The eyes can be affected by several congenital infections. Rubella, cytomegalovirus, toxoplasma, varicella zoster, and herpes simplex virus all cause chorioretinitis, rubella and varicella zoster micro-ophthalmia, and cataracts. Other common features include splenomegaly, rash, anaemia, thrombocytopenia, and leucopenia. Congenital infections are further discussed in The newborn question 12.

e   **False**. Divergent and fixed squints are much more likely to reflect underlying pathology. Conjugate gaze is not always well established before 6 weeks and so may give rise to an intermittent squint, whereas a fixed squint at any age suggests a muscular problem.

The most common cause of strabismus in children is hypermetropia. This is because the accommodation reflex also incorporates convergence. So if a hypermetropic eye is trying to focus, it converges excessively. Other causes in children are listed in Box 5.7.

   6   *These neurological manifestations are commonly associated with the following skin lesions*
         a   infantile spasms and depigmented patches
         b   focal seizures and maxillary capillary haemangioma
         c   neck stiffness and vesicular rash with pustules and crusting
         d   squint and eczema
         e   leg hypotonia and mid-line sacral hairy naevus

Box 5.7   Causes of strabismus

Pseudosquint (prominent epicanthic folds)
Hypermetropia
Cerebral palsy
Paralytic—dysfunction of oculomotor muscles or nerves
Retinopathy of prematurity
Congenital infectious retinopathy
Retinoblastoma

a   **True**. A number of 'neuroectodermal' or neurocutaneous conditions exist, where a neurological abnormality is associated with a skin manifestation. This is because the skin and nervous system have a common origin. The neuroectodermal conditions are neurofibromatosis, tuberose sclerosis and Sturge–Weber syndrome. Tuberose sclerosis is so-called because of the CT appearance of the brain around the ventricles. It may present as developmental delay, infantile spasms, or as convulsions. The skin manifestations vary with age, but include depigmented patches, adenoma sebaceum, subungual fibromas, and shagreen patches.

b   **False**. The Sturge–Weber syndrome incorporates a capillary haemangioma (port wine stain) in the area supplied by the ophthalmic branch of the facial nerve and an angioma on the underlying (ipsilateral) part of the brain. This causes atrophy of the underlying brain and focal convulsions manifest on the opposite side of the body. There must be areas above the eye with the haemangioma or Sturge–Weber cannot be diagnosed.

c   **False**. A vesicular rash with pustules and crusting is strongly suggestive of chicken pox. This can be associated with neurological manifestations, but rarely. The most common of these is encephalitis with cerebellar involvement.

Rash is associated with meningitis, in meningococcal disease and more uncommonly *Haemophilus influenzae* type B (HIB). Meningococcus typically causes a non-blanching purpuric rash, but this may well start with a blanching rash whose spots have a central darker area. HIB is occasionally associated with an erythematous rash.

Herpes simplex virus also causes a vesicular rash and is the most serious cause for encephalitis. It should always be suspected in a child with a focal seizure or unexplained reduction in conscious level.

d   **False**. Eczema has no association with any neurological condition, with the exception of migraine, which can be considered as an atopic condition. Squint has been discussed in question 5, above.

e   **False**. Hypotonia is caused by either anterior horn cell damage, motor nerve damage, or neuromuscular junction disease. All of these are unusual in children, but Werdnig–Hoffmann disease leads to progressive anterior horn cell damage.

Myasthenia gravis may produce hypotonia, but this disease tends to cause ophthalmic and facial nerve manifestations. Paradoxically, CP can also cause hypotonia at certain ages.

Mid-line sacral problems suggest spina bifida. If there is a neurological problem with spina bifida, usually there is hypertonicity, neuropathic bowel and bladder, sensory loss, hydrocephalus, and secondary joint problems (scoliosis, dislocations).

7 *Epilepsy in children*
  a   usually presents as a febrile convulsion
  b   may present as poor school performance
  c   is best treated with phenobarbitone
  d   causes developmental delay
  e   affects 0.5% of the school age population

a **False**. Febrile convulsions are very common and affect 2% of the paediatric population. Three per cent of those with febrile convulsions go on to develop epilepsy, so this cannot be the usual mode of presentation as epilepsy affects 0.5% of children. To confuse matters further, epileptics are more likely to have a convulsion when febrile. This is because the fits can be induced in everyone by raising the temperature and in those with febrile convulsions this threshold is somewhat lower, as it is in those with epilepsy.

b **True**. Generalized absence seizures cause momentary loss of consciousness many times a day. There may be no motor involvement at all or only subtle manifestations, such as flickering of the eyelids. This will disrupt a child's concentration and affect school performance. These are best treated with valproate and have a very good prognosis.

c **False**. Treatment of epilepsy requires balancing the potential benefit and problems of a medication. As about half of the children who have had one convulsion will not go on to have another, so it is reasonable to not start any medicines until there is a second fit. However, some fits invariably return, such as infantile spasms and absence seizures, so should be treated straight away.

Infantile spasms are best treated with vigabatrin or adrenocorticotrophic hormone, partial seizures with carbamazepine. For all other disorders valproate is the best agent to start with, as it is effective and has few side-effects.

Phenobarbitone is only used in the treatment of neonatal seizures, as it often causes lethargy, hyperkinesia, and ataxia.

d **False**. Parents often worry that convulsions cause brain damage. Convulsions increase local oxygen usage in the brain and may affect ventilation causing ischaemia, but permanent damage will not occur for at least 30 min after the start of the convulsion.

Developmental delay is, however, commonly associated with fits as both can be manifestations of underlying brain disease.

e **True**. CP affects 0.2%, neural tube disorders 0.05%, brain tumours 0.05%, and migraine 6% of children.

8 *The anterior fontanelle*
   a   can be felt to pulse
   b   usually bulges when the infant has meningitis
   c   is used for ultrasound scans
   d   is depressed if there is dehydration
   e   closes slowly in infants deficient of vitamin D

a   **True**. As outlined in question 1, the AF is a gap between the bones of the skull. There is no bony obstruction between the skin and the intracranial compartment. Changes in intracranial pressure can therefore be detected at the AF. Both the heart beat and breathing cause pulsation in the AF. Absence of pulsation occurs when there is raised intracranial pressure.

b   **False**. It does bulge as the oedema caused by the infective process increases brain volume. This is, however, a late sign. There may also be neck stiffness and headache in an older child. Hydrocephalus also causes the AF to bulge.

c   **True**. Bone and air are poor at transmitting sound waves, but water is good. Therefore it is difficult to examine the brain by ultrasound once the fontanelle is closed (although the thin bone in the temporal area can allow diagnosis of hydrocephalus). Ultrasound can visualize the ventricles and other fluid collections well. It is less good at looking at the structure of the grey and white matter. The posterior fossa is also difficult to see as it is a long way away from the AF.

d   **True**. Dehydration removes water from cells so can cause depression of the AF. There is also a distinction between different types of dehydration and their effects. Simply, hypernatraemic dehydration causes fluid to leave cells more readily than hyponatraemic dehydration. This preserves circulatory volume at the expense of tissue water. The AF should then be more sunken in a child with hypernatraemic dehydration than in one with the same water loss but a low sodium. This is meant to make the hypernatraemic child more irritable.
   In terms of treatment, shock should always be corrected immediately (0.9% NaCl or 4.5% albumin). All except mildly dehydrated children need their plasma sodium measured. If it is high, 48 h must be taken to rehydrate (0.45% NaCl) compared with other types (24 h with 0.18% NaCl if the sodium is normal and 24 h with 0.45% NaCl if it is low).

e   **True**. The AF is closed by the growth of the surrounding bones. The mean age of closure is 9 months, but it may close by 6–18 months and still be normal. The posterior fontanelle should close by 3 months and the sutures by 6 weeks. If there is delay, there may be bone disease (achondroplasia), a nutritional deficiency (vitamin D, calcium, or phosphate), or metabolic disease. Hypothyroidism also causes delayed closure of the AF.

9   A child is seen because his mother thinks that his muscles are becoming weak

   a   a high blood creatine phosphokinase level implies the child may have muscle disease
   b   Gower's sign (using his hands to assist standing) is a sign specific to Duchenne muscular dystrophy
   c   he may have myasthenia gravis
   d   the weakness may be related to a metabolic disorder
   e   progressive descending weakness over a week is typical of Guillain–Barré syndrome

a   **True.** The symptom of muscle weakness can imply disorders at several different levels. Upper motor neurone lesions make the muscle difficult to use and 'weak'. Anterior horn cell or motor neurone lesions can also cause weakness. Neuromuscular junction problems can occur, and there may also be a problem with the muscle itself. A differential diagnosis is shown in Box 5.8.

Box 5.8   Causes of weakness

Metabolic	Glycogen storage diseases
	Mitochondrial myopathies
Muscular	Duchenne muscular dystrophy
	Becker muscular dystrophy
	Congenital myopathy
	Myotonic dystrophy
	Myositis
Neural	Myasthenia gravis
	Poliomyelitis
	Peroneal muscular atrophy
	Guillain–Barré syndrome
	Werdig–Hoffmann disease
Central	Cerebral palsy
Endocrine	Hypothyroidism

The best way to start evaluating the problem is to take a history and properly examine the child. Of particular interest will be any cause of CP (trauma, meningitis, prematurity, asphyxia), if the problem is worsening (implies ongoing disease, e.g. Guillain–Barré or muscular dystrophy) and if it relates to usage (myasthenia). Examination may distinguish between upper and lower motor neurone problems, and may demonstrate tiring of the muscles. There may be pseudohypertrophy in Duchenne muscular dystrophy (DMD).

Tests can also be used. For possible muscle disease, blood creatine phosphokinase (CPK) will be elevated. It is also elevated after bruising to the muscle. It is useful but non-specific. Muscle biopsy can determine the presence and the type of muscle dystrophy. The edrophonium test causes temporary and immediate improvement in weakness in myasthenia.

b   **False**. Gower's sign is a sign of proximal muscle weakness. It is most often encountered in DMD. This disease is sex-linked recessive, so only is found in boys. It typically presents at the age of 3, but there may be delayed motor milestones before that. Difficulty standing progresses so that the child is usually wheelchair bound by the 10–14 and dies from respiratory failure in his late teens. There are other forms of muscular dystrophy that are less severe (e.g. Becker's) and those that are not progressive.

c   **True**. Myasthenia more usually affects adults, but it can also affect older children. Symptoms and signs are similar. Characteristically, there is a tiring of the muscles. Oculomotor and cranial nerve muscles are most commonly affected. Diagnosis is with the edrophonium test and treatment with pyridostigmine and immunosuppressives.

d   **True**. Several metabolic disorders may involve muscles and so cause weakness such as glycogen storage disorders and muscle lipid disorders. Mitochondrial disorders may also lead to weakness, and present with features suggesting a multi-system disorder (developmental delay, weakness, stroke-like episodes).

e   **False**. Guillian–Barré syndrome is characteristically a progressive ascending weakness that worsens for 3 weeks and then improves gradually. All skeletal muscles are may be affected, and death may occur from respiratory involvement. Treatment is supportive and physiotherapy may be used to maintain joint mobility. There is much less sensory than motor involvement.

Peripheral neuropathy is uncommon is paediatric populations, but if encountered suggests Guillian–Barré syndrome or hereditary motor and sensory neuropathy (HMSN).

10   *The following signs are typically found with these associated conditions*
   a   an abnormal Moro response and Erb's palsy
   b   scissor gait and cerebral palsy
   c   unilateral loss of facial sensation and Bell's palsy
   d   strabismus and tuberculous meningitis
   e   fasciculation and cerebral palsy

a   **True**. In the neonatal examination the Moro (or startle) response can be used to assess the neurology and power of the arms and is also one of the primitive reflexes (see Box 5.2). The reflex is mediated in the brain stem and so may be absent if there is any CNS pathology. A motor nerve or brachial plexus injury will cause an asymmetrical Moro as will a fractured clavicle.

b   **True**. Most CP leads to hypertonia. The hip adductors and calf muscles are particularly affected in the legs. These commonly develop contractures. Adductor hypertonia makes walking more difficult and the child will have to adopt a scissor gait (see Box 5.3).

c   **False.** Bell's palsy is a lower motor neurone seventh nerve palsy. Sensation of the face is mediated by the fifth nerve, and the only sensation carried by the seventh nerve is the taste of the anterior two-thirds of the tongue and cutaneous sensation from the external auditory canal.

Bell's palsy is usually caused by a local viral infection in the nerve itself. It is also associated with hypertension. Prognosis is very good with no treatment, and corticosteroids further improve recovery.

d   **True.** Tuberculous meningitis is now very rare in industrialized countries, but may be encountered in immigrant populations. There may be meningism and cranial nerve palsies with a well-looking child and little fever. CSF is typically turbid with a high protein and white cell count.

e   **False.** Fasciculation occurs when there is denervation of a muscle. In paediatrics this may occur if there is a motor nerve lesion or an anterior horn cell problem (e.g. Werdnig–Hoffmann disease).

11   Ataxia in children
   a   is commonly found in 'clumsy' children
   b   leads to a wide-based gait
   c   is a common presentation of Wilson's disease
   d   is occasionally associated with chicken pox
   e   is usually caused by a primary cerebellar lesion

a   **False.** Ataxia may occasionally be found in 'clumsy' children. Children with cerebellar ataxia may also have intention tremor, overshooting, and a wide based gait. Clumsy children are more likely to be normal neurologically.

b   **True.** This is the typical ataxic gait. Other gaits are outlined in Box 5.3.

c   **False.** Wilson's disease is an autosomal recessive disorder caused by abnormal copper binding and transport. Copper is deposited in the tissues. Copper levels are low and urinary copper excretion high. Copper is deposited in the liver (hepatitis and cirrhosis results) or the brain and in particular the basal ganglia (incoordination, tremor, behavioural change) or the kidneys (causing tubular dysfunction). Caeruloplasmin levels are often low.

d   **True.** A relatively common association of ataxia is with chicken pox (but not the other way around).

Viruses can often affect the brain. Herpes simplex is the most serious of these, which causes encephalitis and can permanently damage the brain. Mumps, chickenpox, and measles can all cause encephalitis, but these almost always have a benign course. Measles is the cause of SSPE (subacute sclerosing panencephalitis), which presents with motor, speech, and visual impairment, progressing to dementia, and eventually death many years after the initial infection.

e   **False.** Cerebellar disease is relatively rare. Commoner causes of ataxia are ataxia telangiectasia, Friedreich's ataxia, and drug or ethanol intoxication.

12   An infant of 3 months with meningitis is likely to have
   a   a rash
   b   a stiff neck
   c   a poor outcome
   d   a fever
   e   a high polymorphonucleocyte count in their cerebrospinal fluid

a   **False.** In a question with *likely* in its stem, the branches must have a chance over 50% of being correct. In this branch, although there may be a rash, most infants will not have a rash. Viral meningitis can be associated with a maculopapular rash and meningococcal meningitis has a purpuric rash.

Box 8.1 shows the commonest organisms at each age.

b   **False.** Older children are more likely to have a rash, but infants have a non-specific presentation, with fever, poor feeding, and lethargy. Septicaemia, urinary tract infection, and upper respiratory tract infection may also present this way. The only specific signs are a bulging fontanelle, but this is usually a late sign, and convulsions, but this may be due to a febrile convulsion.

A stiff neck may be encountered in older children with meningeal irritation (meningitis, subarachnoid haemorrhage) or local pathology (tonsillitis, neck abscess).

c   **False.** Meningitis is a serious infection, but it does not always have a poor outcome. Prognosis depends on the organism responsible, speed of diagnosis and host factors. Meningococcus and group B *Streptococcus* have a relatively good outlook, whereas those infants who have pneumococcal or Gram-negative meningitis are likely to do worse.

Administration of intramuscular penicillin as soon as the diagnosis is suspected before any tests are performed is thought to improve prognosis in meningococcal disease.

d   **True.** A high fever is commonly associated with meningitis. Its absence does not rule out the diagnosis.

e   **True.** CSF samples are interpreted in the light of red and white cell count, protein, and glucose. The conditions that can be identified are bacterial, tuberculous and viral meningitis, cerebral abscess, subarachnoid haemorrhage, and a bloody tap.

The red cell count (normal $<5/mm^3$) is increased if there is inflammation (5–30), as will be the case in all forms of meningitis but much higher if there is a subarachnoid haemorrhage (>100). The red cell count will also be high if there is a bloody tap. If the sample is contaminated with blood the red/white cell ratio will be roughly 550 : 1. Any more white cells than this ratio indicates meningitis. The white cell count is raised (>20) if there is meningitis. It is particularly high in bacterial meningitis. The types of cell can be useful, as polymorphonucleocytes are more often found in bacterial disease whereas lymphocytes are more typical of viral and tuberculous meningitis. Lymphocytes may be the cell type found in early bacterial meningitis.

The protein is normal (0.15–0.4 g/l) in viral disease but elevated in bacterial meningitis and markedly so in tuberculous meningitis.

CSF glucose should be over 50% of blood glucose, which must be taken at the same time as the CSF. Lower levels indicate there is glucose consumption. This may occur in tuberculous disease and bacterial disease.

Data interpretation and reasoning — answers

13(i)   A 14-month-old girl is brought to the emergency department by ambulance. She was found by her mother to be 'shaking', unresponsive with her eyes deviated upwards. The shaking stopped after about 3 min but restarted just before arrival at the emergency department. On arrival she is centrally cyanosed and not breathing. She is moving her limbs at about 3 beats/s. She is unconscious and her temperature is 39.2°C. The doctor should

a first establish intravenous access
b give paracetamol syrup by mouth
c secure the airway by intubating her
d if the seizure is prolonged give diazepam rectally or intravenously
e give antibiotics immediately

a **False** b **False** c **False** d **True** e **False**

As always with a resuscitation question the priorities are Airway, Breathing, and Circulation. With a convulsion 'Don't forget the glucose' is a bit corny, but good advice. With febrile convulsions, early use of antipyretics is warranted as long as there the ABCD are properly taken care of. Antipyretics that can be used are paracetamol and if this has been given, ibuprofen. These can be given rectally, but the oral route should be avoided in the unconscious in case of vomiting.

Intubation is usually not needed as the airways can be maintained using a chin lift (or jaw thrust) with or without a Guedel airway. Oxygen should be given by mask or bag and mask ventilation initiated. Oxygen is given as convulsions often affect respiration and there is also an increased oxygen need. Intubation should only be considered if respiration is suppressed for a prolonged period.

Intravenous access can be a distraction in the resuscitation situation. Airway and breathing can usually be secured without venous access. Only then need access be sought. If this is difficult the intraosseous route can be used. This can be used to obtain blood (it gives an unreliably high white count) and to give all resuscitation drugs, fluids, and glucose.

If the convulsion has lasted over 5 min, diazepam can be given intravenously or rectally (it takes the same time to work). Paraldehyde is the next agent to use (rectal or deep intramuscular injection), and then a loading dose of phenytoin. These agents should be given as soon as it is clear the previous one has not worked to stop the convulsion. If these fail, a clonazepam infusion should be started and then the child anaesthetized with thiopentone.

Antibiotics should be given if *bacterial* infection is suspected. Meningitis is the particular concern here, and the child may be too ill to tolerate a lumbar puncture. If the child has markers of sepsis (poor perfusion, pallor, acidosis) or if the fit is not typical of a febrile convulsion a broad-spectrum antibiotic (e.g. cefotaxime) should be used after blood cultures have been taken.

13(ii)   The convulsion stops. This convulsion is more likely to be a manifestation of another problem rather than a simple febrile convulsion because
   a   she is pale, with a capillary filling time of 4 s
   b   she was unable to sit unsupported before she became ill
   c   her blood sugar is 1.2 mmol/l
   d   she has six café-au lait patches
   e   her 4-year-old brother had febrile convulsions when young

a **True** b **True** c **True** d **True** e **False**
A convulsion at this age is most likely to be a febrile convulsion. Other causes are discussed below. Identifying the febrile convulsion from these other causes is important because the treatment and prognosis is so different. A febrile convulsion itself usually needs no treatment beyond antipyretics (paracetamol or ibuprofen) and cooling measures, such as removal of clothing and tepid sponging when the temperature is high. The febrile convulsion may of course be secondary to an infective process that needs antibiotics (otitis media, urinary tract infection, bacterial upper respiratory tract infection), and these diagnoses should be actively sought and treated if present. The prognosis is excellent, although 30% will have another febrile convulsion. The chance of subsequent development of epilepsy is slightly higher than the rest of the population (3% vs. 0.5%). Therefore, most children with febrile convulsions have no investigations beyond a capillary blood sugar and a urine culture and will receive no specific treatment.

Children with febrile convulsions are typically aged 9–24 months, often have a positive family history and have a short generalized tonic-clonic convulsion. When out of the post-ictal phase they are again alert and interested in their surroundings. They do not look pale or floppy. By contrast, floppy or pale and poorly perfused children may well be septic or have meningitis. Those with a neurocutaneous skin manifestation may be having the convulsion as a result of this disease (neurofibromatosis, tuberose sclerosis, Sturge–Weber). The other important cause of a convulsion at this age is organic brain disease. This is usually associated with delayed development and so a good history is important. Asymmetrical febrile convulsions are also more likely to reflect underlying structural disease (e.g. cerebral abscess, tumour).

Hypoglycaemia is an important cause of convulsions. Identification and rapid treatment is vital as hypoglycaemia can lead to brain damage.

14(i)   A 5-month-old boy is brought to the emergency department. He was found unconscious early that morning by his father who went to wake him up for a feed. He has previously been well. Examining him, he is pink and well perfused. There is no respiratory distress and he has a respiratory rate of 25. His blood pressure is 85/50 and

pulse rate 130. He has no rash. His tone is reduced but there are no other abnormal
neurological findings. Some blood results rapidly become available
Na^+ 131 mmol/l
K^+ 3.7 mmol/l
urea 2.1 mmol/l
glucose 8.9 mmol/l
haemoglobin 9.5 g/dl
white cell count 15.3 × 10^3/mm^3
platelets 179 × 10^3/mm^3

Based on these results and his clinical condition

    a he is unconscious because he is anaemic
    b a convulsion could be the cause
    c his sodium should be corrected urgently
    d he is likely to have had an intracranial bleed
    e he must not have a lumbar puncture if his anterior fontanelle is bulging

a **False** b **True** c **False** d **False** e **False**
The approach to the unconscious patient must be systematic and organized. A list
of common causes in children is in Box 5.9. While keeping this in mind, management is first directed at identifying and 'treating the treatable'—airway, breathing,
and circulatory problems, hypoglycaemia, poisoning with opiates, diabetic coma
and meningitis, encephalitis, or septicaemia.

Box 5.9   Common causes of unconsciousness in children

Postictal
Trauma
Hypoglycaemia
Drugs/poisoning
Shock
Hypoxia
Intracerebral infection
Raised intracranial pressure

Consciousness can be impaired in degrees, ranging from drowsy to unresponsive coma. The Glasgow Coma Scale (GCS) has been developed to try to quantify
consciousness, and to aid communication between medical staff. It scores eye
response (1–4), motor response (1–6), and verbal response (1–5). Hopefully,
anyone reading this has a score of 15, and the score after death would be 3.
    Consciousness requires adequate metabolic provision and a normal intracranial
pressure. Poor blood supply (locally or generally) may impair conscious level, as
happens in shock, cardiac arrest, or with arteriovenous malformations. Renal or
hepatic failure alter the blood chemistry and this can cause coma, as can hypo-

glycaemia, and there may be substances present that depress consciousness (e.g. opiates). Epilepsy, in the post-ictal phase also causes coma. In this scenario this cause is suggested by the high white cell count and hyperglycaemia. Head injury may damage the brain directly, or indirectly by raising intracranial pressure following a bleed. Hypoxia is a common paediatric cause of coma, as a result of airways or breathing problems, but anaemia must be extreme to reduce oxygen delivery so much as to make the brain hypoxic.

Generally speaking, there needs to be a relatively severe insult to cause coma, as the body adapts to accommodate mild degrees of hyponatraemia and hypoxia etc.

An intracranial bleed is a possibility, but an unlikely one. This is more likely to cause some asymmetric neurological signs, and is very unusual in the absence of trauma at this age.

Meningitis and encephalitis should be treated even if no lumbar puncture can be performed. An open fontanelle allows pressure to escape the skull, so there is no risk from coning with this procedure. A lumbar puncture may, however, be inadvisable as the infant may be too unstable.

14(ii) Cerebrospinal fluid is collected and analysed
   red cells 35 mm^3
   white cells 450 mm^3 polymorphonucleocytes
   no organisms seen
   glucose 1.3 mmol/l
   protein 0.8 g/l
Now
   a   bacterial meningitis has been ruled out
   b   the cerebrospinal fluid glucose level has made viral meningitis less likely
   c   he should now be given intramuscular penicillin
   d   the red cell count indicates there has been a subarachnoid haemorrhage
   e   encephalitis is the most likely diagnosis

a **False** b **True** c **False** d **False** e **False**
CSF interpretation is discussed in question 12. It can be seen that this CSF has a low glucose level, raised cell counts, and a high protein. The cell counts indicate that there is meningitis, the glucose level rules out viral meningitis and the protein level is not high enough for tuberculous meningitis. The lack of organisms does not rule out bacterial disease.

A subarachnoid haemorrhage releases blood into the CSF, so there are far more red cells than white (550 : 1).

Treatment should be with a broad-spectrum agent or combination of drugs at high dose. Many units now use cefotaxime or ceftriaxone as single agents. Ampicillin and chloramphenicol is also effective, and ampicillin is added to a third-generation cephalosporin in infants under 3 months to cover the possibility of *Listeria* infection. Dexamethasone is given at the onset of treatment as it is thought to reduce neurological sequelae. Intramuscular benzyl penicillin can be given by a family doctor on the suspicion of meningococcal disease.

15   *A 10-year-old girl is seen by a paediatrician because she has been having recurrent*
      headaches for the past 6 months. The following features make migraine a more likely
      cause for her problem than any other diagnosis

   a   they are worse in the morning
   b   a family history of epilepsy
   c   her aunt has migraine
   d   the headaches are associated with abdominal pain
   e   there is also photophobia

a   **False**   b   **False**   c   **True**   d   **True**   e   **True**

Recurrent headaches are common and can be debilitating for the child. Often the
role of the paediatrician is to exclude serious disease and reassure. The common
causes are migraine, anxiety or depression, space-occupying lesion, refractive
errors, hypertension, or hydrocephalus. Assessment should attempt to identify
those with a tumour (headache in the morning, nausea, neurological signs,
swollen optic disks) so they can be managed appropriately. For the rest, a detailed
history should look into migraine features such as auras and photophobia, trigger
factors, family history, and emotional problems.

Epilepsy and headaches are not associated, but migraine is frequently associated
with abdominal pain, so much so that the term abdominal migraine has been
coined.

The treatment of migraine depends on the severity and frequency of attacks.
Simple analgesia (paracetamol, ibuprofen) is used at first. To stop an attack, suma-
triptan has been used, and as prophylaxis, pizotifen or beta-blockers can be used if
the attacks are disabling or overly frequent.

16   *A 3-year-old girl is seen in outpatients at the request of her family doctor. She has had*
      three episodes of 'twitching' in the last 2 months each lasting several minutes and
      terminating spontaneously. A full neurological examination is normal. Idiopathic
      epilepsy is a more likely cause of her episodes because

   a   she had a febrile convulsion at the age of 13 months
   b   she becomes cyanosed before each attack
   c   they all have occurred during her sleep
   d   her uncle has idiopathic epilepsy
   e   all of the episodes were preceded by an emotional outburst

a   **False**   b   **False**   c   **False**   d   **True**   e   **False**

Investigation of a suspected convulsion is a common cause of referral to paediatric
outpatients. The approach is different from that in adult practice. There are many
additional causes beyond epilepsy (listed in Box 5.10), and a good history is vital to
the evaluation of children with 'funny turns'. Epilepsy is itself classified into several
different types (see question 7). This question is about distinguishing epileptic and
non-epileptic events.

Already having had a febrile convulsions make the subsequent development
of epilepsy statistically more likely, but in such a child the cause for presentation
is even more likely to be further febrile convulsions as they can occur up to the age

---

Box 5.10   The funny turn

Generalized absence seizure
Generalized atonic seizure
Complex partial seizure
Syncope
Breath holding
Reflex anoxic seizures
Pseudoseizures
Arrhythmias
Hypoglycaemia

---

of 6. The child may not always have a fever at the time of the fit as the convulsion tends to occur as the temperature rises. A positive family history of epilepsy makes the diagnosis more likely. Attacks that occur during sleep are unlikely to be either emotionally related (breath holding attacks or reflex anoxic seizures) or pseudo-seizures. Idiopathic epilepsy may cause convulsions during sleep, but if this is the only time fits occur, it is suggestive of benign rolandic epilepsy. Treatment is not usually required.

Cyanosis before attacks suggests reflex anoxic seizures or breath holding. Reflex anoxic episodes are triggered in infants and toddlers in response to a variety of stimuli (cold, accidents) and pallor, anoxia and eventually hypoxic seizures may occur. No treatment is required. Breath holding occurs in response to emotional outbursts in toddlers, usually when the child does not get its own way. Cyanosis, unconsciousness, and eventually convulsions result. These can be difficult to manage, but treatment involves a behavioural approach.

17(i)   A 5-year-old boy is brought into the resuscitation room having fallen 3 m from a tree. He was initially unconscious but then began to speak to the ambulance officers on the way to hospital. Now he is making incomprehensible groans, has a flexor response to pain, and opens his eyes to command. He has a pulse of 130, a blood pressure of 110/70, and a capillary filling (CFT) time of 4 s. He is not cyanosed, but is having difficulty breathing. There is a large contusion on the right side of his head and he has blood coming from his right ear. There are several minor cuts and grazes to the rest of his body. The following steps would now be appropriate

a   he should be nasally intubated
b   a hard neck collar should be applied
c   he should be given 10 ml/kg of colloid intravenously
d   once stabilized, he should have a magnetic resonance imaging of his brain
e   he should be given mannitol

a **False** b **True** c **True** d **False** e **False**
Once the head has been damaged, the aim of treatment is to prevent sec-ondary damage. This may be due to anoxia, hypovolaemia, raised intracranial

pressure, or further trauma during the resuscitation. Intracranial bleeding can lead to raised intracranial pressure, but identification and treatment should only occur once airways, breathing, and circulation are stabilized. When consciousness is impaired, imaging is indicated to identify the cause (diffuse axonal injury, dural tears, cerebral contusions, intracranial bleeds, and raised intracranial pressure).

The CT scan is best for looking for trauma to the skull and bleeding, but magnetic resonance is a better investigation for looking at the structure of the grey and white matter.

The airway is the primary concern, but in all trauma, especially head trauma, a cervical spine fracture should be suspected and a hard collar applied if a fracture cannot be ruled out. This can only be done when a fully conscious child can move his neck freely without pain after X-rays are normal.

As far as the airway is concerned, it may become compromised with local trauma or with a fall in conscious level. A GCS under 7–8 is an indication for intubation. In this scenario his GCS is 9 (see question 14i of this section), but he is having difficulty in breathing. Therefore, the need for intubation cannot be established from the details given. However, if intubation is needed, the oral route must be used, as whenever a base of skull fracture is suspected, nasal intubation is contraindicated. A base of skull fracture is likely as there is blood coming from the ear. Other signs would be blood or CSF coming from the nose, blood behind the tympanic membrane, or racoon eyes.

The cerebral perfusion pressure must be maintained after head trauma. This is the blood pressure minus the intracranial pressure. The blood pressure can be supported with colloid and ionotropic agents. Here however, although the blood pressure is normal, the pulse is raised and CFT prolonged. A child is able to compensate for a much larger blood volume loss than an adult and the only indication may be a rising pulse. The capillary filling time will also increase before the blood pressure falls. So for this child, 10–20 ml/kg of colloid should be given.

17(ii)   The CT shows a base of skull fracture and a small intracranial bleed. Concerning his further management

    a   rising pulse and falling blood pressure indicate rising intracranial pressure
    b   unequal pupils may indicate that his intracranial pressure is rising
    c   a head up posture reduces his intracranial pressure
    d   anticonvulsants should be avoided
    e   he should be fluid restricted

a **False** b **True** c **True** d **False** e **True**

A rising pulse and falling blood pressure indicates impending circulatory collapse, but signs of raised intracranial pressure are a falling pulse and rising blood pressure, unilaterally dilated pupil and opthalmoplegia, and deteriorating conscious level. To reduce intracranial pressure, mannitol can be given, which is an osmotic diuretic. Also the head should be raised 30° and the pCO_2 kept at a low normal level.

Fluid restriction is employed to prevent fluid overload, due to inappropriate antidiuretic hormone secretion. This is discussed further in the Nephrology section, questions 7 and 12. Convulsions increase the intracranial pressure and should be treated with phenytoin.

There is controversy about the use of anticonvulsants following severe head injury, and it is doubtful that prophylactic anticonvulsants are of any benefit. They are of use if convulsions develop after the head injury as convulsions will cause a rise in intracranial pressure.

6 Endocrinology and metabolic disease

Knowledge — questions

1 Glycogen storage diseases
  a usually cause splenomegaly
  b often cause hypoglycaemia
  c are best treated with liver transplantation
  d may lead to death by cardiomegaly and congestive heart failure
  e of some types reduce the capacity for muscular anaerobic work.

2 Rickets in children
  a typically results in a normal calcium and low phosphate level in the serum.
  b will cause enlargement of the radial heads
  c usually requires calcium supplementation for successful treatment
  d is more common among Asians
  e is commonly associated with calcium loss from the kidneys

3 A 10-year-old boy has been stabilized following his first admission with diabetic ketoacidosis and is now being prepared for discharge
  a urine testing is sufficient to monitor his glucose at home
  b he can probably be managed with two insulin injections a day
  c dextrose can be absorbed through the buccal mucosa if he becomes hypoglycaemic
  d oral hypoglycaemics can be useful in reducing his insulin requirement
  e he is likely to develop symptomatic eye or renal disease by the age of 18 years

4 Hypothyroidism following Hashimoto's thyroiditis
  a may be distinguished from hyperthyroidism by the presence of a goitre
  b is associated with delayed skeletal maturation
  c usually presents with poor growth
  d is common in children with Down's syndrome
  e needs short-term L-thyroxine replacement therapy

5 In children who are investigated for thyroid dysfunction
  a a low total thyroxine is often found in nephrotic syndrome

b the thyroid-stimulating hormone level cannot be used in the diagnosis of hyperthyroidism

c a high free triiodothyronine and low thyroid-stimulating hormone may be caused by viral thyroiditis

d a low free triiodothyronine and low thyroid-stimulating hormone may be caused by pituitary dysfunction

e 1-week-old infants with congenital hyperthyroidism have high thyroid-stimulating hormone levels

6 *A 6-year-old girl is referred to the paediatric endocrinologist by her family doctor as she has significant breast development*

a she has premature thelarche if there are no other signs of puberty

b she is more likely to have a tumour than a boy presenting with precocious puberty

c she is likely to have a growth velocity below the average for her age at present

d an adrenal tumour will not cause premature menarche

e puberty could be arrested with a gonadotrophin-releasing hormone analogue

7 *Inborn errors of metabolism*

a by definition present in the neonatal period

b generally occur sporadically

c often cause alkalosis

d can be detected prenatally

e prognosis is usually poor

8 *Cushing's syndrome in children*

a is common in asthmatics

b is usually associated with precocious puberty

c would often present with hypoglycaemia

d is more likely to be primary than in adults

e is best diagnosed with a morning cortisol measurement

Data interpretation and reasoning—questions

9(i) *A 7-year-old boy presents to the emergency department with reduced consciousness. He has been unwell with an increasing temperature for 5 days, vomiting, and excessive thirst. He has been passing large volumes of urine. He has previously been well, and is*

*taking no medications. On examination, he is found to have a dry
tongue and sunken eyes, is peripherally cool and has a heart rate of
150 beats/min and a respiratory rate of 40. There are no added
sounds in the chest. His blood pressure is 80/40 mmHg. Some blood
tests become available*
arterial blood gas:
pH 6.92 (7.35–7.45)
pCO$_2$ 2.6 kPa (4–6)
pO$_2$ 12.4 kPa (10–14)
BE −26.1 mmol/l

This boy

  a has a respiratory alkalosis
  b is likely to have a lower respiratory infection
  c his temperature may be due to hypovolaemia
  d has signs suggesting over 10% dehydration
  e has a large urine output because of an osmotic diuresis

*9(ii)   Following this assessment, an intravenous cannula is inserted. It
would now be important to*

  a rehydrate the boy over 12 h with 0.9% saline
  b start supplemental intravenous potassium
  c give a dose of subcutaneous insulin
  d measure the blood glucose every 6 h to prevent hypoglycaemia
  e use a broad-spectrum antibiotic if the white blood cell count is high

*10   A 6-year-old boy is admitted drowsy and confused. He has been
vomiting profusely over the last day, and was seen by his family
doctor with a mild upper respiratory tract infection 2 days before
that. He is afebrile and has had no head injury. Abdominal
examination reveals a liver edge 4 cm below the costal margin.
Some investigations have been performed, showing a glucose of
1.2 mmol/l and raised levels of liver transaminases. Given this
information*

  a it is likely that his respiratory infection has disseminated
  b clotting studies would be of value
  c. he is likely to be jaundiced
  d his altered conscious level will be corrected by intravenous glucose
  e recent ingestion of aspirin would be implicated in his illness

11   *A 16-year-old girl attends the endocrinology clinic as there is concern that her puberty is delayed. She has Tanner stage 3 breast development and both pubic and axillary hair, but she has had no periods*

a   an imperforate hymen is likely
b   abdominal ultrasound will reveal streak gonads
c   her growth velocity will be low even if she is undergoing a normal, but delayed puberty
d   luteinizing hormone and follicle-stimulating hormone levels will be low
e   her onset of menarche is outside the 95th percentile

12   *A male infant is born at term and weighs 1.9 kg. He is noted to be lethargic and reluctant to feed for the first 4 h and a blood sugar is taken, showing a level of 0.9 mmol/l. In this situation*

a   his hypoglycaemia should be accompanied by a low insulin level
b   he is at risk of a convulsion if untreated
c   rapid correction of hypoglycaemia may cause cerebral oedema
d   glucose should not be given until the cause is known
e   his mother is likely to be diabetic

13   *An infant is born at term following an uneventful pregnancy. However, at delivery it is noticed that the baby has ambiguous genitalia in that there are no testes palpable, a dorsal hypospadias, and a bifid scrotum. Two days later his sodium is 148 mmol/l and his potassium is 2.9 mmol/l. Based on these findings*

a   the blood pressure is likely to be high
b   an abdominal ultrasound scan would be appropriate
c   an absent uterus indicates this child probably has testes
d   the infant may have testicular feminization syndrome
e   the blood cortisol is likely to be high

14   *A 7-year-old girl is taken to the family doctor because her mother is concerned that she has a thyroid disorder, as there is a swelling in the neck and a strong family history of thyroid disease. The following suggest that her problem is associated with hypothyroidism rather than hyperthyroidism*

a   the swelling is tender
b   her pulse rate of 80
c   she is now constipated
d   her school performance has recently deteriorated
e   she has a raised thyroid-stimulating hormone

Knowledge — answers

Endocrinology is often lumped together with metabolic disease because they have common features—both often present with multisystem dysfunction and both require understanding of biosynthetic pathways. This does not mean that a student must know all of the steps or enzymes, just the overall mechanism of the pathway with more detail of the critical and clinically important sections.

In paediatric endocrinology there is not a large range of common diseases as found in adults, and so the student will be expected to have a good understanding of the pathology, investigation, and treatment of diabetes, hypothyroidism, and the disorders of puberty. A reasonable knowledge of the rarer disorders such as hypoparathyroidism, adrenal dysfunction, and Cushing's syndrome will also be expected. Metabolic diseases are important as a group but individually rare. Presentation and an approach to management will be expected for these as a group and specifics should be known for phenylketonuria (see Community paediatrics and development question 4), glycogen storage disease, and organic acidaemias. Hypoglycaemia is an important topic in its own right.

1 Glycogen storage diseases
    a usually cause splenomegaly
    b often cause hypoglycaemia
    c are best treated with liver transplantation
    d may lead to death by cardiomegaly and congestive heart failure
    e of some types reduce the capacity for muscular anaerobic work

a **False.** There are eight glycogen storage diseases (GSDs), all of which are caused by a defect in the synthesis of glycogen or its degradation to produce glucose. The diseases are distinguished by the deficient enzymes, and the presentation of each disease depends on the tissue distribution and function of the missing enzyme. Broadly speaking either the liver is affected, the muscle, or both, as it is these tissues that participate in glycogen metabolism. All of the commoner GSDs are inherited in an autosomal recessive manner.

If the liver glycogen degradation is affected, then there will be a tendency to hypoglycaemia, especially in the neonatal period. This is especially a problem with type 1 (von Gierke), where there is a deficiency of glucose-6-phosphatase and type 3 (Forbes), with no debranching enzyme and type 6 (Hers), where there is deficiency of liver phosphorylase. If the liver glycogen degradation is affected, hepatomegaly will also develop, but enlargement of other organs does not occur (except the in type 2, as discussed in part d). Type 4 (Andersen), a deficiency of the branching enzyme is rare and presents with progressive liver failure from cirrhosis.

If muscle glycogen metabolism is affected then the presentation will include fatigue or myopathy. This group includes type 3 (Forbes), with debranching enzyme deficiency, type 5 (McArdle), with muscle phosphorylase deficiency, and type 7 (Tarui), which has deficient muscle phosphofructokinase. If muscle alone is affected prognosis is good, although activity will be limited.

b   **True**. As indicated above, hypoglycaemia is found with diseases that affect liver glycogen metabolism. Neonatal hypoglycaemia is further discussed in question 12 and its management in The newborn question 20(ii).

Hypoglycaemia may be a presenting feature of many diseases other than metabolic disease, including hyperinsulinism, Beckwith—Wiedemann syndrome, glucagon or corticosteroid deficiency, poisoning with alcohol or salicylate, sepsis, extreme malnutrition, and the growth retarded neonate. If there is a metabolic cause the low glucose is found with an otherwise normal fasting response—raised ketones, triglycerides, and free fatty acids. Commonly there is also a lactic acidosis.

A specific diagnosis can be made by examining the response to glucagon, assaying white blood cell enzymes and occasionally a liver biopsy or electromyograph.

c   **False**. The aim of treating children with GSD that affects the liver is to prevent the need for glycogen storage or degradation, by providing a steady supply of glucose, often with nocturnal gastric feeding. There is no treatment for muscle disorders, but a liver transplant could be considered for the fatal type 4 GSD.

d   **True**. One of the important GSDs is Pompe's disease (type 2), because it is one the commoner forms and it results in death. All organs are affected, particularly the heart and liver. There is a deficiency of lysosomal α-glucosidase, leading to a build up of glycogen in lysosomes. This leads to hepatomegaly and cardiomegaly, and eventually cardiac failure.

e   **True**. Inability to break down muscle glycogen reduces the capacity for anaerobic work. This applies to all the muscle types of GSD (3, 5, 7). This feature can be used as a diagnostic test, as during anaerobic exercise children with these types of GSD will not show the normal rise in lactic acid.

2   *Rickets in children*
   a   typically results in a normal calcium and low phosphate level in the serum
   b   will cause enlargement of the radial heads
   c   usually requires calcium supplementation for successful treatment
   d   is more common among Asians
   e   is commonly associated with calcium loss from the kidneys

a   **True**. There are two main mechanisms to control the blood calcium. Parathyroid hormone (PTH), secreted by the parathyroid glands maintains blood calcium levels. It moves calcium into the blood by causing release from bony stores, reduces excretion of calcium in the kidneys and to avoid precipitation of calcium, this hormone at the same time increases excretion of phosphate. It also increases 1,25 hydroxyvitamin D production.

1,25 hydroxyvitamin D is the active hormone product of vitamin D. It is converted by the liver and then the kidneys from vitamin D that is either ingested or made by sunlight in the skin. It increases absorption of calcium from the gut.

Rickets has different aetiologies, but all result in undermineralization of the bone. The effects are discussed in (b). This can be due to inadequate absorption of calcium, or due to a diet deficient in vitamin D or calcium. To maintain normocalcaemia, parathyroid hormone (PTH) is released and so calcium is lost from the bones and phosphate from the kidneys. Calcium will thus be normal and phosphate low.

Occasionally, rickets is caused by a low blood phosphate resulting from a genetic (X-linked *dominant*) defect in phosphate reabsorption in the kidneys, leading to defective bone mineralization. This is vitamin D resistant rickets.

As with all diseases causing increased bone activity, alkaline phosphatase (ALP) levels are increased.

b   **True**. Poor mineralization of the bone can be seen as reduced growth, bowed legs, and thickened wrist and ankles. A rachitic rosary is enlargement of the costochondral junctions. On X-rays, a widened epiphyseal plate and cupping and fraying of the metaphysis is seen.

c   **False**. The most common cause for rickets is inadequate vitamin D in the diet or inadequate sunlight exposure, with adequate calcium in the diet. Here there will be a low level of 25-hydroxyvitamin D in the blood and treatment with calciferol (unhydroxylated vitamin D) along with a dietary review is needed. For those children with inadequate calcium intake or excessive phosphate loss, supplementation of these elements is needed. In the rare instance of a defect in the metabolism of vitamin D calciferol will be less effective than calcitriol (1,25-hydroxyvitamin D), which needs no metabolism before it is active.

Treatment should be monitored with regular measurements of calcium, phosphate, and ALP, which should all become normal. Wrist X-rays should also normalize.

d   **True**. Vitamin D deficiency is most likely to occur in breast-fed infants born to vitamin D deficient mothers. Asians are especially at risk because dark skin reduces vitamin D synthesis and their traditional diet is low in vitamin D and high in cereals. Phytates are high in the West African diet and these bind calcium, causing rickets.

Other non-nutritional causes of rickets include rickets of prematurity (malabsorption and inadequate intake of calcium, phosphate, and vitamin D), kidney disease (vitamin D is not synthesized, calcium is lost, and acidosis liberates calcium from the bones), and malabsorption (e.g. coeliac disease).

e   **False**. Usually calcium excretion is reduced as discussed above to maintain calcium levels, but excessive calcium loss and phosphate retention may occur in chronic renal disease.

3   *A 10-year-old boy has been stabilized following his first admission with diabetic ketoacidosis and is now being prepared for discharge*
   a   urine testing is sufficient to monitor his glucose at home
   b   he can probably be managed with two insulin injections a day
   c   dextrose can be absorbed through the buccal mucosa if he becomes hypo-glycaemic
   d   oral hypoglycaemics can be useful in reducing his insulin requirement
   e   he is likely to develop symptomatic eye or renal disease by the age of 18 years

a   **False.** In addition to understanding of the management of acute diabetic complications (ketoacidosis and hypoglycaemia), knowledge is expected of the maintenance treatment of children with diabetes. This requires control of the blood sugar, screening and prevention of complications, education, and attention to the psychological implications of growing up with a chronic disease.

There is now increasing evidence that scrupulous attention to glycaemic control reduces the long-term complications of diabetes. However, this increases the risk of hypoglycaemia causing drowsiness, coma, permanent brain damage, and death. Therefore, the blood sugar must be carefully monitored. The best way to do this at home uses capillary blood and a portable analyser. Blood is dropped on to a stick (e.g. Dextrostix), which produces a colour change proportional to the blood sugar.

There are various different ways to time measurement to get information about a patient's glycaemic status. If hypoglycaemia is a concern pre-feed measurements are best, but to get a good profile over a day, measurements before meals should be done. As this is impractical to do every day, one or two measurements can be done every day to ensure control is maintained.

The urine only contains glucose when the blood sugar exceeds the renal glucose reabsorbing ability, typically about 10 mmol/l, although this may be less in disease states. This makes it an unsuitable method for monitoring glucose except possibly in elderly patients with diet-dependent diabetes.

b   **True.** To control blood sugar, a balance between the type and amount of food and insulin must be achieved. This requires a carefully controlled diet, rich in complex carbohydrates, and low in fats and refined sugars.

The minimum number of injections should be given that effectively controls the blood glucose. More injections might improve control at the expense of an increased risk of hypoglycaemia and discomfort. Adequate control is usually possible with two injections a day, by mixing short-, medium-, and long-acting insulins.

Some older children prefer to use an 'insulin pen'. This is an injection device filled with short-acting insulin that enables the child to alter the dose and timing of the insulin to fit with the size and timing of their meals.

c   **True.** In the short term the most serious complications of diabetes are keto-acidosis, hypoglycaemia, and infections. Families should be educated so that they are able to recognize and manage these. A 'hypo' may present with poor behaviour, hunger, sweating, pallor, drowsiness, reduced consciousness, or none of these.

Dextrose should be given immediately as a sugary drink, or a dextrose gel can be given that is absorbed through the buccal mucosa. Also glucagon for intramuscular injection can be issued.

When a diabetic becomes ill and stops eating, often parents will omit the insulin, but this leads to ketoacidosis. In this situation insulin should still be given and the glucose monitored closely.

d   **False.** Oral hypoglycaemics are of no use in managing children with diabetes. They are of use in some adults where there is insufficient insulin secretion for maintaining normoglycaemia. By control of the diet and boosting insulin release (sulphonylureas such as glibenclamide) or cell response to insulin (biguanides such as metformin), the glucose level can be kept near normal in these patients.

Diabetic children are all insulin-dependent diabetics and have no insulin production. Without exogenous insulin, blood sugar and ketones will rise and cause ketoacidosis.

e   **False.** The long-term micro- and macrovascular complications of diabetes relate to the length of the disease, patient factors, and the control during that time. Few will ever develop significant eye, renal, or cardiac complications less than 10 years after diagnosis or before puberty, but most will have developed them after 20 years. So, although children will rarely have these, screening ophthalmology assessment, renal function measurement, and attention to glucose control is important. Haemoglobin A_{1C} measurement allows assessment of control over several months.

More commonly encountered complications are injection site lipohypertrophy and scarring.

4   Hypothyroidism following Hashimoto's thyroiditis

    a   may be distinguished from hyperthyroidism by the presence of a goitre
    b   is associated with delayed skeletal maturation
    c   usually presents with poor growth
    d   is common in children with Down's syndrome
    e   needs short-term l-thyroxine replacement therapy

a   **False.** Hypothyroidism in childhood is most commonly due to a congenital defect in the thyroid gland or to Hashimoto's thyroiditis, an autoimmune disorder most likely to affect older girls. A full list of causes for hypothyroidism is in Box 6.1.

A goitre is caused by either the effect of thyroid-stimulating hormone (TSH) on the thyroid gland (as in inborn errors of thyroid hormone metabolism) or inflammation that is normally long term and caused by antibodies (Hashimoto's and Graves' disease). Occasionally, a viral thyroiditis will also cause a goitre. So, although there are many ways to distinguish hyper- and hypothyroid conditions, the presence of a goitre is not one. Graves' goitres may have a bruit that can be heard over the swelling.

Box 6.1   Causes of hypothyroidism

Congenital	Thyroid agenesis
	Abnormal descent of the thyroid
	Enzyme deficiency
	Deficiency of TSH or TRH
Acquired	Hashimoto's (lymphocytic) thyroiditis
	Viral (subacute) thyroiditis
	Iodine deficiency
	Drugs (amiodarone, carbimazole)

---

b   **True**. Skeletal maturation can be measured using a wrist X-ray. Here the ossification centres of the bones of the wrist appear in a predictable manner during childhood and allow a radiologist to give a 'bone age'. This will be delayed in hypothyroid children. The bone age can be thought of as the developmental age of the bones, and can also indicate how much growth is still possible when the hypothyroidism is corrected.

c   **True**. The thyroid gland is important in the control of growth from infancy up to puberty. Hypothyroid children are typically short and plump, as are children with other endocrine disorders (growth hormone deficiency, Cushing's syndrome).

Other symptoms and signs of hypo- and hyperthyroidism are listed in Box 6.2.

d   **True**. Children with Down's more commonly are hypothyroid or are insulin-dependent diabetics. Hypothyroidism will worsen their intellectual progress, as

---

Box 6.2   Symptoms and signs of thyroid dysfunction

Hyperthyroidism	Hypothyroidism
Heat intolerance	Cold intolerance
	Jaundice
Advanced growth and bone age	Poor growth, delayed bone age
Behavioural problems	Intellectual delay
Tremor	Slow relaxing reflexes
Diarrhoea	Constipation
Sweaty skin	Dry skin and coarse hair
	Umbilical hernia in infant
Tachycardia	Bradycardia
Eye signs	

---

will undiagnosed myopia and hearing loss, both of which are more common in Down children.

e   **False.** The majority of thyroid conditions need continuous treatment. On the other hand, a viral thyroiditis may cause a temporary hyperthyroidism followed by a short term period of hypothyroidism.

L-thyroxine (T4) is needed for hypothyroidism, and for hyperthyroidism carbimazole is the treatment of choice. For both conditions dose should be adjusted according to the TSH, T4, and growth velocity, which will be normal if the thyroid status has been normalized.

> 5   *In children who are investigated for thyroid dysfunction*
>   a   a low total thyroxine is often found in nephrotic syndrome
>   b   the thyroid-stimulating hormone level cannot be used in the diagnosis of hyperthyroidism
>   c   a high free triiodothyronine and low thyroid-stimulating hormone may be caused by viral thyroiditis
>   d   a low free triiodothyronine and low thyroid-stimulating hormone may be caused by pituitary dysfunction
>   e   1-week-old infants with congenital hyperthyroidism have high thyroid-stimulating hormone levels

a   **True.** To answer this type of question, you need knowledge of both the physiology of the thyroid axis and the conditions that affect it. Thyrotrophin-releasing hormone (TRH) is secreted from the hypothalamus and has its action in the pituitary. The TRH stimulates secretion of TSH from the cells in the anterior pituitary. TSH has its action on the thyroid, and control of TSH production is achieved by negative feedback at both pituitary and hypothalamic level. The thyroid gland secretes mainly T4 and less (20%) triiodothyronine (T3). T4 is converted to the active T3 or inactive rT3. All of these substances are largely protein bound by thyroid-binding globulin (TBG) and albumin and only the free hormones have any action.

In protein loosing states, particularly cirrhosis and nephrotic syndrome there is less binding capacity. Total hormone levels will be low but free levels normal. Oestrogens and pregnancy increase the TBG levels so increase total hormone levels. Chronic illness reduces the peripheral conversion so that free T3 is low but T4 and TSH normal.

Tests that measure thyroid function all have their problems and must be interpreted with clinical and other data. The TRH cannot routinely be measured. TSH is easy to measure, and will provide an assessment of the hypothalamic/pituitary response to the thyroid status. Levels will be high if the thyroid gland is under functioning and are also high in the first few days of life. TSH is low if there is hyperthyroidism or a hypothalamic or pituitary problem that is causing hypothyroidism. These can be distinguished using the TRH stimulation test.

Total T3 and T4 are not nearly as useful as the levels of free hormones, as there can be a variable amount of protein binding. However, in conjunction with the

TSH, most disorders can be diagnosed with total T3 and T4. As the hormones have long half-lives, the timing of a sample is not important.

b **False**. TSH levels can be used in the diagnosis of hyperthyroidism, but must be supplemented with a high T3 level. TSH is easier to measure when high, but modern assay techniques can now reliably detect a low TSH.

c **True**. A high free T3 and low TSH indicates there is hyperthyroidism, and this is one of the presentations of a viral thyroiditis. This condition is caused by a variety of viruses, including mumps. It may also present as a tender swelling, hypothyroidism, or hyperthyroidism, and is usually temporary.

d **True**. As indicated above, pituitary or hypothalamic dysfunction will reduce TSH and therefore thyroid activity, causing secondary or tertiary hypothyroidism. This may be congenital or caused by tumours or trauma, but is much less common than other causes of hypothyroidism. The Guthrie card used for neonatal hypothyroid screening measures TSH and so this type of hypothyroidism will not be detected.

Thyroid hormone replacement is usually needed in conditions that affect the hypothalamus (craniopharyngioma, gliomas) and the pituitary stalk (trauma).

e **False**. Congenital hyperthyroidism is rare, but interesting. It is caused by TSH receptor antibodies (IgG) from a mother with Graves' disease passing into the fetus and stimulating release to thyroid hormones in the fetus. No practical treatment for the mother will alter the production of these antibodies. TSH in both mother and fetus will thus be low.

The condition may present antenatally as hydrops fetalis, which in this situation is high output cardiac failure. The newborn will also be tachycardic, irritable, and have poor weight gain.

Treatment during pregnancy should aim to normalize the for the fetal heart rate, using carbimazole, as this crosses the placenta. The mother's thyroid levels may then need supplementation with thyroxine. After birth the infant may need propranolol and propylthiouracil.

6 *A 6-year-old girl is referred to the paediatric endocrinologist by her family doctor as she has significant breast development*

    a she has premature thelarche if there are no other signs of puberty
    b she is more likely to have a tumour than a boy presenting with precocious puberty
    c she is likely to have a growth velocity below the average for her age at present
    d an adrenal tumour will not cause premature menarche
    e puberty could be arrested with a gonadotrophin-releasing hormone analogue

a **True**. Puberty is a complex process and delay or precocious puberty are common. Sexual development beginning before 8 years in girls and 9 years in boys is defined as precocious. Lack of development at 13 in females and 15 years in boys is delayed. Thelarche is the development of breast tissue in the female, adrenarche the appearance of pubic hair, and menarche the start of menstruation. Puberty is a slow process and to help describe the physical changes that occur, there is the Tanner staging for breasts, male genitalia, and pubic hair. Stage 1 is prepubertal and stage 5 adult.

When assessing a child with precocious pubertal development, examination and investigations aim to determine if the changes are early but physiological or caused by abnormal synthesis of hormones. If there is abnormal hormone synthesis, there may be discordance of pubertal features (e.g. pubic hair and a growth spurt without breast development), and the process is likely to be abrupt.

As breast development is the first sign of puberty, this girl is most likely to be going into a normal puberty. Younger girls (under 3 years) sometimes have precocious and asymmetrical breast development. If there are no other signs of puberty, no treatment is necessary.

In boys puberty begins with testicular enlargement, measured using an orchidometer, before penile enlargement and growth of pubic hair.

b   **False**. Puberty is initiated by increased secretion of gonadotrophin-releasing hormone (GnRH) pulses, causing an increase in the pulses of follicle-stimulating hormone (FSH) and luteinizing hormone (LH). This stimulates gonadal development and the secretion of oestradiol or testosterone. These hormones cause breast and penile growth and the pubertal growth spurt

Precocious puberty is divided into pituitary dependent (with high GnRH and FSH/LH) or pituitary independent (low GnRH, FSH, and LH). Pituitary-dependent causes include constitutional or idiopathic and intracranial pathology, particularly hamartomas and other tumours of the hypothalamus. Pituitary-independent causes include congenital adrenal hyperplasia (CAH; see question 13) and adrenal, ovarian or testicular tumours, and drug use such as the contraceptive pill.

Statistically, a girl with precocious puberty is most likely to have a benign cause but boys have about a 50% chance of an underlying tumour.

c   **False**. The pubertal growth spurt is caused by oestrogen and testosterone. These hormones also close the growth plate. The growth velocity should be appropriate for the stage of puberty, and is maximal early in female puberty (stage 3 breasts) but later in male puberty (stage 5 penis). This accounts for some of the difference in height between the sexes, as boys have longer to grow before the pubertal growth spurt and also there is more growth for boys during the spurt.

Therefore, although her growth velocity may not be above normal, it should not be low.

Other endocrine disorders often result in alteration in growth rate, both decrease (hypothyroidism, growth hormone deficiency) or an increased rate (hyperthyroidism). Other aspects of growth are discussed in the Growth and nutrition chapter.

d   **True**. Adrenal tumours secrete sex steroids and so cause the development particularly of pubic hair and growth, and to a lesser extent breast tissue. Cycling levels of FSH and LH are required to stimulate ovarian development and to start menstruation.

e **True.** With precocious puberty, after eliminating and treating a non-idiopathic cause, the priorities of treatment are to delay the pubertal growth spurt and closure of the epiphyses. There are also psychological problems for affected children.

If the precocious puberty is pituitary dependent, exogenous GnRH can suppresses the secretion of FSH and LH as a pulsatile secretion of GnRH is needed to stimulate FSH and LH. Hence sex steroid levels will be reduced and closure of the epiphyses delayed, so while the GnRH is being given growth will continue.

  7 Inborn errors of metabolism
  a by definition present in the neonatal period
  b generally occur sporadically
  c often cause alkalosis
  d can be detected prenatally
  e prognosis is usually poor

a **False.** Inborn errors of metabolism can present at any age. The most common times for presentation are in the first week of life or during a viral illness during the first year.

The neonatal presentation is similar to that of neonatal sepsis, necrotizing enterocolitis or even a coarctation. The baby is likely to be shocked and lethargic and if there is acidosis there will also be tachypnoea (see The newborn question 20).

Inborn errors of metabolism can be placed in several groups. There are defects in amino acid metabolism (e.g. phenylketonuria, tyrosinaemia, maple syrup urine disease, homocysteinuria), organic acidaemias (lactic or propionic acidosis), carbohydrate disorders (galactosaemia, fructosaemia), urea cycle defects (ornithine transcarbamylase deficiency), and storage disorders.

b **False.** Most inborn errors show autosomal recessive inheritance, and there are a few X-linked recessive mutations. This is because these defects are all caused by an absent or poorly functioning enzyme. As an enzyme can be produced from either chromosome if it is an autosomal gene, two absent genes are needed for the child to have an inborn error, making the disorder follow recessive inheritance. Parents are likely to be related.

On the other hand, most dominant conditions are characterized by the production of a faulty protein that interferes with normal cell function (e.g. hypercholesterolaemia, Duchenne muscular dystrophy).

c **False.** Acidosis is a fairly common finding in children presenting acutely with an inborn error. When there is a enzyme defect, there is a build up of the precursor to its reaction and low levels of the reaction product. Glucose is often low and ammonia high.

d **True.** If the gene has been identified and cDNA made or if a linked marker is present in a family, prenatal diagnosis is possible using chorion villus sampling.

Amniocentesis is not useful unless the chromosomal number is in doubt. Screening would not be of value prenatally because the chance of picking up a defect would be far lower than the risk of miscarriage attributable to the procedure. Also the number of possible defects is high and so the programme would be exceedingly expensive. However, early diagnosis can help to improve prognosis, particularly by avoiding hypoglycaemia and collapse.

The only metabolic disease for which screening is carried out is phenylketonuria. This is done at 7 days with a TSH level on the Guthrie card. This disease is selected because it is asymptomatic in its early stages but causes mental retardation if untreated (see Community paediatrics and development question 4).

e   **False.** Prognosis is usually fairly good, depending on the condition. Cure is not possible without liver transplant or perhaps gene therapy. The effects of many inborn errors can be avoided by dietary manipulations. For any defective enzyme, the precursor will be at high levels and the reaction product at low levels. The aim of a diet will be to reduce the amount of precursor by decreasing flux through the pathway and occasionally supplement levels of the product. Dietary manipulations for various inborn errors are shown in Box 6.3.

Box 6.3   Dietary treatment of metabolic disorders

	Enzyme defect	Diet
Phenylketonuria	Phenylalanine hydroxylase	Low phenylalanine
deficiency	Ornithine transcarbamylase	Protein restriction, benzoate, citrulline
Glycogen storage diseases	Various	Regular carbohydrate feeds
Maple syrup urine disease	branched chain a-ketoacid dehydrogenase	Diet low in branched chain amino acids (leucine, isoleucine, valine)
Hurler syndrome	α-L-iduronidase	No diet helpful
Galactosaemia	Galactose-1-phosphate uridyl transferase or galactokinase	Galactose-free

---

8   Cushing's syndrome in children

   a   is common in asthmatics
   b   is usually associated with precocious puberty
   c   would often present with hypoglycaemia
   d   is more likely to be primary than in adults
   e   is best diagnosed with a morning cortisol measurement

a   **False.** Cushing's syndrome is the name given to the clinical picture associated with high corticosteroid levels. Cushing's disease is the syndrome caused by pituitary overproduction of adrenocorticotrophic hormone (ACTH) and is very rare in children. Much more common is the syndrome associated with systemic steroid medications, and adrenal tumours. Cushingoid children then are likely to have either bronchopulmonary dysplasia, a tumour requiring chemotherapy, nephrotic syndrome, or an arthritis. It is very rare for a child to take enough steroid in the course of asthma treatment to become cushingoid. Short courses of oral steroids can be used to supplement inhaled steroids. Neither usually cause adrenal suppression.

b   **False.** The adrenal cortex secretes several hormones (cortisol, aldosterone, sex steroids). All are synthesized in a common pathway. Enzymatic disorders of this pathway are discussed in question 13 and below. There is close regulation of the levels of corticosteroids with negative feedback at the pituitary level via corticotrophin-releasing hormone and ACTH. Aldosterone too is carefully regulated by a feedback loop incorporating blood pressure, angiotensin, and the kidneys. Sex steroids are also regulated with a separate feedback loop.

As there are three separate feedback loops for these three types of hormones, a defect in one does not always alter the levels of another. The exception to this is in CAH. Here there is a defect in the biosynthetic pathways for glucocorticoids, mineralocorticoids, and sex steroids. The commonest defect is 21-hydroxylase deficiency, an enzyme in the cortisol synthesis pathway. Deficiency leads to a high level of ACTH secretion. This hormone, in attempting to normalize the corticosteroid level, causes adrenal hyperplasia. It also stimulates the whole pathway and so there will be high levels of sex steroids (causing precocious puberty in the male or ambiguous genitalia in the female). Aldosterone is also synthesized using 21-hydroxylase and so a salt losing state may result or hypertension if the defect is less severe. Other enzyme defects can cause high or low aldosterone or sex steroid levels, but the cortisol is only ever normal or deficient.

Hence Cushing's syndrome is unlikely to be found in association with precocious puberty. However, both will lead to closure of the epiphyses.

c   **False.** Presentation of Cushing's syndrome in children is similar to that in adults, with a characteristic moon face, central obesity and short stature, muscle wasting, acne, and striae. Blood pressure and glucose are likely to be high.

Adrenal cortical insufficiency is less common, and may present with circulatory collapse due to sodium loss and hypoglycaemia. Skin pigmentation develops if the disorder is long-standing due to the action of high levels of ACTH, as this hormone is structurally related to melanocyte-stimulating hormone.

d   **False.** The pituitary adenoma that secretes ACTH and causes primary Cushing's disease is very unusual in children.

e   **False.** Normally, cortisol is high in the morning and low at midnight. This diurnal pattern is lost in Cushing's, so the best time to measure the cortisol is late at night. (The urinary free cortisol can also be measured which should be high.) Conversely, the best time to make a diagnosis of adrenal cortical insufficiency is the morning.

The dexamethasone suppression test can be used to help determine the aetiology of a high cortisol level. The low dose suppression test identifies that there is excessive secretion of cortisol as there is inappropriate synthesis after a synthetic steroid is given. The high dose test will suppress some sources of cortisol, such as adrenal tumours, but not the very rare ectopic ACTH production.

Data interpretation and reasoning—answers

9(i)   A 7-year-old boy presents to the emergency department with reduced consciousness. He has been unwell with a increasing temperature for 5 days, vomiting, and excessive thirst. He has been passing large volumes of urine. He has previously been well, and is taking no medications. On examination, he is found to have a dry tongue and sunken eyes, is peripherally cool and has a heart rate of 150 beats/min and a respiratory rate of 40. There are no added sounds in the chest. His blood pressure is 80/40 mmHg. Some blood tests become available
arterial blood gas:
pH 6.92 (7.35–7.45)
pCO_2 2.6 kPa (4–6)
pO_2 12.4 kPa (10–14)
BE −26.1 mmol/l

This boy

 a has a respiratory alkalosis
 b is likely to have a lower respiratory infection
 c his temperature may be due to hypovolaemia
 d has signs suggesting over 10% dehydration
 e has a large urine output because of an osmotic diuresis

a **False** b **False** c **True** d **True** e **True**
This boy has a typical presentation for diabetic ketoacidosis (DKA). He has polyuria despite dehydration with vomiting and polydipsia. He also has a severe metabolic acidosis.

The polyuria is caused by the presence of glucose beyond the proximal tubule in the kidney. It is there because the glucose reabsorbing capacity of the proximal tubule has been exceeded by the large amount of glucose being filtered in the glomerulus. The glucose causes an osmotic diuresis in the same way that mannitol is used to cause a diuresis in a patient with raised intracranial pressure.

This boy also has evidence of hypovolaemic shock (cool peripheries, tachycardia, and reduced consciousness) that would suggest that he is over 10% dehydrated. The sunken eyes and dry tongue alone would make him 5–10% dehydrated.

Another DKA feature is Kussmaul's breathing, which is deep, fast, and regular, and is caused by acidosis. There are typically no other respiratory signs in DKA.

DKA may occasionally be confused with other causes of vomiting and dehydration (especially as there is often central abdominal pain in DKA). The respiratory signs may also lead to confusion. Here any respiratory problem is unlikely because there are no other respiratory signs other than tachypnoea. Patients with DKA often have an underlying infection and upper respiratory tract infections (URTIs), lower respiratory tract infections and urinary tract infections are common. Such infections, by stimulating stress hormones can raise blood glucose and precipitate DKA. As DKA causes a raised white blood cell count, it is more important to use clinical criteria to identify a patient that would benefit from antibiotics.

Stress hormones can also raise the blood glucose as can be also seen in sepsis, after convulsions and after surgery, but they will be near the normal range (3–5.5 mmol/l). A high temperature is usually caused by an infection, but often occurs where there is severe hypovolaemia as heat cannot be lost from the vaso-constricted skin.

The blood gas results show a partially compensated metabolic acidosis. The severe acidosis is caused by the large negative base excess (this is the measurement of free base in the body, and a negative value implies an excess of acid). Respiratory compensation can be seen from the attempts of the body to reduce the acidosis by lowering the CO_2. Further information about blood gases can be found in The newborn question 18.

9(ii) *Following this assessment, an intravenous cannula is inserted. It would now be important to*

a rehydrate the boy over 12 h with 0.9% saline
b start supplemental intravenous potassium
c give a dose of subcutaneous insulin
d measure the blood glucose every 6 h to prevent hypoglycaemia
e use a broad-spectrum antibiotic if the white blood cell count is high

a **False** b **True** c **False** d **False** e **False**

The management of DKA simply corrects the fluid and electrolyte disturbances, at the same time supplying insulin which corrects the underlying problem.

The most important disturbance is fluid depletion, caused by vomiting, poly-uria, and hyperventilation. If there is shock, as in the above scenario, it should be corrected relatively quickly with 0.9% saline; 0.9% saline is a safe and useful fluid for use in resuscitation before any electrolytes are available. A bolus of 10–20 ml/kg is usually required. Following fluid resuscitation, fluid therapy should aim to re-place the deficit over 36–48 h; 0.45% saline is used until the blood glucose reaches 10–14 mmol/l when dextrose/saline is used. Fluids are given at a rate to replace the deficit and allow for ongoing losses (especially urine) and give maintenance fluid.

A lack of insulin causes potassium and hydrogen ions to leave cells. The potas-sium is then lost into the urine under the influence of aldosterone. Aldosterone levels are high as there is hypovolaemia and the kidney is trying to retain sodium. Although blood potassium may be normal or even high, the total body potas-sium will be low, and the level will fall rapidly once insulin is started. In order to compensate for this, intravenous potassium should be given. Some recommend only starting this once urine is passed, in case the hypovolaemia has caused renal failure.

Insulin needs to be given to correct the hyperglycaemia and reduce the production of ketones. A sliding scale is usually used to match insulin given with blood sugar. The subcutaneous route is not useful if there is shock, and control of the insulin delivery rate will not be possible with only one injection. Therefore an infusion of insulin is used.

The two most serious problems commonly encountered during DKA treatment are cerebral oedema caused by overly rapid rehydration and hypoglycaemia. To avoid this the glucose must initially be monitored hourly and changes made based on these findings in the rate of insulin and glucose given

As discussed in part (i), the white count is unreliable as evidence for infection in DKA.

Catheterization and insertion of a gastric tube have been recommended but are not needed in all children.

10   *A 6-year-old boy is admitted drowsy and confused. He has been vomiting profusely over the last day, and was seen by his family doctor with a mild upper respiratory tract infection 2 days before that. He is afebrile and has had no head injury. Abdominal examination reveals a liver edge 4 cm below the costal margin. Some investigations have been performed, showing a glucose of 1.2 mmol/l and raised levels of liver transaminases. Given this information*

     a   it is likely that his respiratory infection has disseminated
     b   clotting studies would be of value
     c   he is likely to be jaundiced
     d   his altered conscious level will be corrected by intravenous glucose
     e   recent ingestion of aspirin would be implicated in his illness

a **False**   b **True**   c **False**   d **False**   e **True**

This boy's presentation contains several unusual features—his confusion, an enlarged liver, elevated transaminases, and a low glucose. While drowsiness can be caused by a wide range of diseases (sepsis, head injury, subarachnoid haemorrhage), it is also often found in association with drug ingestion or a metabolic disturbance. Reye's syndrome, a hepatic encephalopathy, is strongly suggested by this scenario. Reye's is now rare, but remains important as it may be precipitated by aspirin. Aspirin is now avoided in the treatment of pyrexia in children under the age of 12 years. This disease commonly follows an URTI and features include hepatomegaly, abnormal liver function, clotting disturbance, and hypoglycaemia. Consciousness is impaired because of the severe metabolic derangement and raised intracranial pressure. Jaundice is unusual because the disease is of acute onset and there is insufficient time for the bilirubin to build up.

URTIs may disseminate, but would not cause this presentation. However, they may lead to arthropathy or renal disease, and the organisms may invade and cause septicaemia.

Treatment is supportive aimed at controlling the raised intracranial pressure and hypoglycaemia.

11   A 16-year-old girl attends the endocrinology clinic as there is concern that her puberty is delayed. She has Tanner stage 3 breast development and both pubic and axillary hair, but she has had no periods

   a   an imperforate hymen is likely
   b   abdominal ultrasound will reveal streak gonads
   c   her growth velocity will be low even if she is undergoing a normal, but delayed puberty
   d   luteinizing hormone and follicle-stimulating hormone levels will be low
   e   her onset of menarche is outside the 95th percentile

a **False** b **False** c **False** d **False** e **True**

No signs of puberty at 13 years in a girl and 15 years in a boy is abnormal. A lack of menarche at the age of 16 with other signs of pubertal development present is also abnormal. Menstruation typically starts 1–2 years after breast development begins.

The aetiology can be divided into those causes with high and low gonadotrophin levels. High levels indicate there is gonadal resistance (Turner's, Klinefelter's, and following gonadal disease). Low gonadotrophin levels associated with delayed puberty indicates that there is constitutional delay, which is more common in boys, systemic disease (e.g. cystic fibrosis or anorexia), or a hypothalamopituitary disorder. An imperforate hymen typically presents with delayed menarche is associated with an otherwise normal puberty and regular lower abdominal pain. When colposcopy is attempted, blood can be seen behind the hymen.

A normal puberty requires a rise in the levels of FSH and LH. These hormones stimulate the ovaries or testicles and these hormones then give rise to secondary sexual characteristics. As this girl has breast development and pubic hair, she must be undergoing a normal puberty and have normal ovaries. This does not rule out Turner's syndrome. Although most Turner's have streak gonads, many have ovaries that can produce hormones and allow some secondary sexual characteristics. So, although it is possible her FSH and LH are high, they will not be low.

As maximum growth occurs when the breasts are Tanner stage 3, this girl should be growing rapidly despite her delayed puberty.

The abdominal ultrasound is a useful investigation for precocious or delayed puberty in girls, as information about the uterus, ovaries, and the adrenals (which may have a tumour) can be obtained. FSH and LH can also identify the organ that is functioning poorly.

Treatment of delayed puberty is not always needed if constitutional delay is the cause or the delay is secondary to another disease. Oestrogens or testosterone can be used to bring on secondary sexual characteristics in constitutional delay or Turner's. Pulsatile GnRH can be given if there is hypothalamic or a pituitary defect and this can allow fertility if ovarian function is normal.

12   *A male infant is born at term and weighs 1.9 kg. He is noted to be lethargic and reluctant to feed for the first 4 h and a blood sugar is taken, showing a level of 0.9 mmol/l. In this situation*

    a   his hypoglycaemia should be accompanied by a low insulin level
    b   he is at risk of a convulsion if untreated
    c   rapid correction of hypoglycaemia may cause cerebral oedema
    d   glucose should not be given until the cause is known
    e   his mother is likely to be diabetic

a **True** b **True** c **False** d **False** e **False**

This infant is hypoglycaemic (the normal range is in dispute, and levels under 2.4 mmol/l may be associated with an poorer neurological outcome. Over 2.0 mmol/l is usually acceptable). This is a common situation in infancy and this boy is particularly at risk, being growth retarded. Owing to placental insufficiency, his liver glycogen will be low and fat and muscle energy reserves will also be depleted. Hypoglycaemia will prompt glucagon secretion and inhibit insulin production, but will not be enough to raise the blood glucose. In a non-growth-retarded infant, the lack of insulin will increase ketone body formation from fat, and ketone bodies can be used as a fuel. If there is 'non-ketotic hypoglycaemia', this is suggestive of a metabolic disorder or hyperinsulinism (e.g. Beckwith–Wiedemann syndrome, infant of a diabetic mother). In this case this is unlikely as hyperinsulinism promotes growth and this infant is very small. Sepsis and in-born errors are also important causes of hypoglycaemia.

Treatment must not wait for a specific diagnosis, as hypoglycaemia can make a baby jittery, floppy, and cause coma, fits, and brain damage, and it is important to return the glucose to the normal range as fast as possible. A bolus of feed should be tried if the glucose is 1.7–2.5 mmol/l. Intravenous glucose will be needed if the glucose is under 1.7 mmol/l or there is no response to enteral feed or if there are symptoms of hypoglycaemia. A bolus of glucose is only indicated if there is a severe complication, such as a convulsion.

There is no risk of cerebral oedema from rapid correction of the glucose. This can only occur if there is rapid infusion of a fluid more hypotonic than the brain. This is most likely in children with hypernatraemic dehydration. Here the brain has become used to a high sodium and osmolality and the infusion of a fluid of lower osmolality will cause an osmotic shift of water into the brain, which can result in cerebral oedema and coning.

13   *An infant is born at term following an uneventful pregnancy. However at delivery it is noticed that the baby has ambiguous genitalia in that there are no testes palpable, a dorsal hypospadias, and a bifid scrotum. Two days later his sodium is 148 mmol/l and his potassium is 2.9 mmol/l. Based on these findings*

    a   the blood pressure is likely to be high
    b   an abdominal ultrasound scan would be appropriate
    c   an absent uterus indicates this child probably has testes
    d   the infant may have testicular feminization syndrome
    e   the blood cortisol is likely to be high

a **True** b **True** c **True** d **False** e **False**

The birth of an intersex child can be devastating for the parents and difficult for the doctors as the diagnosis and sex is sought. The question is whether the baby is a masculinized girl or a feminized boy. Here there is some additional detail about the blood sodium and potassium that makes CAH likely (see question 8). The differential diagnosis of an intersex child includes CAH, hermaphroditism, androgen exposure during pregnancy, and partial testicular feminization syndrome.

In assessing an intersex baby, examination should first describe the genitalia. If there are palpable masses in the groin, these are probably undescended testes and the baby is genetically a boy. There may be a large clitoris or a phallus, rugosity of the labia or the appearance of a bifid scrotum. The urethra will usually not discharge from the end of the enlarged clitoris.

The most useful investigation is the abdominal ultrasound. If performed in the first week it is possible to see the uterus as it is still enlarged following the effects of maternal hormones. If it is not there it is because Müllerian structures have regressed under the influence of testosterone. Ovaries or undescended testes may also be seen. A karyotype can determine genetic sex and a β-human chorionic gonadotrophin stimulation test may provoke the secretion of testosterone if there is testicular tissue present.

CAH may present in a variety of different ways. If the biosynthetic pathways for aldosterone and testosterone are unaffected, ACTH stimulation of the gland will raise the levels of aldosterone, causing sodium retention, potassium loss, and hypertension (e.g. 11β-hydroxylase deficiency). Boys will have precocious puberty and girls will be virilized. If there is a common defect of corticosteroid and aldosterone synthesis, there will be a loss of salt in the kidneys, leading to hypotension and collapse. If there is poor synthesis of testosterone, boys will be incompletely masculinized (e.g. 5α-reductase deficiency).

Here the child has a high sodium and low potassium, so he will have a high aldosterone and as a result a high blood pressure. Blood cortisol will be low or normal if he has CAH, as the ACTH is trying to bring the cortisol up to normal.

14 *A 7-year-old girl is taken to the family doctor because her mother is concerned that she has a thyroid disorder, as there is a swelling in the neck and a strong family history of thyroid disease. The following suggest that her problem is associated with hypothyroidism rather than hyperthyroidism*

   a the swelling is tender
   b her pulse rate of 80
   c she is now constipated
   d her school performance has recently deteriorated
   e she has a raised thyroid-stimulating hormone

a **False** b **False** c **True** d **False** e **True**

Swellings of the thyroid gland may be associated with hyperthyroidism (Graves' disease), hypothyroidism (Hashimoto's, iodine deficiency), and with normal thyroid function (viral thyroiditis, simple colloid goitre, thyroid cyst, carcinoma, abscess). In this scenario, Hashimoto's is suggested by the family history, although iodine deficiency used to be endemic in certain areas and therefore certain families.

In examining a child with a possible thyroid problem, attention must be paid to the gland itself and to distant effects that may reveal the thyroid status. The neck should be palpated from behind and the effect of swallowing and of tongue extension noted. The purpose of this is to see if the swelling is in the thyroid gland and to feel if the swelling is smooth or nodular. Nodular goitres are most often found with carcinomas and Graves' disease, when there may be a bruit over the gland. Tenderness is suggestive of a viral thyroiditis, which can be associated with low, normal, or high thyroid hormone levels.

The distant effects of hyperthyroidism are increased growth, diarrhoea, poor concentration, sweating, tachycardia, tremor, and the eye signs of Graves' disease. Hypothyroidism manifests with poor growth, constipation, cold intolerance, bradycardia, and slow relaxing reflexes. Because the child often becomes less distractible, school performance is usually not so badly affected with hypothyroid conditions as with hyperthyroid ones.

The tests used to investigate thyroid dysfunction are discussed in question 4.

7 Haematology and oncology

Knowledge — questions

1 *Henoch–Schönlein purpura*
   a is associated with meningococcal septicaemia
   b is associated with an arthropathy
   c occurs in clusters
   d should be treated with intravenous immunoglobulins
   e needs follow-up because of the risk of glomerulonephritis

2 *Sickle cell disease*
   a is a recognized cause of haemolytic disease of the newborn
   b all patients should receive regular transfusions to reduce the sickle percentage
   c usually affects renal function
   d can cause splenic atrophy
   e patients are prone to infection with *Streptococcus pneumoniae*

3 *Idiopathic thrombocytopenic purpura*
   a often presents with a haemarthrosis or bleeding after surgery
   b is caused by the production of antiplatelet antibodies
   c usually relapses and remits over several years
   d should be treated with platelet transfusions
   e has a risk of intracranial haemorrhage

4 *Leukaemia in childhood*
   a is most likely to be acute myeloblastic in type
   b usually presents with pallor
   c is associated with vitamin K given at birth
   d a normal full blood count rules out the diagnosis
   e is more common in Down's syndrome

5 *Paediatric brain tumours*
   a are most likely to be neuroblastomas
   b can be usefully treated with radiotherapy
   c may cause precocious puberty
   d often cause a communicating hydrocephalus
   e are a common cause of convulsions

6   *Thalassaemia in children*

   a   always results from deletion of the gene coding for the α or β haemoglobin chain

   b   is usually asymptomatic in β-thalassaemia trait

   c   is often treated with bone marrow transplantation

   d   will cause the development of frontal bossing and hepatosplenomegaly
in untreated β-thalassaemia major

   e   should be treated with supplementation of iron, folic acid, and vitamin
B_{12}

7   *Neoplasia in children*

   a   is increasing in incidence

   b   now has a overall five year survival over 85%

   c   is more common in children with Turner's syndrome

   d   should not be treated with long-term steroids

   e   does not present before birth

8   *A child with haemolytic anaemia*

   a   will probably have a high reticulocyte count

   b   will usually have antibodies against the red cells

   c   may present during treatment for malaria

   d   will have a high serum bilirubin

   e   will often have splenomegaly

9   *When treating children with cancer*

   a   thrombocytopenia commonly develops as a result of the treatment

   b   combinations of chemotherapeutic drugs should be avoided

   c   cyclophosphamide may cause deterioration in pulmonary function

   d   radiotherapy is useful in preventing recurrence of lymphoma

   e   bone marrow transplantation has not been shown to be of any benefit

Data interpretation and reasoning—questions

10   *An Asian boy is reviewed at his 3-year check. His mother reports
that his appetite is poor and most of his daily intake is cow's milk.
On examination he has a soft systolic murmur loudest over the
precordium with no radiation and is noted to have pale conjunctivae
and nail beds. Thalassaemia is more likely to be the cause of his pallor
rather than any other cause because he is also found to have*

  a   a macrocytic anaemia
  b   a low ferritin and a high transferrin (iron binding capacity)
  c   an enlarged liver
  d   frontal bossing
  e   Heinz bodies

11   *A previously well 5-year-old child is seen by his family doctor with*
     recurrent pharyngitis. His full blood count result is
     Hb 6 g/dl
     WCC 35 × 10³/mm³
     platelets 55 × 10³/mm³
  a   he needs antibiotics to treat his infection
  b   his full blood count should be repeated after 1 week of observation
  c   he should be admitted for a bone marrow aspirate
  d   blood products are contraindicated
  e   he is at high risk of haemorrhage

12   *A child is admitted for elective surgery. On questioning his mother*
     preoperatively, he had a large bleed following extraction of a tooth.
     Clotting studies are performed
     platelet count 265 × 10³/mm³
     PTT 15.6 s (11.0–15.0 s)
     INR 1.2
     APTT 75 s (27–39 s)
  a   this is a typical presentation of von Willebrand's disease.
  b   with these results, a history of purpura would be more usual
  c   a history of bleeding in his mother would be expected
  d   fresh frozen plasma should ideally be given prior to the procedure
  e   vitamin K will not correct his clotting

Knowledge — answers

Paediatric haematology is dominated by several fairly common conditions—iron deficiency anaemia is the most common red cell problem, with other haemo-globinopathies (sickle cell, thalassaemia) being important in certain populations. Clotting disorders may be encountered too, particularly immune thrombocyto-penic purpura, and also haemophilia is important because of the genetic aspect. Although less common, an approach to haemolytic anaemia should also be under-stood. Oncology is a very complex subject and the student is not expected to know about more than the presentation of cancers, their epidemiology, and the broad principles of treatment.

1 Henoch–Schönlein purpura

a   is associated with meningococcal septicaemia
b   is associated with an arthropathy
c   occurs in clusters
d   should be treated with intravenous immunoglobulins
e   needs follow-up because of the risk of glomerulonephritis

a   **False.** Henoch–Schönlein purpura (HSP) is not strictly a haematological disease but rather a vasculitis but is included is this section as purpura is a often seen as a clotting disorder. Purpura and petechiae are the names given to larger and smaller leaks of blood into the tissues respectively. By definition they will not blanch. The leak of blood will be caused by either a low platelet count, platelet dysfunction (see question 3), a high venous pressure (e.g. whooping cough), or vascular disease. HSP and meningococcal septicaemia are the most common causes of vasculitis in paediatric populations, but are separate entities. Meningococcal vasculitis is caused by endotoxin on the wall of the organism. The lesions may be petechiae or larger purpura and at worst large vessels are thrombosed leading to amputation. Other features of meningococcal infection are discussed in Immunology and infectious diseases question 10. HSP rarely produces large lesions but they are distributed on extensor surfaces 'especially the legs' more than other areas.

b   **True.** Other features of HSP include abdominal pain—this is typically central and colicky. Occasionally, HSP may be complicated by intussusception or gastrointestinal bleeding. Arthralgia and arthropathy are common, but resolve leaving no residual lesion. The kidneys are also affected, as outlined in part e).

Diagnosis is clinical and any investigations are usually normal except for the urine microscopy, which will demonstrate haematuria in 90% of children.

c   **True.** Although no infectious agent has been identified as the cause of HSP, the disease often occurs after a viral upper respiratory tract infection (URTI). The disease is more common in contacts and families.

d   **False.** Treatment of HSP is largely supportive with analgesia. No therapy has been shown to alter the course of the disease unless there is severe renal involvement.

Intravenous immunoglobulins (IVIG) are used in several immune mediated diseases in children including immune thrombocytopenic purpura (see question 3), Kawasaki disease, chronic atopic sinusitis, and Guillian–Barré syndrome. Patients with immunodeficiencies have been shown to have less bacterial infections with IVIG treatment (HIV, premature neonates, hypogammaglobulinaemia).

e   **True.** The only serious long-term effect of HSP involves the kidneys. Of those children with the disease, 10% will have long-term renal impairment and may develop progressive renal failure. Children with haematuria in the acute phase should be followed up. Blood pressure should be measured regularly and urine tested for protein or blood to detect deterioration.

 2 *Sickle cell disease*
   a is a recognized cause of haemolytic disease of the newborn
   b all patients should receive regular transfusions to reduce the sickle percentage
   c usually affects renal function
   d can cause splenic atrophy
   e patients are prone to infection with *Streptococcus pneumoniae*

a **False**. Sickle cell disease (SCD) is caused by a mutation in the gene encoding the β-chain of haemoglobin. This makes the tetramer less soluble and prone to precipitation within the red cell. This distorts the cell (sickle cells are seen in addition to target cells and Howell-Jolly bodies) and thus obstructs capillary blood flow. Hypoxia, acidosis, and hypovolaemia increase this tendency. β-chains are not synthesized at birth at a high rate and so SCD does not present until 6 months at the earliest. All of the complications of the disease are either related to anaemia (tiredness, pulmonary flow murmur) or infarction (crises, stroke, functional asplenia, renal impairment, splenic sequestration) and the high red cell turnover (jaundice, aplastic crises).

  Haemolytic disease of the newborn (HDN) is recognized by the combination of jaundice and anaemia. The spleen and liver are often enlarged. The causes are either due to intrinsic red cell enzyme defects (glucose 6 phosphate dehydrogenase (G6PD) deficiency, pyruvate kinase deficiency), cell membrane defects (spherocytosis, eliptocytosis) or alloimmune diseases (rhesus, ABO incompatibility).

b **False**. There is much variation between patients with sickle disease that in part are related to the rate of synthesis of fetal haemoglobin ($\alpha_2\gamma_2$). Patients with high levels will have a higher haemoglobin and a lower sickle percentage of their haemoglobin.

  The serious complications of SCD are all related to the sickle percentage (sickle crisis, infarctions, stroke, sickle chest). A regular transfusion programme would make these less likely, but is not warranted in most children unless they have already had a stroke or chest crisis before or suffer very severe crises.

  The likelihood of sickle complications can also be reduced by maintaining hydration and oxygenation when the child is unwell.

c **True**. Renal function is reduced when children with SCD are several years old. Infarcts to the renal medulla reduce the concentrating ability. This impairs the ability of the kidney to retain water if there is reduced fluid intake. SCD also leads to renal papillary necrosis.

d **True**. Repeated splenic infarcts eventually lead to splenic atrophy. This reduces the immune response to certain organisms, particularly *Haemophilus* and streptococci. Conversely, splenic venous obstruction is a particular complication under the age of 5 causing splenic sequestration of blood. This leads to shock and abdominal distention as blood is pooled in the spleen.

e   **True.** Because of the risk of infection, children without functional spleens should be given daily penicillin prophylaxis. Immunization with Pneumovax is also indicated.

3   *Idiopathic thrombocytopenic purpura*
   a   often presents with a haemarthrosis or bleeding after surgery
   b   is caused by the production of antiplatelet antibodies
   c   usually relapses and remits over several years
   d   should be treated with platelet transfusions
   e   has a risk of intracranial haemorrhage

a   **False.** As discussed in question 1, a low platelet count leads to leaks of blood from capillaries causing petechiae and purpura. A reasonable platelet count is required for coagulation and so a low count results in easy bruising and haemorrhage from operations and other cuts. Most children will be asymptomatic until the count is under $20 \times 10^9/l$.
   Low levels of clotting factors present less with bruising but more with haemarthroses and bleeding into tissues.
   Von Willebrand's disease behaves as a combination of a platelet disorder and a clotting factor problem. This is because von Willebrand factor acts both as a carrier preventing factor VIII degradation and also aids platelet adhesion.

b   **True.** This disease is autoimmune. It typically occurs 1–4 weeks after a viral infection. Children over 2 years are most often affected, girls as often as boys. Platelet levels are often below $10 \times 10^3/mm^3$ and a bone marrow aspirate, if performed, will show active megakaryocytes. The rest of the blood count and blood film should be normal.
   The main differential diagnosis is with leukaemia, and children who are an unusual age or have an abnormal blood film should have a bone marrow aspirate before treatment is begun. The bruising in children with idiopathic thrombocytopenic purpura (ITP) may also lead to the suspicion of non-accidental injury.

c   **False.** The paediatric type of ITP differs from the adult type which typically relapses and remits over several months and years whereas the paediatric type has usually resolved after 3 months.

d   **False.** Platelet transfusions are almost useless as the platelets given are immediately removed from the circulation by antiplatelet antibodies. Platelets can only be used for short-term cover for procedures. IVIG can be used to reduce the destruction of platelets. An alternative is steroid therapy but both treatments should only be used to treat active bleeding.

e   **True.** This is the most serious complication of ITP, fortunately affecting under 1%.

4 *Leukaemia in childhood*

   a   is most likely to be acute myeloblastic in type
   b   usually presents with pallor
   c   is associated with vitamin K given at birth
   d   a normal full blood count rules out the diagnosis
   e   is more common in Down's syndrome

a **False**. Leukaemia is the most common group of paediatric neoplasias. Acute lymphoblastic leukaemia (ALL) is much more common than the myelocytic type (AML). Chronic leukaemia is very rare in children. ALL and AML have a similar presentation but differ in treatment and prognosis.

    ALL is a cancer of the lymphoid elements of the marrow. It will present with the effects of anaemia, thrombocytopenia, or defective immune function. A high white count can cause hyperviscosity phenomena and the high cell turnover may cause hyperuricaemia. Infiltration may also cause lymphadenopathy, hepatosplenomegaly, and other effects. It can affect any age. Prognosis is generally good with long-term survival over 75% in the more favourable groups (low white cell count, over 1 year, female, no CNS involvement).

    AML presents similarly, the only characteristic feature being gingival hypertrophy. Liver and spleen are usually more enlarged. The prognosis is worse for AML, and a bone marrow transplant is now recommended at first or second relapse for both ALL and AML, depending on other risk factors.

b **True**. Pallor may be caused by a low haemoglobin or poor skin perfusion. In leukaemia the low haemoglobin, platelet count, and immune dysfunction are the result of the filling of the bone marrow with neoplastic cells. Later, chemotherapy will suppress the bone marrow and reduce haematopoiesis.

c **False**. One study from Bristol, UK suggested that infants receiving intramuscular vitamin K at birth might have a higher incidence of childhood cancer. This increase did not apply to those receiving oral vitamin K. Although there was no explanation offered for the observation, many hospitals switched to using vitamin K orally unless there was bleeding or reason to suspect that the gut might not absorb the vitamin K. Subsequent studies have not found an increase of cancer in the intramuscular group.

    Vitamin K is given in the early neonatal period to prevent haemorrhagic disease of the newborn. This disease affects 1% of neonates who are not given vitamin K are is due to reduced levels of clotting factors. It is more common if the mother is taking anticonvulsants or the baby has cystic fibrosis, but is prevented by vitamin K administration, preferably parenterally. Skin, gastrointestinal, and umbilical bleeding are common but intracranial bleeding can be fatal even though it is rare.

d **False**. A normal full blood count makes it unlikely, but will miss 'aleukaemic leukaemia'. Although with this ALL variant there is a normal full blood count, a blood film will demonstrate abnormal white cells or blasts.

e **True**. Most problems are more common in Down's syndrome, including leukaemia. Down's syndrome is also discussed in The newborn, question 13

5 *Paediatric brain tumours*
  a are most likely to be neuroblastomas
  b can be usefully treated with radiotherapy
  c may cause precocious puberty
  d often cause a communicating hydrocephalus
  e are a common cause of convulsions

a **False**. Brain tumours are the second most common type of malignant disease in children, making up 20% of cases. In contrast to adult brain tumours most paediatric brain tumours are primary and over half are infratentorial. The commonest types are astrocytomas and medulloblastomas.

Neuroblastomas are not brain tumours and originate from tissue of the neural crest—that is, they usually originate from paravertebral tissue or within the adrenal glands.

b **True**. Overall prognosis for brain tumours is about 50% for long-term survival, depending on tumour type and site of the primary and the presence of metastases. Some have a worse prognosis, particularly brainstem gliomas.

Treatment is with surgical excision where possible and radiotherapy. The role of chemotherapy is still being evaluated. Surgery and radiotherapy are both known to be bad for the developing brain and intellectual impairment, behavioural problems and endocrine disorders are common following treatment.

c **True**. The presentation of children with brain tumours is similar to that of adults, with early morning headache and vomiting, ataxia if there is a cerebellar tumour and signs of raised intracranial pressure (papilloedema, VIth nerve palsy). Headache is an unusual complaint in young children and should prompt a thorough examination. In older children the headache of a brain tumour is usually symptomatically different from that of a migraine. Serious concerns should prompt an MRI scan, as this is the best investigation for viewing the posterior fossa.

d **False**. As paediatric brain tumours are often found in the posterior fossa, hydrocephalus is a common complication, but of the non-communicating type. The communicating type is usually caused by dysfunction of the arachnoid granulations or a lack of subarachnoid channels, caused by blood or previous infection. Drainage of the CSF is possible by performing a lumbar puncture. By contrast the non-communicating or obstructive type is caused by obstruction within the ventricular system, and this usually occurs at the aqueduct of Sylvius or the fourth ventricle. A drain (shunt) from the lateral ventricles to the abdomen or the right atrium is necessary to remove the fluid.

Another complication that may develop is endocrine disturbance, particularly if the hypothalamus is involved. Poor growth and precocious puberty are often found with craniopharyngiomas, tumours that may also cause visual field defects.

e **False.** Tumours rarely present with convulsions, but convulsions may develop after surgery and during radiotherapy. Focal fits that are difficult to control are more likely to be caused by a brain tumour.

6 *Thalassaemia in children*

    a always results from deletion of the gene coding for the α or β haemoglobin chain
    b is usually asymptomatic in β-thalassaemia trait
    c is often treated with bone marrow transplantation
    d will cause the development of frontal bossing and hepatosplenomegaly in untreated β-thalassaemia major
    e should be treated with supplementation of iron, folic acid, and vitamin B_{12}

a **False.** Haemoglobin is encoded by four α and two β chain genes, half of which come from the father and half from the mother. All forms of thalassaemia are caused by deletion of some or all of these genes or mutation resulting in low levels of expression. α-thalassaemia is more often caused by deletion of gene, whereas β-thalassaemia is more likely to be caused by a low level of chain synthesis. A non-synthesizing gene is denoted $\beta thal^{0}$ and one with reduced function $\beta thal^{+}$. All of the manifestations of thalassaemia result from low levels of expression of one chain type and the response of the body to the resulting anaemia.

b **True.** One of the problems with thalassaemia is the terminology. Thalassaemia minor or trait is usually asymptomatic and identified as a hypochromic microcytic anaemia in a blood count, similar to iron deficiency anaemia. The genotype will be heterozygous for the defect. β-thalassaemia intermedia is the result when there is some, but little β chain synthesis, usually homozygous for the $\beta thal^{+}$ gene. HbH disease is the a chain equivalent of $\beta thal$ intermedia, with 1 of the 4 α chain genes present. β-thalassaemia major is more serious with almost no synthesis of that chain. α-thalassaemia major is not seen as the a chain is needed to make fetal haemoglobin. A fetus with this genotype develops hydrops fetalis due to anaemia and rarely survives to birth. β-thalassaemia major does not present until adult haemoglobin is needed (after 6 months).

c **False.** As all the symptoms are caused by anaemia, regular blood transfusions enable a near normal life. Desferrioxamine is needed to reduce iron overload, which can lead to cardiac, liver, and pancreatic failure.

    Bone marrow transplantation is now being tried as an alternative treatment in selected individuals if there is a well matched sibling. This form of treatment is also gaining acceptance in severe sickle cell disease.

d **True.** Frontal bossing and enlargement of the maxilla develop as the body increases the haemopoietic capacity in an attempt to compensate for the poor quality of red cells produced. These are signs of long-term untreated thalassaemia major. Hepatosplenomegaly will also be found in a child with extramedullary haematopoiesis.

e **False.** Laboratory features of thalassaemia include iron overload (high ferritin, low iron binding capacity).

Although iron is needed to make red cells, it is recycled and in children with thalassaemia iron overload is usual. High red cell turnover (sickle cell, thalassaemia, spherocytosis, etc.) are more likely to cause folic acid depletion.

7 Neoplasia in children
   a is increasing in incidence
   b now has a overall 5-year survival over 85%
   c is more common in children with Turner's syndrome
   d should not be treated with long-term steroids
   e does not present before birth

a **False.** Despite many health scares, the overall incidence of cancer in children is not increasing.

b **False.** Survival for paediatric malignancies has improved dramatically over the last 10 years and is better than adult tumours. This is partially because the type of tumour is more amenable to treatment and because there are usually no other diseases that might make therapy more hazardous. For instance cure from ALL survival is now over 60% and even for a stage IV lymphoma over 50%.

Staging systems have been developed for all the common tumours and should be known in outline. Stage I is disease within the organ of origin, stage II local invasion to surrounding tissues. Stage III is disseminated but within one part of the body (e.g. abdomen, above the diaphragm) and stage IV widespread dissemination. Other letters may be used to denote a particular organ that the disease has spread to, such as neuroblastoma stage IVS, where there is spread to the skin only. This particular type of neuroblastoma is interesting as the tumour will spontaneously regress and eventually disappear even without treatment.

c **False.** There is no increased incidence of malignancy associated with Turner's. This is a feature of Down's syndrome, ataxia telangiectasia, Bloom syndrome, and neurofibromatosis type 1.

d **False.** Steroids are an important part of the treatment of leukaemias, lymphomas and brain tumours, and Cushing's syndrome frequently develops.

Other agents used in treatment include alkylating agents (e.g. cyclophosphamide) which inhibit DNA polymerase, antimetabolites (methotrexate) which deprive dividing cells of substrate, antibiotics (adriamycin) which bind to DNA, enzymes (asparaginase) which breaks down asparaginine, and the vinca alkaloids (e.g. vincristine) which affect microtubule formation. All of these agents inhibit or interrupt cell division, and so have most effect on tissues in which there is rapid cell division. The most aggressive tumours are therefore more responsive to treatment than less aggressive ones as they are more sensitive to chemotherapy. Such agents also affect normal tissue with a high cell turnover (e.g. gut, bone marrow) and this causes serious side-effects (mucositis, neutropenia, thrombocytopenia).

e   **False**. Most cancers that children have are unusual outside the paediatric age group. Sacrococcygeal teratomas are often diagnosed antenatally while the 'blastomas' usually present under 4 years. ALL is far more common in children than adults and Wilm's tumour is rare over the age of 8. AML and the lymphomas on the other hand occur more in older children as well as adults.

8   *A child with haemolytic anaemia*
   a   will probably have a high reticulocyte count
   b   will usually have antibodies against the red cells
   c   may present during treatment for malaria
   d   will have a high serum bilirubin
   e   will often have splenomegaly

a   **True**. Anaemia is either caused by lack of production of red cells or their excessive destruction. In the haemoglobinopathies both processes are important. Excessive destruction that results in anaemia is called haemolytic anaemia. The key features of all types of haemolytic anaemia is evidence of high red cell synthesis (high reticulocyte count, active bone marrow, reticulocytosis on the blood film) and cell destruction (high bilirubin, red cell fragments, bite cells). If the haemolysis is intravascular there will be free haemoglobin in the blood and haemoglobinuria, but if extravascular there will be none. The spleen enlarges to remove the cells from the circulation.

b   **False**. Many of the causes of haemolytic anaemia are inherited, including the enzyme defects, cell membrane defects, and the haemoglobinopathies. Because the red cell is a much more complex and larger entity than the platelet, there is more scope for non-immune destruction and immune-mediated anaemia is numerically less important. Immune involvement is found in allo-immune disease (rhesus, ABO incompatibility), associated with mycoplasma and Epstein–Barr viral infection, lymphoma, and with the use of certain drugs.
   Red cells can also be damaged by prosthetic valves (unusual in children) and angiopathic processes.

c   **True**. Malaria treatment (and also sulphonamides, nitrofurantoin, and the fava bean) exposes the red cell to oxidative stress. Normally, the red cell is able to protect itself from this, but is not able to do this if there are defective enzymes in the respiratory chain. Glucose-6-phosphate dehydrogenase and pyruvate kinase deficiency are the commonest red cell enzyme defects and can present either as an acute or chronic haemolytic anaemia. They are also causes of a neonatal jaundice.
   Glucose-6-phosphate dehydrogenase deficiency is inherited in an X-linked recessive fashion, whereas pyruvate kinase deficiency is autosomal recessive.

d   **True**. A raised bilirubin is one of the hallmarks of haemolytic anaemia. Other causes of bilirubinaemia include liver disease, biliary obstruction, and the various causes of neonatal jaundice (see The newborn, question 10).

e   **True**. The spleen is the site of removal of red cells from the circulation and so it is enlarged in haemolytic anaemia. Other common paediatric causes of spleno-megaly include infection, portal hypertension, and malignancy.

9   *When treating children with cancer*
   a   thrombocytopenia commonly develops as a result of the treatment
   b   combinations of chemotherapeutic drugs should be avoided
   c   cyclophosphamide may cause deterioration in pulmonary function
   d   radiotherapy is useful in preventing recurrence of lymphoma
   e   bone marrow transplantation has not been shown to be of any benefit

a   **True**. While detail of chemotherapeutic agents should not be memorized, understanding of their mode of action and the common complications of the more widely used agents is useful. As outlined above in question 7, inhibition of cell division results in bone marrow suppression. This first affects the neutrophil count and then the platelet count, and lastly the haemoglobin due to differences in the turnover of these cell types. Packed cells and platelets can be given, but neutropenia cannot be directly corrected. Infection with Gram-positive organ-isms (staphylococcus and streptococcus), Gram negatives as well as fungi can be life threatening, and fevers in neutropenia should be investigated thoroughly and treated with broad-spectrum antibiotics.

b   **False**. Combinations of drugs have proved successful in reducing mortality from cancers. By interrupting cell division in different ways, the drugs can act synergistically. For instance, one ALL induction combination employs vincristine (microtubules), asparaginase (inhibits cell metabolism), intrathecal methotrexate (inhibits CNS cell division), and prednisolone.
   Chemotherapy can also be subdivided into remission induction, consolidation and maintenance, and CNS prophylaxis. All of these steps require different agents.

c   **True**. All chemotherapy agents have multiple side-effects, particularly bone marrow suppression, although vincristine, adriamycin, and asparaginase do not. In addition, cyclophosphamide causes cystitis and pulmonary fibrosis, vincristine causes peripheral neuropathy and adriamycin cardiomyopathy.

d   **True**. Lymphomas are sensitive to radiotherapy and so this is used, often in combination with chemotherapy and surgery to reduce recurrence of the disease. Radiotherapy is ineffective in neuroblastoma and little used in leukaemia, but useful for children with Hodgkin's lymphoma and brain tumours.

e   **False**. Bone marrow transplantation (BMT) allows high doses of chemo-therapy and radiotherapy that ablates the original bone marrow. After a period without bone marrow, it can then be put back in hopefully with no malignant cells left in the body. Autologous BMTs require separation of the tumour cells from the normal bone marrow harvested during a remission.
   BMTs carry a mortality of 10–20%, and are used in situations where mortality from the cancer is well above this. These include first or second relapses of AML

and ALL, depending on other factors. This treatment is also used for serious inherited marrow related disorders including severe sickle cell disease and thalassaemia.

Data interpretation and reasoning — answers

10 *An Asian boy is reviewed at his 3-year check. His mother reports that his appetite is poor and most of his daily intake is cow's milk. On examination he has a soft systolic murmur loudest over the precordium with no radiation and is noted to have pale conjunctivae and nail beds. Thalassaemia is more likely to be the cause of his pallor rather than any other cause because he is also found to have*

   a a macrocytic anaemia
   b a low ferritin and a high transferrin (iron binding capacity)
   c an enlarged liver
   d frontal bossing
   e Heinz bodies

a **False** b **False** c **True** d **True** e **False**

This boy looks pale and has a systolic murmur, which is probably a pulmonary flow murmur, even though it might be an innocent murmur (see Heart disease, question 13i). It is likely that he is anaemic, although clinical pallor is an insensitive test for anaemia and a formal haemoglobin measurement should be done. He has risk factors for several causes of anaemia—he is Asian, so may have thalassaemia. α-thalassaemia is common in Asians and β-thalassaemia in those from the Mediterranean and the Middle East. He will not be asymptomatic at the age of 3 if he has thalassaemia major, but he may have thalassaemia minor. He is also likely to have iron deficiency, based on his poor diet and the high prevalence at his age. Studies have reported that the incidence of iron deficiency anaemia is 3–25% and iron deficiency twice that, depending on the population.

Clinical signs of iron deficiency other than pallor are uncommon, although such children may have mild developmental delay, muscle weakness, and occasionally, koilonychia. Frontal bossing, maxillary hypertrophy, and hepatosplenomegaly are signs consistent with thalassaemia.

Blood tests can be helpful, but most common causes of anaemia in childhood result in a microcytic hypochromic anaemia (iron deficiency and thalassaemia). A macrocytic anaemia would suggest a folic acid or vitamin B_{12} deficient anaemia, both of which are much less common but can be found with malabsorption, poor diet, and folate antagonists. Phenytoin also causes a megaloblastic anaemia.

Red cell inclusions include Heinz bodies and Howell-Jolly bodies. The latter are found in hyposplenic patients. Heinz bodies are areas of denatured haemoglobin bound to the red cell membrane. Before the cell is removed from the circulation, the Heinz body may be phagocytosed leaving a bite cell. They are found principally in children with G6PD deficiency and unstable haemoglobins.

Measuring the levels of red cell folate, B12 and ferritin indicate stores of these haematinics, and the transferrin (iron-binding capacity) should be high if iron deficiency is present.

If this child has iron deficiency he will need a dietary review and iron supplementation for several months. Depending on severity he may need regular transfusion if he has thalassaemia.

11   *A previously well 5-year-old child is seen by his family doctor with recurrent pharyngitis. His full blood count result is*
   Hb 6 g/dl
   WCC 35 × 10³/mm³
   platelets 55 × 10³/mm³

   a   he needs antibiotics to treat his infection
   b   his full blood count should be repeated after 1 week of observation
   c   he should be admitted for a bone marrow aspirate
   d   blood products are contraindicated
   e   he is at high risk of haemorrhage

a **True** b **False** c **True** d **False** e **False**

'Recurrent' pharyngitis is very common, and occasionally is caused by immuno-deficiency. Here the full blood count shows a low haemoglobin and platelet count but a very high white count. This cannot be an artefact and the only likely cause is acute leukaemia. Isolated high white counts (up to $30 \times 10^3/mm^3$) or high platelet counts (up to $1000 \times 10^3/mm^3$) are common in children with infection.

This boy will need chemotherapy but first he needs intravenous antibiotics to treat his throat infection and packed cells to correct his anaemia. He is not at high risk of haemorrhage at present, so platelets will not be needed. As a guide, a count under $50 \times 10^3/mm^3$ in association with bleeding or a count under $20 \times 10^3/mm^3$ should be treated. The count should be over $100 \times 10^3/mm^3$ in those being prepared for surgery.

Although the diagnosis can be made on the history and blood film, a bone marrow aspirate gives more information about type and prognosis.

12   *A child is admitted for elective surgery. On questioning his mother preoperatively, he had a large bleed following extraction of a tooth. Clotting studies are performed*
   platelets 265 × 10³/mm³
   PTT 15.6 s (11.0–15.0 s)
   INR 1.2
   APTT 75 s (27–39 s)

   a   this is a typical presentation of von Willebrand's disease
   b   with these results, a history of purpura would be more usual
   c   a history of bleeding in his mother would be expected
   d   fresh frozen plasma should ideally be given prior to the procedure
   e   vitamin K will not correct his clotting

a **False** b **False** c **False** d **False** e **True**

Before elective surgery, a preoperative assessment aims to identify problems that may make the operation more difficult or dangerous. Blood tests are not routinely done. Reactions to previous anaesthetics and allergies to antibiotics or respiratory disorders may cause anaesthetic problems. Anaemia or a clotting defect will make the surgery more difficult and hazardous.

Here questions have raised a concern about a child's clotting and studies have shown a raised APTT. This is the intrinsic clotting pathway that is being measured, as opposed to the PTT which measures the extrinsic pathway. The INR is simply the PTT of the patient divided by the normal for the laboratory. Prolongation of clotting tests is usual in young children and neonates.

The APTT is raised in conditions in which there are low levels of factors VIII, IX, XI, or XII, usually as a result of an inherited deficiency. Haemophilia A (X-linked recessive) is a deficiency of factor VIII and is the commonest defect. This would be inherited from the mother, a heterozygote carrier. Christmas disease, also termed haemophilia B (also X-linked recessive) is associated with low factor IX. The factors themselves can be measured and supplemented as necessary using concentrate which is heat or detergent treated to get an adequate level. Cryoprecipitate and fresh frozen plasma are not treated and so carry a risk of infection. However, if there is bleeding, the clotting is deranged and the cause is not known, fresh frozen plasma is effective at achieving haemostasis.

The PTT is prolonged when there are deficient factors II, V, VII, or X, as in liver disease. The PTT and INR are good markers of synthetic liver function and rapidly become abnormal if the liver fails. The PTT is also prolonged in vitamin K deficiency, caused rarely by dietary deficiency and commonly by fat malabsorption. Parenteral vitamin K will improve the PTT in this situation.

Defects in clotting factors may cause bruising but more commonly there is a history of haemorrhage into muscle, joints, and delayed surgical haemostasis.

Von Willebrand's disease is discussed in question 3.

8 *Immunology and infectious diseases*

Knowledge — questions

1 *Other individuals should be screened or treated if the index case*
   a has had *Mycobacterium tuberculosis* isolated from a lymph node
   b has epiglottitis
   c had streptococcal meningitis
   d has *Salmonella* dysentery
   e is a newborn baby with chlamydial conjunctivitis.

2 *For a previously well child in a developed country*
   a *Listeria* can cause neonatal septicaemia
   b the Epstein–Barr virus usually affects children under the age of 2
   c Gram-negative organisms are unlikely to cause meningitis outside the neonatal period
   d group B streptococcus most commonly affects children in the first week
   e Streptococcus pneumoniae is the most frequent cause of meningitis under the age of 5

3 *The body is able to counteract infectious agents because*
   a complement is able to opsonize bacteria
   b viruses are mostly phagocytosed by neutrophils
   c complement is able to lyse bacteria directly
   d *Candida* is effectively killed by IgG
   e natural killer lymphocytes destroy cells without antibody interaction

4 *Fungal infection*
   a often involves the mouth in immunocompetent infants
   b by *Candida* will often cause invasive infection
   c can involve the scalp in childhood
   d usually requires amphotericin B for effective treatment
   e may colonize central venous catheters

5 *A 4-year-old boy has a fever and a erythematous rash*
   a the presence of conjunctivitis suggests that he has mumps
   b that the rash started behind the ears and has now spread to the rest of the body is suggestive of measles

c he may have typhoid fever
d as he also has cataracts, rubella is a more likely cause
e a rash on his cheeks alone is typical of fifth disease (erythema infectiosum)

6 *Herpes simplex*

a lesions are often superinfected with *Staphylococcus aureus*
b infections usually require treatment with acyclovir
c type II cannot cause stomatitis
d infection may complicate eczema
e encephalitis may present with focal seizures

7 *Lower respiratory tract infections in childhood caused by*

a *Strep. pneumoniae* are the commonest acquired in the community
b staphylococci are usually associated with a severe illness
c *Mycoplasma pneumoniae* are uncommon in children
d respiratory syncytial virus will only affect those under 18 months
e *Haemophilus influenzae* can be effectively prevented by *Haemophilus
   influenzae* type B vaccination.

8 *Streptococci*

a are the commonest cause of abscesses
b are usually resistant to penicillins in the UK
c cause over 50% of urinary tract infections
d cause about a third of cases of pharyngitis
e can cause meningitis in the newborn period

9 *Tuberculosis in children*

a is decreasing in incidence
b is more frequently extrapulmonary than in adults
c can be reliably diagnosed using the Mantoux test
d can be screened for with chest X-rays
e can be cultured from stomach aspirates in affected individuals

Data interpretation and reasoning — questions

10 *A previously well 3-year-old girl is brought to the emergency
    department. She has become increasingly lethargic and unresponsive
    over the past 8 h. She has a widespread purpuric rash, and looks pale.
    Her heart rate is 150 beats/min and blood pressure 70/30 mmHg. An
    intravenous cannula is sited and some blood tests taken*

haemoglobin 12.1 g/dl
WCC 1.3 × 10³/mm³
platelets 28 × 10³/mm³

Based on these results and her presentation

    a the patient's main problem is meningococcal meningitis
    b this result may be artefactual
    c clotting times are likely to be prolonged
    d treatment with white cells and platelets is needed
    e leukaemia should be excluded with a bone marrow aspirate

11   *Infection with human immunodeficiency virus*

    a can be diagnosed with HIV IgG levels in the infant at birth
    b may be transmitted by breast feeding from an HIV positive mother
    c is a contraindication for diphtheria/pertussis/tetanus immunization
    d often presents with failure to thrive
    e can cause dementia

12   *A 9-month- old girl is admitted to the children's ward with a temperature of 38.6°C, pallor, and vomiting. She is more likely to have a bacterial rather than another cause for her fever because she has*

    a had a febrile convulsion
    b a fine blotchy erythematous rash on her trunk that comes and goes
    c her pulse is 150, blood pressure 85/35, and a capillary filling time of 4 s
    d a marked improvement following the administration of paracetamol
    e a white cell count of 1.5 × 10³/mm³

13   *A 7-month-old child has been admitted for further investigation. He is well known to the ward as he has already been an inpatient with a chest infection at 4 months, and diarrhoea at 6 months. The following features make it more likely that he has an immunodeficiency*

    a his neutrophil count is 3.5 × 10³/mm³
    b he has crossed from the 75th to below the third centile since birth
    c he is a sub-Saharan African
    d he had a lump at the site of his diphtheria, pertussis, and tetanus injection
    e his umbilical cord separated at 3 weeks of age

14   *A 2-year-old girl is undergoing chemotherapy for leukaemia. She is now unwell and has a temperature of 38.9°C. A full examination does not reveal any focus of infection, although the site of insertion*

of her indwelling central venous catheter is red. A full blood count
is taken
haemoglobin 8.9 g/dl
white cell count $0.7 \times 10^3/mm^3$
platelets $130 \times 10^3/mm^3$

a   a chest X-ray should be avoided as it may cause further malignant trans-
    formation
b   she may have *Pneumocystis carinii* pneumonia
c   she should be started on broad-spectrum antibiotics and an antifungal
    agent immediately
d   she should be given a platelets infusion
e   the venous catheter should be removed urgently

15   *A 7-month old is admitted with a high fever, pallor, and tachycardia.
     A full septic screen is performed, and this shows a leucocytosis, but no
     excess of white cells in urine or cerebrospinal fluid. Cefotaxime, a
     third-generation cephalosporin, is started and the infant clinically
     improves. Four days later, the blood culture results become available*
     Staph. epidermidis, *growing in one of two bottles
     sensitive to chloramphenicol, vancomycin
     resistant to cephalosporin, penicillin*

a   the infant may have had a viral infection
b   this organism is a commonly found in the blood
c   this blood culture result is good evidence of septicaemia
d   the antibiotics should be changed to a combination of chloramphenicol
    and vancomycin
e   this organism is usually a skin commensal

16   *A 5-year-old African boy has returned 3 days ago from Nigeria
     where he had been visiting relatives. He is now unwell with a fever
     and rigors. His examination is unremarkable, and some blood tests
     are performed*
     haemoglobin 8.1 g/dl
     white cell count $19.3 \times 10^3/mm^3$
     platelets $490 \times 10^3/mm^3$
     Na^+ 134 mmol/l
     K^+ 4.2 mmol/l
     urea 9.5 mmol/l
     creatinine 82 μmol/l

Given these data

    a *Campylobacter* is a likely cause for his illness
    b typhoid fever is unlikely as he has had no diarrhoea
    c a thick film would now be appropriate
    d the high white cell count could be caused by the rigors
    e he has evidence of dehydration

Knowledge — answers

Changes in disease patterns, antibiotic use, and research have made this a fast moving and exciting subspeciality. From a clinical viewpoint, the diseases are varied and dramatic. For an exam student, knowledge will be expected of all the common diseases and organisms. Understanding of the changes in prevalence of the various diseases with age is expected. Interpretation and management questions will focus particularly on the febrile child or one with a rash. Students are also expected to have some understanding of immune function and immunodeficiency.

1 Other individuals should be screened or treated if the index case

    a has had *M. tuberculosis* isolated from a lymph node
    b has epiglottitis
    c had streptococcal meningitis
    d has *Salmonella* dysentery
    e is a newborn baby with chlamydial conjunctivitis

a **True**. Contact tracing applies to infectious diseases and aims to identify and give prophylactic treatment to those likely to get the disease and discover those with the disease in an early (pre-clinical) stage so that early treatment is possible. This in turn reduces the spread of the disease. Disease that merit contact tracing are those that have effective treatment or prophylaxis, are serious and also, for practical reasons, not very prevalent. Contact tracing is undertaken for tuberculosis (TB), meningococcus, and *Haemophilus influenzae* type B (HIB).

    TB in children is frequently extrapulmonary, although it is still acquired through the pulmonary route and can be spread further by the index case. Screening for contacts involves a Heaf test and, if this is positive, a Mantoux test and a chest X-ray. Further evidence of infection then prompts specimen collection for culture and treatment.

b **True**. Epiglottitis is only caused by HIB. This is now much less common than before the HIB immunization was available. HIB is an encapsulated organism, and is capable of invasive infection. It also causes septicaemia and meningitis. Unencapsulated *Haemophilus* does not cause these infections, causing bronchitis, sinusitis, and upper respiratory tract infections (URTIs) instead.

HIB infection in a child should lead to identification of 'close' contacts and their treatment with Rifampicin. This is usually defined as those living with the index case, but children play closely with each other and so whole playgroups may need prophylaxis!

c   **False**. Streptococcal meningitis is caused by *Strep. pneumoniae* (also called pneumococcus). This is now the second most common cause of meningitis behind meningococcal disease, but more serious in terms of neurological sequelae. More often it causes lobar pneumonia, can cause septicaemia, and is a particular problem for children with nephrotic syndrome (peritonitis) and with sickle cell disease.

Contact tracing is not used as the organism is prevalent in the community, so the contacts are at little more risk than the rest of the population. Instead, those particularly at risk because of reduced immunity can be given penicillin prophylaxis or immunized with Pneumovax.

d   **False**. Contacts are not always sought, and treatment is rarely indicated. Contact tracing is appropriate when a common source is suspected, such as a food outlet. Treatment may prolong bacterial carriage, and indicated only for invasive disease and severe cases (see Gastroenterology question 2). Ciprofloxacin is an effective agent.

e   **True**. Early neonatal infections are almost always acquired from the mother during birth. Chlamydia causes a severe conjunctivitis in the neonate and pneumonitis, which can be life threatening. The contact in question is the mother, for whom the chlamydia is a sexually transmitted disease. The baby needs systemic erythromycin. The mother and her partner will need evaluation in a genitourinary clinic.

2   *For a previously well child in a developed country*
   a   *Listeria* can cause neonatal septicaemia
   b   the Epstein–Barr virus usually affects children under the age of 2
   c   Gram-negative organisms are unlikely to cause meningitis outside the neonatal period
   d   group B streptococcus most commonly affects children in the first week
   e   *Strep. pneumoniae* is the most frequent cause of meningitis under the age of 5

a   **True**. One of the distinctives of paediatric infectious diseases is that the agents responsible change with time. This is because the immune system is changing and the exposure to organisms tends to occur at specific times. As shown in Box 8.1, *Listeria* is one of the organisms that can cause neonatal illness.

All of these neonatal infectious agents are unusual at any other time of life, and occur then because of exposure during labour. Prolonged rupture of membranes allows more time for ascending infection, and this may show as a maternal fever during labour.

The neonate is also relatively immunodeficient. IgG is passively transferred from the mother to fetus from about 30 weeks reaching normal levels by term.

Box 8.1   Age and common organisms causing septicaemia or meningitis

Neonate	group B streptococcus
	Listeria
	Gram negatives e.g. *Escherichia coli*
Premature neonate	As above
	Staph. epidermidis (usually not meningitis)
	Candida (usually not meningitis)
0–5 years	*Neisseria meningitidis*
	Strep. pneumoniae
	Haemophilus influenzae type B (HIB)
Over 5 years	*Neisseria meningitidis*
	Strep. pneumoniae

This renders the preterm infant especially susceptible to infection. Other immuno-globulins are at low levels for the first few months, and the immunoglobulin response to infection is reduced. Complement is lower than adult levels and phagocytes show reduced chemotaxis and killing capacity.

Listeria may cause septicaemia or late onset (over 1 week) meningitis. Presentation, in common with other causes of neonatal sepsis is usually with lethargy, poor feeding, pallor, and respiratory distress (see The newborn, question 23). *Listeria* can sometimes cause a rash and is associated with meconium staining of the liquor in premature infants. After a full septic screen, it is treated by a combination of ampicillin or penicillin with gentamicin.

b   **False.** This virus causes infectious mononucleosis. Exposure in the developed world tends to occur in the teens, but occurs earlier in less affluent circumstances.

In older children the Epstein–Barr virus causes a febrile illness with tonsillitis and widespread tender lymphadenopathy. In addition, there is commonly spleno-megaly, hepatomegaly, jaundice, and a rash. In younger children, the disease is more likely to present as a non-specific febrile illness. Blood tests often show atypical lymphocytes and positive Monospot or Paul–Bunnell tests.

This illness may be indistinguishable from a cytomegalovirus (CMV) infection.

c   **True.** Gram-negative organisms, especially *Escherichia coli* and *Klebsiella* sp. are a serious cause of meningitis in the newborn period, and are also acquired from the birth canal. After the neonatal period they are a common cause of urinary tract infection (UTI), and a cause of septicaemia in the immunocompromised.

d   **True.** This is another of the common neonatal organisms that can cause early-onset septicaemia or late-onset meningitis (1–4 weeks).

Streptococci are often confusing organisms as they are classified in three different ways, each of which tends to be used in different situations!

α-, β- and γ-haemolytic refers to how the colony haemolyses red cells on a plate, determined by the production of haemolysin. β-haemolysis is complete, α is partial and γ no haemolysis at all. This gives a clue as to the organism, as *Strep. pyogenes* is β-haemolytic, *Strep. viridans* (an important cause of endocarditis) α-haemolytic and *Strep. faecalis* γ (or non) haemolytic.

β-haemolytic streptococci are further separated based on their cell wall components, giving rise to Lancefield groups (A–K). Group A is better known as *Strep. pyogenes* and group B is *Strep. agalactiae*. Streptococci are usually sensitive to penicillins.

e   **False.** This organism is one of the commoner causes of bacterial illness in older children. Meningitis is now most commonly caused by meningococcus at all ages except in the neonate, although prior to the introduction of HIB immunization, *Haemophilus* caused more cases in the under 5 age group than *Strep. pneumoniae*.

3   *The body is able to counteract infectious agents because*
   a   complement is able to opsonize bacteria
   b   viruses are mostly phagocytosed by neutrophils
   c   complement is able to lyse bacteria directly
   d   *Candida* is effectively killed by IgG
   e   natural killer lymphocytes destroy cells without antibody interaction

a   **True.** Complement has two pathways and two functions. There is the classical pathway (C1, C2, and C4) and the alternative pathway (factors B and D). They come together to make C3b, which is the pivotal substance in the system. The complex C5b6789 is then formed which lyses cells. Opsonization is achieved by this complex and C3b. The classical pathway is activated by antibody–antigen complexes and C-reactive protein, whereas the alternative pathway is activated by fungal and bacterial substances. Cleavage by-products have roles in the immune reaction, such as chemotaxis.

b   **False.** Viruses can be inactivated by antibody binding, and the cells in which they are dividing are killed by natural killer (NK) cells, but phagocytosis is not an important part of the body's defence against viruses.

c   **True.** As outlined above, complement is able to lyse bacteria directly, and defence against *Neisseria* is particularly dependent on this system. Deficiency of the complement factors C5, 6, 7, or 8 thus presents as repeated episodes of septicaemia with meningococcus.

d   **False.** Although antibodies against *Candida* are made, fungal infection is mainly prevented by cell-mediated immunity—neutrophils and T cells. While superficial fungal infection is common, invasive infection occurs only with immunodeficiency or when there are indwelling cannulae.

e   **True.** NK cells are able to lyse target cells without prior antigenic stimulation or antibody interaction. K (killer) cells require the cell to be coated with antibody before lysis. Cytotoxic cells require antigen stimulation before lysis occurs. All of these are T-cell subtypes.

4   *Fungal infection*
     a   often involves the mouth in immunocompetent infants
     b   by *Candida* will often cause invasive infection
     c   can involve the scalp in childhood
     d   usually requires amphotericin B for effective treatment
     e   may colonize central venous catheters

a   **True.** Candidal infection of the nappy area and mouth is common in infants. Candidal nappy rash is distinguished by satellite lesions around the area of rash. The oral infection is identified by a buccal mucosa that is red with white plaques. Topical antifungals (miconazole or nystatin) should be used.

b   **False.** Candidal septicaemia is most likely in the premature neonate and the child undergoing chemotherapy. Children who have conditions reducing cell-mediated immunity or phagocytic defects (e.g. chronic granulomatous disease) may also have invasive disease or abscesses. Treatment is with systemic antifungals —amphotericin or 5-flucytodine.

c   **True.** Skin infection with dermatophyte fungi is common. This gives rise to the diseases of tinea pedis (athlete's foot), tinea corporis (ringworm), and tinea capitis (scalp ringworm). After puberty this is much less common. Treatment with topical antifungals is usually effective.

d   **False.** Amphotericin B is an effective anti-yeast agent that is only used where topical treatment is ineffective. However, it also causes fever and hypokalaemia. The side-effects are minimised by the use of liposomal amphotericin. Here the drug is encapsulated in such a way that the liposome binds to the yeast and delivers the drug specifically to the yeast cell. Other useful antifungals are ketoconazole, which can be given orally to treat systemic infections and miconazole, which is not absorbed, so is useful for oral infections.

e   **True.** The infection is then difficult to clear until the cannula is removed.

5   *A 4-year-old boy has a fever and a erythematous rash*
     a   the presence of conjunctivitis suggests that he has mumps
     b   that the rash started behind the ears and has now spread to the rest of the body is suggestive of measles
     c   he may have typhoid fever
     d   as he also has cataracts, rubella is a more likely cause
     e   a rash on his cheeks alone is typical of fifth disease (erythema infectiosum)

a   **False.** Fever, a rash, and conjunctivitis suggests either measles or Kawasaki disease (KD). Distinguishing features of diseases with a fever associated with a rash are listed in Box 8.2.

Box 8.2   Differential diagnosis of rash with a fever

	Distinguishing features
Enterovirus	Mild reticular rash on trunk, well child
Measles	Rash from behind ears, conjunctivitis, Koplik spots
Rubella	Rash spreading from face
Exanthem subitum	Fever 4–5 days which subsides as rash appears
Erythema infectiosum	'Slapped cheeks' progressing to body
Systemic-onset juvenile rheumatoid arthritis	Salmon-pink rash, dramatic swinging fever, hepato- splenomegaly, lymphadenopathy
Scarlet fever	Generalized rash, strawberry tongue
Kawasaki disease	Conjunctivitis, lymphadenopathy, oral changes, erythematous and oedematous extremities, later peeling of fingers
Scalded skin syndrome	Epidermis separates on gentle pressure

b   **True**. This progression of the rash is typical of measles, whereas a rash spreading down from the face is more suggestive of rubella. Chicken pox is centripetal in distribution and 'crops' rather than 'spreads' as such. Exanthem subitum (also called roseola infantum), caused by herpesvirus type 6, is characterized by a rash that suddenly appears after 5 days of high fever, while erythema infectiosum presents as a florid rash on one or both cheeks before spreading to the rest of the body. There is no rash associated with mumps.

c   **True**. Although *Salmonella typhi* is rare in developed countries, other *Salmonella* species such as *paratyphi* and *enteritidis* are more common and give rise to a similar but less severe illness. The child is toxic and febrile, may have a rose coloured rash, be constipated, and have abdominal distension. The bloody diarrhoea will then occur.

d   **False**. Congenital rubella and childhood rubella have completely different manifestations and importance. Childhood rubella is a self-limiting illness with no long-term consequences. Those with the disease should be kept away from non-immune pregnant women.

Congenital rubella is discussed in The newborn, question 12.

e   **True**. This disease is caused by parvovirus B19. This virus also causes aplastic crises in those with chronic haemolysis.

6   *Herpes simplex*

    a   lesions are often superinfected with *Staph. aureus*
    b   infections usually require treatment with acyclovir
    c   type II cannot cause stomatitis
    d   infection may complicate eczema
    e   encephalitis may present with focal seizures

a   **True.** This virus most commonly presents with gingivostomatitis, and later reactivates as a cold sore. Other primary infections may be with conjunctivitis, whitlows, meningitis, or encephalitis. Lesions may be superinfected by *Staph. aureus* and streptococci. As the lesions are severe even without superinfection, the child can become very ill and unable to tolerate fluids. If there is superinfection, hospitalization for fluids, antibiotics, and antivirals (acyclovir) is needed.

b   **False.** Most infections are asymptomatic or self-limiting and need no treatment.

c   **False.** Although type II is more commonly associated with adult genital herpes, it can cause gingivostomatitis and encephalitis. It is also a cause of neonatal infection and encephalitis, acquired during vaginal delivery from lesions around the birth canal. In this situation, Caesarean section delivery and treatment with acyclovir is indicated.

d   **True.** The broken, dry skin of children with eczema allows rapid establishment of infections. The herpes viruses can cause severe infection in these children requiring treatment with acyclovir.

e   **True.** Herpes simplex and varicella zoster viruses are neurotropic, so tend to involve neural tissue in the infection. This allows latency and reactivation from sensory ganglia causing cold sores and shingles. More seriously these viruses can affect the brain, with varicella zoster causing cerebellar dysfunction and herpes simplex encephalitis. This may present as altered consciousness with focal signs and acyclovir should be started immediately for such patients.

7   *Lower respiratory tract infections in childhood caused by*
    a   *Strep. pneumoniae* are the commonest acquired in the community
    b   staphylococci are usually associated with a severe illness
    c   *Mycoplasma pneumoniae* are uncommon in children
    d   respiratory syncytial virus will only affect those under 18 months
    e   *Haemophilus influenza* can be effectively prevented by *Haemophilus influenza* type B vaccination

a   **True.** The commonest causes of pneumonia in childhood are *Strep. pneumoniae* (pneumococcus), *Haemophilus influenzae*, *Mycoplasma*, and viruses such as influenza A and B, respiratory syncytial virus, and adenovirus. In hospitals staphylococcal pneumonia is more common.

   Strep. pneumoniae usually causes lobar pneumonia. *Klebsiella* also tends to do this, and swelling of the affected lobe on the X-ray can be seen.

b   **True.** Staphylococcus is a cause of pneumonia, but is unusual unless there is a pre-existing problem, such as cystic fibrosis or cerebral palsy. Patients are usually very ill. It characteristically causes air−fluid levels on the chest X-ray.

c   **False.** It is one of the commonest causes in those over 5 years. *Mycoplasma* often causes a more diffuse 'atypical' picture in terms of signs and radiographic appearances. Other causes of atypical pneumonia are viruses and *Chlamydia trachomatis*. These organisms are mainly not sensitive to penicillins, and a macrolide such as erythromycin is needed for resolution.

d   **False**. Under 18 months it usually causes bronchiolitis, but it may cause a runny nose, cough, and a chest infection at any age. In fact viruses cause over 70% of pneumonias.

e   **False**. Sadly not! HIB is an encapsulated form of *Haemophilus* responsible for invasive disease and sometimes pneumonia. More commonly, unencapsulated types cause URTIs and bronchitis.

> **8   *Streptococci***
>   a   are the commonest cause of abscesses
>   b   are usually resistant to penicillins in the UK
>   c   cause over 50% of urinary tract infections
>   d   cause about a third of cases of pharyngitis
>   e   can cause meningitis in the newborn period

a   **False**. Staphylococci are more commonly found in abscesses. Together staphylococci and streptococci cause most skin infections. Cellulitis is usually caused by *Strep. pyogenes* and both may cause periorbital cellulitis, although HIB is also an important agent. For these reasons, flucloxacillin does not have a broad enough spectrum when treating skin infections and another antibiotic, such as amoxycillin should be added.

b   **False**. Streptococci are still almost entirely sensitive to penicillins in the UK, although some parts of southern Europe have resistant forms. Even these organisms are sensitive to third-generation cephalosporins.

Staphylococci are often resistant to penicillins in the community, and much more so in hospital, so agents such as flucloxacillin, fucidic acid, vancomycin, and teicoplanin must be used.

c   **False**. *Strep. faecalis* causes fewer UTIs than *E. coli* and other Gram-negative organisms. Therefore, a penicillin is unlikely to resolve the infection. Instead, trimethoprim or a cephalosporin can be used.

d   **True**. The commonest cause is viral, but *Strep. pyogenes* is also an important cause. The pharyngitis tends to be worse, perhaps with pustules in the pharynx or the tonsils, although infectious mononucleosis (IM) may give a similar appearance. If a bacterial throat infection is suspected benzylpenicillin should be started after a swab, as other antibiotics are likely to cause a rash if it is IM. This is discussed further in Respiratory disease, question 17.

Certain subtypes of *Strep. pyogenes* cause distant, immune related effects, such as the rash of scarlet fever from erythrotoxin, rheumatic fever, glomerulonephritis, arthritis, and erythema nodosum.

e   **True**. Group B *Streptococcus* is the most common cause of neonatal sepsis.

9 *Tuberculosis in children*
   a is decreasing in incidence
   b is more frequently extrapulmonary than in adults
   c can be reliably diagnosed using the Mantoux test
   d can be screened for with chest X-rays
   e can be cultured from stomach aspirates in affected individuals

a **False.** World-wide, and even in developed countries the incidence is rising. Over 40% of the world's population will have had TB infection at some time, and the annual incidence is about 0.2% for Africa and South-east Asia. In the developed world, socially deprived children, immigrants, and those with HIV infection are particularly at risk.

b **True.** About 40% of children present with an extrapulmonary manifestation. As in adults, the disease enters the body through the lungs and sets up a Ghon focus, which is the initial pulmonary lesion with associated hilar lymphadenopathy. If not contained, further lymphatic or haematogenous spread can occur. Common sites of further infection are the lungs (bronchopneumonia or miliary TB), lymph nodes, the kidney, bone, gut, and central nervous system. Tuberculous meningitis is unusual but severe.

c **False.** The Mantoux test requires a T-cell-mediated immunological reaction to the purified protein derivative (PPD). False positive results may occur if the child has had TB or another mycobacterial infection, but is now cured, or even if he has had a BCG vaccination in the past. False negative results may occur if he is immunodeficient. The main role for this test is in following up those likely to have TB, along with a history and chest X-ray.

   The Heaf test is used as a screening test for TB, as it is less specific than the Mantoux test, but easier to administer.

d **False.** The chest X-ray may be normal even with active TB. However, abnormalities on the film, depending on the context, can be good evidence of TB.

e **True.** Children do not readily cough up sputum for the microbiologist to culture until they are at least 5 years. Instead, stomach aspirates, containing swallowed sputum can be used to culture the organism. Biopsy of enlarged lymph nodes or infected tissue (e.g. pleura) is more likely to enable culture, but fluids (pleural aspirate, early morning urine) can also be used

Data interpretation and reasoning — answers

10 *A previously well 3-year-old girl is brought to the emergency department. She has become increasingly lethargic and unresponsive over the past 8 h. She has a widespread purpuric rash, and looks pale. Her heart rate is 150 beats/min and blood pressure 70/30 mmHg. An intravenous cannula is sited and some blood tests taken*

haemoglobin 12.1 g/dl
WCC 1.3 × 10³/mm³
platelets 28 × 10³/mm³

Based on these results and her presentation

    a the patient's main problem is meningococcal meningitis
    b this result may be artefactual
    c clotting times are likely to be prolonged
    d treatment with white cells and platelets is needed
    e leukaemia should be excluded with a bone marrow aspirate

a **False** b **False** c **True** d **False** e **False**

The important features in her presentation are the rapid progression with deteriorating conscious level, features of shock and purpuric rash. Her blood count shows a low white count and thrombocytopenia. The neutropenia reflects neutrophils rapidly leaving the circulation and is a feature of overwhelming sepsis. The low platelet count is also due to consumption, and is evidence for disseminated intravascular coagulation (DIC). This is a consumptive coagulopathy, consuming platelets and coagulation factors, which gives rise to increased clotting times. Common causes of DIC in paediatrics are sepsis, asphyxia, shock, burns, and respiratory distress syndrome, as discussed in Newborn question 22.

There is no possibility of artefact as the haemoglobin level is normal for a child of this age, so dilution could not have caused the white count and platelet count to be this low. Although such a count may be found rarely at the presentation of non-leukaemic leukaemia and more commonly during chemotherapy, the clinical situation in this scenario is very much against this diagnosis.

Purpuric spots found with both meningococcal septicaemia and meningitis, but are less extensive in the latter condition. The systemic features (widespread rash and shock) indicate that this child is septicaemic. This is bad for her prognosis (mortality is 20–50% as against 3% for meningitis), but if she survives she is likely to have no neurological sequelae.

Treatment is with supportive care (ventilation, large volumes of colloid, ionotropes, clotting factors, and platelets) as well as antibiotics. Third-generation cephalosporins such as cefotaxime are commonly used, but the combination of ampicillin and chloramphenicol is effective. As the systemic effects (shock and rash) are caused by endotoxin on the cell wall of the bacteria, antibiotics initially can make the child worse as they cause bacterial cell lysis.

White cells are rarely infused, but can be used as a diagnostic test (technetium-labelled cells can identify the site of inflammation), and granulocytes can be used in specific immunodeficiencies.

Close contacts of children with meningococcal infections should receive rifampicin prophylaxis.

11 Infection with human immunodeficiency virus

    a can be diagnosed with HIV IgG levels in the infant at birth
    b may be transmitted by breast feeding from an HIV-positive mother

    c is a contraindication for diphtheria/pertussis/tetanus immunization
    d often presents with failure to thrive
    e can cause dementia

a **False** b **True** c **False** d **True** e **True**
Paediatric HIV is a growing area, particularly as the affected children are now living longer. Once again there are important differences in presentation and diagnosis compared with the adult disease.

Almost all cases in children are vertically acquired from the mother. Transmission can occur in utero, perinatally, or from breast feeding. Caesarean section is the route of choice for delivery as the transmission rate is lower. It is lowered more by the use of zidovudine during the procedure. Breast feeding is discouraged in the developed world, but in the developing world, benefits from breast feeding (reduced mortality, particularly from gastroenteritis) outweigh the risks. Transmission from blood products has occurred in the past, but is less common now.

Presentation may be early or delayed. Early-onset *Pneumocystis carinii* pneumonia (PCP) has a bad prognosis. Other modes of presentation include failure to thrive, chronic diarrhoea, dementia, opportunistic infections, parotid gland swelling, generalized lymphadenopathy, or lymphocytic interstitial pneumonitis.

Diagnosis can be difficult. Maternally acquired HIV IgG will give a positive 'HIV test' in all infants, but this test should become negative in uninfected infants by 18 months. HIV IgM will be made by the infant and so, if present, is good evidence of infection, but may not be synthesized even in infected infants. Polymerase chain reaction (PCR) for HIV RNA from peripheral blood is more sensitive than IgM, but still has a high false negative rate. Other useful tests include viral culture and antigen testing.

Prognosis for children with HIV is variable, with some children living beyond 10 years and others dying in the first year. Prognosis is now much improved with the use of antiretroviral agents.

Both parents are often also HIV positive, so the child may be orphaned.

12   *A 9-month-old girl is admitted to the children's ward with a temperature of 38.6°C, pallor, and vomiting. She is more likely to have a bacterial rather than another cause for her fever because she has*

    a had a febrile convulsion
    b a fine blotchy erythematous rash on her trunk that comes and goes
    c her pulse is 150, blood pressure 85/35, and a capillary filling time of 4 s
    d a marked improvement following the administration of paracetamol
    e a white cell count of $1.5 \times 10^3/mm^3$

a **False** b **False** c **True** d **False** e **True**
The majority of infants with fevers do not have bacterial infections. Many vomit as a result of the fever and may be pale as their temperature rises. Most of these children do not need investigations beyond a urine culture and are best treated

with paracetamol. There are few specific signs of bacterial infection to help decide if antibiotics should be used.

A tachycardia is expected in fever, but a prolonged capillary filling time is not, and should prompt the taking of blood, urine, and possibly CSF for culture and administration of broad-spectrum antibiotics. Leucopenia or neutropenia are also indicators of severe infection. There may be clinical signs suggestive of bacterial infection, such as neck stiffness, a purpuric rash, or cloudy urine.

As the high temperature itself will make the child look and feel sick, paracetamol can be used to see how well the child is without the fever. If there is little improvement, a serious (bacterial) illness is more likely.

A fine blotchy erythematous rash is non-specific and frequently accompanies viral illnesses, particularly those caused by enteroviruses.

Febrile convulsions are most often caused by viral infections, but can be a manifestation of meningitis, viral encephalitis, or cerebral abscess. When the infant has had recovered from the convulsion and the temperature has been reduced by paracetamol, she should be alert and responsive to her surroundings. If she is, a viral aetiology is most likely.

13 *A 7-month-old child has been admitted for further investigation. He is well known to the ward as he has already been an inpatient with a chest infection at 4 months, and diarrhoea at 6 months. The following features make it more likely that he has an immunodeficiency*

   a   his neutrophil count is $3.5 \times 10^3/\text{mm}^3$
   b   he has crossed from the 75th to below the 3rd centile since birth
   c   he is a sub-Saharan African
   d   he had a lump at the site of his diphtheria, pertussis, and tetanus injection
   e   his umbilical cord separated at 3 weeks of age

a **False** b **True** c **True** d **False** e **True**

There are a number of inherited immunodeficiency syndromes and some acquired ones. The commoner ones are shown in Box 8.3.

Here the boy has had a chest infection and diarrhoea both severe enough for hospitalization. IgA or IgG subclass deficiency are suggested, but almost any type of immunodeficiency may cause this presentation. He may even have cystic fibrosis.

His neutrophil count is normal. This should be over $2 \times 10^3/\text{mm}^3$. If it is lower it may be an autoimmune neutropenia, cyclical neutropenia, marrow dysfunction, congenital neutropenia, or HIV.

That his umbilical stump took 3 weeks to separate is abnormal (usually it falls off about day 7). This is suggestive of a chemotaxis defect or leucocyte adhesion problem. However, these defects tend to present with skin infections.

Failure to thrive is common is severe immunodeficiencies, owing to the frequency of illnesses.

His sub-Saharan origins make HIV a more likely diagnosis than in a Caucasian child.

Box 8.3 Commoner immunodeficiencies

	Deficient in	Infecting organisms
Selective IgA deficiency	IgA	Gastrointestinal and respiratory infections
IgG subclass deficiency	IgG_2	Gastrointestinal and respiratory infections
Common variable immunodeficiency	Any	*Strep. pneumoniae*, *Haemophilus*, *staphylococcus*
DiGeorge syndrome	Lymphocytes	*Listeria*, viruses, fungi, *Pneumocystis*
HIV infection	Lymphocyte function	*Listeria*, viruses, fungi, *Pneumocystis*
Severe combined immunodeficiency	Lymphocyte, antibody	Fungi, viruses, bacteria
Chronic granulomatous disease	Neutrophil function	Skin and lung fungi and *staphylococcus*
Hyposplenism	Response to sepsis	*Strep. pneumoniae*, *Haemophilus*, *Neisseria*, *E. coli*

14 *A 2-year-old girl is undergoing chemotherapy for leukaemia. She is now unwell and has a temperature of 38.9°C. A full examination does not reveal any focus of infection, although the site of insertion of her indwelling central venous catheter is red. A full blood count is taken*
haemoglobin 8.9 g/dl
white cell count 0.7 × 10³/mm³
platelets 130 × 10³/mm³

a a chest X-ray should be avoided as it may cause further malignant transformation
b she may have *Pneumocystis carinii* pneumonia
c she should be started on broad-spectrum antibiotics and an antifungal agent immediately
d she should be given a platelets infusion
e the venous catheter should be removed urgently

a **False** b **True** c **False** d **False** e **False**
Chemotherapy and immunosuppression in a child with leukaemia can affect the immune system in a variety of ways. The child is particularly at risk of bacterial and fungal infection, and the venous catheter may be the source of this infection. Common organisms include *Staph. aureus* and *epidermidis*, Gram-negatives such as *Pseudomonas*, *Candida*, and *Aspergillus*, and *Pneumocystis carinii*.

After a full examination, which may suggest at particular focus, blood and urine cultures should be taken and broad-spectrum antibiotics started. Chest infection especially with PCP can be identified with a chest X-ray, and the tiny increase in risk of malignancy is far outweighed by the information gained. For initial therapy, a penicillin with activity against *Pseudomonas* (piperacillin) and an aminoglycoside (gentamicin) is used. If there is no improvement, fungal infection is more likely and amphotericin added. Removal of indwelling cannulae may eventually be needed, but they can often be preserved.

Supportive therapy may be needed, but platelets are only needed if the count is very low (under $20 \times 10^3/mm^3$) or under 50 when there is bleeding.

15 *A 7-month-old is admitted with a high fever, pallor, and tachycardia. A full septic screen is performed, and this shows a leucocytosis, but no excess of white cells in urine or cerebrospinal fluid. Cefotaxime, a third-generation cephalosporin, is started and the infant clinically improves. Four days later, the blood culture results become available*
Staph. epidermidis, *growing in one of two bottles*
sensitive to chloramphenicol, vancomycin
resistant to cephalosporin, penicillin

a the infant may have had a viral infection
b this organism is a commonly found in the blood
c this blood culture result is good evidence of septicaemia
d the antibiotics should be changed to a combination of chloramphenicol and vancomycin
e this organism is usually a skin commensal

a **True** b **False** c **False** d **False** e **True**
Any result needs to be taken in the context of the clinical situation. The initial presentation is typical of bacterial sepsis, but a viraemia could also cause these features. An appropriate antibiotic has been started and the child has got better, despite the fact that the organism cultured is resistant to the antibiotic used. This implies that either there was a viral illness in the first place, the organism has some sensitivity to the antibiotic, or the organism identified in culture is a contaminant. This last interpretation is further suggested by only one blood culture bottle growing the organism and the organism being an unusual cause of septicaemia at this age. It is usually found as a skin commensal, but is an important cause of septicaemia in immunocompromised patients and of late-onset neonatal infection in premature infants.

So, as far as treatment is concerned, the antibiotics should not be changed as there is clinical improvement and the result is likely to be a contaminant.

16 *A 5-year-old African boy has returned 3 days ago from Nigeria where he had been visiting relatives. He is now unwell with a fever and rigors. His examination is unremarkable, and some blood tests are performed*
haemoglobin 8.1 g/dl
white cell count 19.3 × 10³/mm³
platelets 490 × 10³/mm³
Na⁺ 134 mmol/l
K⁺ 4.2 mmol/l
urea 9.5 mmol/l
creatinine 82 μmol/l

Given these data
a *Campylobacter* is a likely cause for his illness
b typhoid fever is unlikely as he has had no diarrhoea

    c a thick film would now be appropriate
    d the high white cell count could be caused by the rigors
    e he has evidence of dehydration

a **False** b **False** c **True** d **False** e **True**

A child returning from abroad may well have an unusual infection. Following a full history, including contacts and precise details of the area visited and any prophylaxis, and a full examination (anaemia, jaundice, splenomegaly, rash), investigations should be performed. Beyond a full blood count, looking for haemolysis, raised white cells and a blood culture, malaria should be excluded with at least three thick films. If these are positive (thick films show the presence of plasmodia), thin films will identify the type of malaria.

Salmonella typhi can be cultured from blood or urine before it is present in the stool. This is useful, as he will still be in the septicaemic phase of the illness, when there is constipation rather than diarrhoea.

A high white cell count can be caused by factors other than infection. Convulsions, pregnancy, corticosteroid therapy, and trauma can all raise the white count, but not rigors. His urea and creatinine are both at high levels, suggestive of intravascular depletion and dehydration. Even though there is no mention of vomiting or reduced intake, fever and tachypnoea can lead to dehydration.

Campylobacter, *Shigella*, *E. coli*, and *Entamoeba* can all cause fevers in those returning from tropical countries, but are accompanied by diarrhoea and dysentery. If the child is systemically unwell with these symptoms, ciprofloxacin is the most useful agent.

9 Rheumatology and orthopaedics

Knowledge — questions

1 *Kyphoscoliosis*

    a is more common in children with spina bifida
    b if severe usually compromises respiration
    c is always present if there are hemivertebrae
    d usually becomes more pronounced on bending forward
    e can be treated by the insertion of rods alongside the spine

2 *Congenital dislocation of the hip*

    a should be suspected in a child with an abducted, flexed, and externally rotated hip
    b can lead to osteoarthritis
    c often delays walking
    d should be treated by splinting
    e is more common in infants born after an oligohydramniotic pregnancy

3 *Juvenile chronic arthritis*

    a does not present under 1 year
    b with eye involvement is common in the polyarticular form
    c should be treated with non-steroidal anti-inflammatory agents and systemic steroids if necessary
    d is almost never rheumatoid factor positive
    e rarely persists into adulthood.

4 *In children fractures*

    a of the distal radius are uncommon
    b are more common in children with rickets
    c across the growth plate can cause asymmetrical growth
    d should not be treated with internal fixation in order to preserve growth
    e need not be realigned exactly as remodelling will occur

5 *Skull fractures in children*

    a even if linear the child should be closely observed
    b if depressed require evaluation with a CT scan
    c usually need surgical treatment

d   may occur after forceps delivery
e   of the temporal bone are usually associated with intracranial haemor-
     rhage

6   *It is likely that treatment is required for*
     a   a 2 year old with a medial longitudinal arch that disappears when he is
          not on tiptoe
     b   genu valgum in a $3\frac{1}{2}$ year old
     c   overlapping sutures in a newborn
     d   a clicky hip in a newborn
     e   talipes calcaneovarus

Data interpretation and reasoning — questions

7   *A 10-year-old boy is referred to the paediatric rheumatology clinic*
     because he has been experiencing increasing pain in his right knee and
     hip over the last 2 weeks. Three days prior to the onset of the pain he
     had a fall during a game of football. On examination he is afebrile
     and his leg is held slightly flexed, externally rotated, and abducted at
     the hip. He is able to move at the hip but this movement is painful both
     actively and passively. The knee is normal to examination
     a   this would be a typical presentation of polyarticular juvenile chronic
          arthritis
     b   avascular necrosis of the hip is unlikely to be the cause unless he also has
          a haemoglobinopathy
     c   an anteroposterior X-ray of the pelvis will not exclude a slipped upper
          femoral epiphysis
     d   a septic arthritis can be ruled out with a neutrophil count
     e   if all his X-rays and blood tests are normal, he would be best treated with
          bed rest and gentle traction

8   *A 3-year-old girl is brought to her family doctor with a swollen knee*
     and an effusion
     a   septic arthritis must be excluded with a normal aspirate of joint fluid.
     b   a long history of painless swelling in the knee is suggestive of juvenile
          chronic arthritis
     c   an immobile joint makes septic arthritis more likely
     d   osteomyelitis can be excluded by plain X-rays
     e   a recent pharyngitis may have led to a reactive arthritis

9   A 2-year-old boy is admitted to the children's ward for further
    evaluation of a fever that has failed to respond to a 1 week course of
    Amoxil, prescribed for a sore throat. In the time he has been on the
    antibiotic, his leg has become painful, especially when moved. On
    examination he has a tender swelling over the proximal fibula. A
    bone scan is performed, showing increased radionucleotide uptake in
    the proximal third of the fibula. This boy
    a   may not have changes visible on his plain X-ray of the limb
    b   should be effectively treated by a third-generation cephalosporin with
        flucloxacillin
    c   should be investigated for an immunodeficiency
    d   will usually have positive blood cultures
    e   may subsequently have poor growth in the affected limb

Knowledge — answers

1   *Kyphoscoliosis*
    a   is more common in children with spina bifida
    b   if severe usually compromises respiration
    c   is always present if there are hemivertebrae
    d   usually becomes more pronounced on bending forward
    e   can be treated by the insertion of rods alongside the spine

a   **True**. The spine should be straight when viewed from behind but should
deviate in the anterior–posterior (AP) plane at the neck, chest, and in the lumbar
region (known as the cervical, thoracic, and lumbar lordoses). Scoliosis is an
abnormal lateral deviation and kyphosis deviation in the anterior-posterior direction. (You can think of this as S for scoliosis looks like a twisted spine from the
back. Once you know that kyphosis must be an AP deviation). These conditions
often coexist and may be idiopathic or caused by underlying bony or non-bony
pathology. Almost any long-standing pathology affecting the spine or spinal cord
can result in kyphoscoliosis.
    Idiopathic kyphoscoliosis is usually painless. If there is pain, an idiopathic cause
is less likely and other aetiologies such as tumour or osteomyelitis should be
considered.

b   **True**. Kyphoscoliosis can cause mechanical embarrassment and neurological
dysfunction. When curvatures are up to 90°, the breathing is restricted and so
cor pulmonale and respiratory failure may result. Neurological problems may
be associated with the cause of the deformity (e.g. spina bifida) or result from the
deformity itself, so affected children should have a full neurological assessment.

Skin changes over the spine (hair or pigmentation) might suggest spina bifida oculta or diastematomyelia. Bladder and bowel function should also be checked.

c   **False.** Maintaining a normal spine a during growth depends on normal growth and tone in the muscles that support the spine. As all of the vertebral bodies grow, particularly during puberty, deformities tend to worsen as the child ages, especially around the time of puberty.

Congenital causes, such as hemivertebrae and fused vertebrae are often diagnosed incidentally on a X-ray. Also two hemivertebrae may cancel out each other. On the other hand the deformity may be rapidly progressive in which case early surgery is indicated. Another common cause is adolescent idiopathic scoliosis, which is usually benign. Some individuals have rapid progression (mainly girls) during puberty and require surgery.

d   **True.** When assessing a child with a spinal problem, the important questions to ask are: At what level is the problem, how bad is it, is it progressing and is there any underlying cause or complication? Therefore the angle of scoliosis is measured (this is the angle of deviation between the spine above and below the curvature) and the degree of twisting. Twisting can be determined by leaning forward and measuring the size of the hump on one side that is seen.

Bending forward to touch the toes is the best way to screen for spinal problems, even though it will identify children who have benign kyphoscoliosis not requiring treatment.

e   **True.** Treatment options include doing nothing (as many mild forms resolve), spinal braces, and surgery. Surgery is required for children with compromised chest function or severe kyphoscoliosis. For this metal rods are secured alongside the vertebrae and can be fused into the pelvis to provide extra rigidity. Before this is performed, diastematomyelia or spinal cord tethering must be excluded (MRI or a myelogram) because otherwise the procedure can damage the spinal cord.

   2   *Congenital dislocation of the hip*
      a   should be suspected in a child with an abducted, flexed, and externally rotated hip
      b   can lead to osteoarthritis
      c   often delays walking
      d   should be treated by splinting
      e   is more common in infants born after an oligohydramniotic pregnancy

a   **False.** Progressive congenital dislocation of the hip (CDH) affects 1/600 infants. It is further subdivided into dislocatable and dislocated hips. The condition is caused by the femoral head not remaining in the acetabulum during growth, being in a dislocated position. The acetabulum may be too shallow or the leg in an abnormal posture (see part e).

CDH may not be noticeable at birth, but later the affected limb has limited abduction and has apparent shortening. The posture described in the question is that of least pressure on the hip joint, adopted when there is a joint effusion.

The condition is screened for at birth and at 6 weeks with the Barlow and Ortolani tests. The Barlow test attempts to elicit a clunk as the femoral head is dislocated by pushing the adducted and flexed hip posteriorly. This is a test for a dislocatable hip. The Ortolani test attempts to relocate a dislocated hip by abducting the flexed hip and pushing the femoral head anteriorly.

When performing these tests, abnormal hips 'clunk' in and out of the acetabulum. Normal hips frequently 'click' but this is normal and is caused by ligaments and tendons around the hip joint.

b **True.** If the femoral head is not in the true acetabulum during growth, the acetabulum does not develop properly and instead a new acetabulum forms around the femoral head posterior and superior to the true acetabulum. Such a hip is unstable and likely to develop osteoarthritis.

c **True.** The abnormal mechanics and shortening on one side leads to a delay in walking. Other complications include an increased lumbar lordosis and toe walking.

d **True.** In the neonatal period, clunky hips should be investigated with ultrasound and plain pelvic X-ray. Splinting the legs with the dislocation reduced (legs abducted and flexed at the hip) allows normal growth of the acetabulum and frequently cures the problem. If the diagnosis is missed in the first six months, open reduction and fixation is normally required.

e **True.** Various conditions predispose to CDH. If there is limitation to the movement of the hips in utero, they may become dislocated. This applies to breech infants and those born following oligohydramniotic pregnancies, and the problem is more common in girls than boys perhaps because of a hormone-related laxity. Neurological problems also increase the risk of dislocation due to imbalance of muscular tone, as would be the case in cerebral palsy or spina bifida.

3 *Juvenile chronic arthritis*
    a does not present under 1 year
    b with eye involvement is common in the polyarticular form
    c should be treated with non-steroidal anti-inflammatory agents and systemic steroids if necessary
    d is almost never rheumatoid factor positive
    e rarely persists into adulthood

a **False.** Juvenile chronic arthritis (JCA) can occur at any age, but the subtype and manifestations are related to the age and sex of the child. As indicated in question 7, infants with JCA are most likely to have the systemic onset (Still's disease) form of the condition. Young children may have any type, including the pauciarticular form, the polyarticular form, and the systemic-onset type. Older boys with pauciarticular onset are more likely to have an ankylosing spondylitis-like disease and be human leucocyte antigen B27 positive. Older girls with polyarticular disease may have a rheumatoid arthritis-like disease and be rheumatoid factor positive.

b   **False**. Manifestations other than joint involvement can occur with almost any joint disorder typically of other serosal or collagenous tissue.

In children with systemic-onset disease, features include a salmon-pink rash, lymphadenopathy, hepatosplenomegaly and pericarditis can occur. Other forms have less extra-articular features. The pauciarticular form is particularly associated with chronic iridocyclitis when the child is antinuclear antibody (ANA) positive. This is important because it is a reversible cause of blindness.

Joint complications of JCA include muscle wasting, contractures, and growth failure or unilateral leg overgrowth if only one knee is affected.

c   **True**. Management of JCA is not easy because it requires long-term involvement with a family and a disease that relapses and remits and has a variable prognosis. As the disease burns out in most children, the goal is to minimize contracture formation and growth delay during the course of the illness. Contractures form when a joint is held still for a prolonged period, so physiotherapy and hydrotherapy can be used to ensure the joint is moved properly. 'Resting' splints place the joint in a good and functional position when the child is asleep and at other times.

Drug therapy is also important. Non-steroidal anti-inflammatory drugs are used for pain control and sometimes steroids for acute exacerbations. Longer-term therapy avoids steroids (one of the causes of growth failure in these children) and instead uses agents such as methotrexate, antimalarials, gold, and sulphasalazine. Intra-articular steroids are useful for pauciarticular disease.

d   **False**. All children presenting with joint disease should be tested for rheumatoid factor (RF), as it is a predictor of a worse prognosis, especially in older girls.

e   **True**. As indicted, most children with JCA do not have active disease in adulthood, with the important exception of those RF positive and with polyarticular disease.

4   *In children fractures*
    a   of the distal radius are uncommon
    b   are more common in children with rickets
    c   across the growth plate can cause asymmetrical growth
    d   should not be treated with internal fixation in order to preserve growth
    e   need not be realigned exactly as remodelling will occur

a   **False**. The commonest sites for fractures in children are the distal radius and other long bones. Rib fracture is less common than in adults and is suggestive of non-accidental injury. Skull fractures are also relatively common. Children do not tend to have fractures of the neck of the femur.

When breaking a bone a child is likely to have a 'greenstick' fracture, in which there is disruption of the bone but not a clean break. These differences all reflect the increased flexibility and cartilage in children's bones.

b   **True**. Rickets weakens the bones and makes them more flexible. Bones are easily deformed (e.g. craniotabes) and break with greenstick fractures. Other conditions that predispose to fractures include metabolic bone disease of prematurity, osteopetrosis, untreated thalassaemia, and osteogenesis imperfecta.

c   **True**. Growth occurs when the chondrocytes in the cartilage of the physis or growth plate divide. The cartilage is then mineralized and becomes part of the metaphysis and eventually the diaphysis. If there is a fracture across the growth plate (described by the Salter–Harris classification) this can disrupt growth. Such fractures need to be realigned and fixed accurately.

d   **False**. As most fractures occur in the region of the metaphysis or diaphysis, there is no problem with internal fixation as this part of the bone is not elongating. Fixation across the growth plate will reduce growth on that side of the bone. This is used therapeutically in conditions in which there is asymmetric growth, such as Blount's disease.

e   **True**. When a bone is broken, the first sign is a periosteal reaction. Next callus is formed and this mineralizes. When the callus has fixed the two parts of the bone together, remodelling allows the bone to return to its normal shape. This process takes several months.

5   *Skull fractures in children*
   a   even if linear the child should be closely observed
   b   if depressed require evaluation with a CT scan
   c   usually need surgical treatment
   d   may occur after forceps delivery
   e   of the temporal bone are usually associated with intracranial haemorrhage

a   **True**. With fractures in any site, management aims to not only heal the bone but also anticipate and deal with likely complications related to the injury. For instance, with fractures of the calf, the bones must be left in a position in which healing is possible, but also compartment syndrome can develop and cause ischaemia of the calf muscles and foot. For the humerus, damage to the radial nerve can also occur. For skull fractures the fracture itself often does not need any treatment itself, depending on its type. However, associated brain injury and intracranial bleeding is more likely when there is a fracture. For this reason children who have had a head injury should all be monitored by hospital staff or parents for signs of deterioration.

Most children seen after a head injury have no fracture or intracranial problem. Symptoms suggesting a more serious injury include vomiting, dizziness or drowsiness, and reduction in level of consciousness. Such children without fractures should be admitted for observation. Those with fractures are likely to have had a more severe injury and so should also be admitted. Deterioration (rising blood pressure, falling pulse and conscious level, change or asymmetry in pupils, and their response to light) suggests a rising intracranial pressure and should prompt treatment with mannitol and a CT scan to see if there is a surgically treatable cause for the deterioration.

b **True**. Skull fractures can be divided into those that are linear, depressed, or diastatic (spreading the sutures). They may also be compound or closed. There are also certain sites that are more likely to be associated with damage to other structures, as discussed in part e.

Closed linear fractures are least likely to cause complications. Depressed fractures commonly damage the underlying brain and so should be evaluated with a CT scan and then the depressed part of bone elevated. Children with open fractures should be given antibiotics to try and prevent intracranial infection.

c **False**. Most children with fractures of the skull need no intervention. The indications for surgery include a depressed fracture, evacuation of a haematoma, and the insertion of an intracranial pressure monitoring device. These can also be used to drain CSF if there is a blockage to the flow of CSF, such as intraventricular haemorrhage. Surgery may also be indicated for specific injuries, such as those of the orbit, where fractures may prevent binocular vision.

d **True**. Birth is a traumatic procedure for the infant (and the mother). Commonly associated with birth are fractures of the clavicle and skull, occurring at a high rate with instrumental delivery and may be asymptomatic. Cephalhaematomas are common, which are haematomas enclosed by the periosteum, and therefore lie entirely over one of the bones of the skull. This helps distinguish the swelling from caput succedaneum, which is tissue swelling and can straddle the sutures between the bones of the skull. Nerve damage can also occur, particular Erb's palsy and a VIIth nerve lower motor neurone lesion, particularly after forceps delivery.

e **False**. Fractures of the temporal area can damage the middle meningeal artery and lead to an extradural haematoma. This is still not the usual consequence of a temporal fracture.

Fractures of the base of skull require relatively more force than other areas of the skull, so the brain injury is likely to be worse and bleeding also more common. Furthermore, other structures such as the cranial nerves and the brainstem may be directly damaged. Such fractures may manifest as CSF leakage from nose or ear or blood behind the tympanic membrane or bruising over the mastoid process.

6 *It is likely that treatment is required for*
    a a 2 year old with a medial longitudinal arch that disappears when he is not on tiptoe
    b genu valgum in a $3\frac{1}{2}$ year old
    c overlapping sutures in a newborn
    d a clicky hip in a newborn
    e talipes calcaneovarus

a   **False.** There is a large range of normal in a child's skeleton. Many unusual features resolve spontaneously as the child grows. Other abnormalities remain but do not interfere with function.

In the feet common anomalies include talipes (see part e) and flat feet. Flat feet are common is toddlers when the appearance is exacerbated by fat on the feet at this age. If it is not associated with any other problem and the arch reappears when the child stands on tiptoes, the problem will not need treatment.

b   **False.** A valgus deformity describes deviation away from the mid-line and varus is a deviation towards the mid-line. Genu valgum is therefore better known as knock-knees. The problem is likely to resolve.

Genu varum is better known as bow legs. In most children it is a normal finding but it may be due to rickets (see Endocrinology and metabolic disease, question 2) or Blount's disease.

c   **False.** Overlapping sutures in the newborn are needed to fit the head out of the maternal pelvis. If fused they will require treatment as brain growth will be restricted.

d   **False.** As discussed in question 2, the finding of clicky hips in a newborn is a normal finding that does not need treatment. By contrast clunky hips are abnormal require splinting to ensure the normal development of the hip joint.

e   **False.** Talipes is a common finding in the newborn. The most common abnormalities seen are talipes calcaneovarus (the foot is deviated to the mid-line and extended at the ankle) and talipes equinovarus (the foot is deviated outwards and flexed at the ankle). Both abnormalities can be divided into positional and fixed deformities depending on whether the foot can be manipulated back into a normal position. Both are caused by the lack of room in utero but some children also have malformation of the bones of the ankle. This is associated with other bony malformations, such as CDH and spina bifida.

Most talipes is positional and needs no treatment. If the foot cannot be returned to the normal position by manipulation, it needs treatment with strapping or casts to encourage growth into a more normal position. If this is not successful, operative repair will be needed.

Data interpretation and reasoning — answers

7   *A 10-year-old boy is referred to the paediatric rheumatology clinic because he has been experiencing increasing pain in his right knee and hip over the last 2 weeks. Three days prior to the onset of the pain he had a fall during a game of football. On examination he is afebrile and his leg is held slightly flexed, externally rotated and abducted at the hip. He is able to move at the hip but this movement is painful both actively and passively. The knee is normal to examination*

a   this would be a typical presentation of polyarticular juvenile chronic arthritis

b   avascular necrosis of the hip is unlikely to be the cause unless he also has a
    haemoglobinopathy
c   an anteroposterior X-ray of the pelvis will not exclude a slipped upper femoral
    epiphysis
d   a septic arthritis can be ruled out with a neutrophil count
e   if all his X-rays and blood tests are normal, he would be best treated with bed rest
    and gentle traction

a **False** b **False** c **True** d **False** e **True**

The possible causes of a painful hip are irritable hip, avascular necrosis (AVN)
of the femoral head (Perthes disease), slipped upper femoral epiphysis, septic
arthritis, and JCA. These can usually be distinguished by careful examination
and X-rays.

JCA is divided into that with a systemic presentation, also known as Still's
disease, polyarticular (over four joints) and pauciarticular (with four or less
joints). The systemic presentation is easily confused with that of sepsis in an infant
or toddler. Still's is identified by a high fever, malaise, splenomegaly, and a salmon-
pink rash but any joint involvement at presentation may be subtle or absent.
Progression to chronic articular involvement does not always occur.

The polyarticular form of the disease tends to affect small joints and is usually
symmetrical. RF is more often positive in older girls with a polyarticular presentation, and this disease then behaves similarly to adult rheumatoid arthritis. Other
than this subgroup the prognosis is good.

The pauciarticular form typically affects large joints, particularly the knee. In
older boys the disease may progress to a spondyloarthropathy, but otherwise its
prognosis is good. If the child is ANA positive, there is a higher risk of developing
chronic iridocyclitis, also known as chronic anterior uveitis. This complication
can lead to blindness, and so such children should have regular slit-lamp examinations and be treated with topical steroids and pupil dilators. The other notable
complication of pauciarticular JCA is overgrowth in the affected limb, leading to
a limp.

AVN of the hip is an important cause of a painful hip in the years preceding puberty, and is much more common in children with sickle cell disease. The
femoral head is supplied by blood vessels that pass through the femoral neck and
this leaves the head vulnerable to AVN if there is trauma (fractured neck of femur),
a slipped epiphysis, infarction (making AVN more common in sickle cell disease),
or without an underlying cause. The presentation of AVN of the hip is usually a
gradual onset of pain in the hip and thigh and a plain X-ray of the hip is usually
diagnostic showing flattening and reduced bone density in the femoral head.
Traction, with or without femoral osteotomy is required to allow remoulding of
the bone. The condition may result in arthritis of the hip in early adulthood.

Slipped epiphysis typically occurs during puberty and may be acute or chronic.
Pain may be absent, but the leg is externally rotated and shortened. Diagnosis is
by plain X-ray, but the AP view may not demonstrate the slip if it is in the wrong
plane. A frog leg lateral view is often better to make the diagnosis. Treatment is

with internal pinning or occasionally osteotomy and fixation if the slip is more long-standing.

This presentation cannot be that of a septic arthritis. Although this is an important diagnosis to exclude, immobility of the joint and a septic presentation is needed for septic arthritis to be considered unless the child is immunocompromised. The neutrophil count will be elevated in most children with septic arthritis, but will also be raised in JCA. Septic arthritis is discussed further in question 8.

If X-rays and antibody screen are normal, the most likely diagnosis is an 'irritable hip'. This term refers to a synovitis of the hip joint. An effusion is present and whenever this is the case, the child preferentially places the leg in the position that reduces the pressure within the hip joint—slight abduction, flexion, and external rotation. If there is an irritable hip, the child should not be toxic, and although there will be pain, passive movement will be possible. A history of recent viral infection is sometimes found. Treatment is with traction, rest, and non-steroidal analgesics.

8   *A 3-year-old girl is brought to her family doctor with a swollen knee and an effusion*

   a   septic arthritis must be excluded with a normal aspirate of joint fluid

   b   a long history of painless swelling in the knee is suggestive of juvenile chronic arthritis

   c   an immobile joint makes septic arthritis more likely

   d   osteomyelitis can be excluded by plain X-rays

   e   a recent pharyngitis may have led to a reactive arthritis

a **False**   b **True**   c **True**   d **False**   e **True**

A septic arthritis is the most serious cause of swelling or pain in any joint. Other possible causes include recent trauma, an idiopathic or reactive synovitis, JCA presenting in one joint, osteomyelitis in the bone near the joint, and a haemarthrosis.

Septic arthritis is serious because it rapidly destroys the articular surface and results in arthritis after the infection has cleared. Other joint disorders that cause swelling either do not cause articular destruction (synovitis, trauma) or do so more slowly (JCA, haemarthrosis). The risk of this complication of septic arthritis is reduced by prompt diagnosis and effective treatment. So in any child with a swollen joint this diagnosis must be excluded. This can usually be done with history and examination. A child with a septic arthritis will be febrile and toxic. The history will be short, and in some a previous source of haematogenous spread may be revealed (e.g. an abscess). On examination the joint will be hot and tender and erythematous. It will be fixed and attempts to move it passively will be very painful. If this is the case, synovial fluid aspiration should be performed. In the inflammatory and infective conditions the fluid is turbid, but if there is infection microscopy will reveal organisms on Gram stain in addition to the white cells. Culture will most commonly isolate *Staphylococcus aureus*, but *Haemophilus* and *Streptococcus pneumoniae* may instead be the cause.

Although a short history of swelling and pain is found in children with septic arthritis, a longer history is usually present in those with JCA. Pauciarticular JCA in particular is not so destructive to the joint, so there is less attendant pain, making the time to presentation longer. Reactive synovitis tends to present 1–2 weeks after a viral upper respiratory tract infection (URTI).

Osteomyelitis is painful and associated with swelling. Although this is an infection of the bone, the commonest site is in the metaphysis near the growth plate. Closer examination will usually demonstrate that a child with osteomyelitis has an swelling over the bone, not over the joint. In addition to these symptoms, there may be a longer history of malaise. In an infant, diagnosis is more difficult, with no visible local changes, just that the baby will not move the affected limb.

Following evaluation of the child with history and examination, special investigations can be of some use. Joint aspiration is of use only to exclude septic arthritis. Blood tests may show a raised white count (infection, polyarticular JCA, osteomyelitis) but the white count is likely to be normal in pauciarticular JCA or reactive synovitis. The erythrocyte sedimentation rate and other acute phase reactants such as C-reactive protein will be particularly raised in osteomyelitis and polyarticular JCA. Antibody tests can be used if there is suspected JCA and results can dramatically alter the prognosis. RF-positive children are much more likely to have a prolonged and debilitating illness and ANA positive children much more likely to have chronic iridocyclitis (see question 7)

Plain X-rays performed in this situation are frequently unhelpful. Osteomyelitis may not be detected on plain X-ray for up to 2 weeks after presentation, when bone hypodensities will be seen. If osteomyelitis is seriously suspected, a radionucleotide bone scan should be performed, which will show increased uptake in the affected bone.

Reactive or idiopathic synovitis frequently occurs after a viral URTI. The typical course is that of a short history of arthralgia and swelling that limits movement. The joint can be moved with little pain passively. X-rays and blood tests are normal. The hip is more commonly affected than the knee.

This condition is sometimes confused with the rare (in the developed world) rheumatic fever. This condition follows infection by a *Strep. pyogenes* subtype in the throat or elsewhere. Antigen–antibody complexes form and cause manifestations throughout the body, classified according to the Jones criteria. These include polyarthritis, carditis, chorea, erythema marginatum, and subcutaneous nodules.

9 *A 2-year-old boy is admitted to the children's ward for further evaluation of a fever that has failed to respond to a 1 week course of Amoxil, prescribed for a sore throat. In the time he has been on the antibiotic, his leg has become painful, especially when moved. On examination he has a tender swelling over the proximal fibula. A bone scan is performed, showing increased radionucleotide uptake in the proximal third of the fibula. This boy*

   a   may not have changes visible on his plain X-ray of the limb
   b   should be effectively treated by a third-generation cephalosporin with flucloxacillin
   c   should be investigated for an immunodeficiency

d will usually have positive blood cultures

e may subsequently have poor growth in the affected limb

a **True** b **True** c **False** d **True** e **True**

Children that do not respond to antibiotics either have a non-infective cause (e.g. systemic onset of JCA), a viral infection, a bacterial infection not sensitive to the antibiotic given, or a site of infection that is not adequately penetrated by the antibiotic. The latter is important cause and is responsible for partially treated meningitis, abscesses, and osteomyelitis.

In this scenario a throat infection is most likely to be viral (at least two out of three) and if bacterial will be streptococcal and therefore well treated by Amoxil. Another site is suggested by the painful leg and the swelling over the fibula. This could be either a cellulitis, an abscess or an osteomyelitis.

Plain X-rays will usually be normal in the early stages of osteomyelitis. Later, bone cysts and areas of lucency within the bone will be seen. A radionucleotide scan should be performed unless the swelling clearly is in the tissue overlying the bone.

Blood tests other than blood cultures will be of little diagnostic help, but will show a neutrophilia.

The commonest organisms responsible are *Staph. aureus*, *Haemophilus influenzae* type B, *Strep. pneumoniae*, and *Salmonella*. Antibiotics should cover all the likely organisms, but the use of broad-spectrum agents should be avoided where possible to reduce antibiotic resistance. A third-generation cephalosporin will cover Gram-negative organisms well and offers some Gram-positive cover for streptococcus but less for Staph. Flucloxacillin and fusidic acid are useful anti-staphylococcal agents. Treating osteomyelitis requires prolonged (up to 6 weeks) administration at sufficiently high levels. Even despite these agents, surgical debridement is sometimes needed.

Osteomyelitis usually has no underlying cause, but may complicate immuno-deficiencies, particularly chronic granulomatous disease. Another site of staphylococci infection may be found. Sickle cell disease, by causing bone ischaemia also predisposes to osteomyelitis. Fractures and even insertion of intravenous cannulae in children can also introduce infection into the bone.

Growth may be affected. Other complications include amyloidosis, chronic sinus, and abscess formation.

10 Gastroenterology

Knowledge — questions

1 *The following sections of the gastrointestinal tract are commonly directly affected by the associated conditions*

   a   the pancreas and coeliac disease

   b   the rectum and cystic fibrosis

   c   the liver and thalassaemia

   d   the small intestine and rotavirus gastroenteritis

   e   the stomach and Hirschsprung's disease

2 *Diarrhoea caused by*

   a   *Rotavirus* is often watery and greenish

   b   *Campylobacter* should not be treated with antibiotics

   c   *salmonella* food poisoning is not infectious

   d   *Giardia* is caused by colonic invasion

   e   *shigella* may contain blood and pus

3 *Infants with gastro-oesophageal reflux*

   a   typically present at 4–6 weeks

   b   can be improved by postural manipulation

   c   commonly develop an alkalosis

   d   are at higher risk of sudden infant death syndrome

   e   usually fail to thrive

4 *Hepatitis occurring in children*

   a   is most commonly caused by the hepatitis B virus world-wide

   b   cannot be acquired from a correctly screened blood transfusion

   c   can be congenitally acquired

   d   raises the aspartate transaminase level

   e   usually causes excessive bruising and deranged clotting

5 *Coeliac disease*

   a   can be diagnosed on history and examination alone

   b   may present with irritability

   c   is usually accompanied by serum antibodies to gliadin and reticulin

   d   typically presents in the weeks after birth

   e   often causes anaemia

6   **When examining a child**

    a spider naevi may be caused by autoimmune hepatitis

    b clubbing is likely to be associated with cirrhosis

    c wasting of the buttocks is diagnostic of coeliac disease

    d a rectal examination should always be performed if there are gastro-intestinal symptoms

    e hepatomegaly is present in over 90% of those with liver disease

7   **In a patient with malabsorption, the following statements are correct**

    a stools that are offensive indicate that there is bacterial overgrowth

    b cystic fibrosis causes malabsorption by making the small bowel lining mucus more viscid

    c Cotrimoxazole (septrin) will improve children with bacterial overgrowth

    d anaemia in coeliac disease is usually caused by iron deficiency

    e faecal fat globule estimation can detect fat malabsorption

8   **In children with constipation**

    a dietary factors are usually important

    b Hirschsprung's disease can be ruled out if there was no delayed passage of meconium

    c a full neurological examination will often reveal upper motor signs in the legs

    d the possibility of child sexual abuse should be considered more than in other children

    e urinary tract infections are more common

Data interpretation and reasoning — questions

9   **A child is brought to the family doctor as he has had loose stools for over a month. He has two to seven motions a day which are sometimes watery and sometimes semiformed**

    a in an otherwise thriving 2 year old intestinal hurry is the most likely cause

    b a history of recent travel would be needed for *Giardia lamblia* to be a potential cause

    c only children with neurological problems are likely to develop overflow diarrhoea

    d lactose intolerance often develops temporarily after a viral gastroenteritis

    e cystic fibrosis is unlikely if his weight is normal

10   *A 6-week-old boy is brought to his family doctor because he is*
      vomiting. The doctor thinks that pyloric stenosis is a more likely
      cause than any other because
      a   he has not gained weight since birth
      b   he vomits every time he coughs
      c   the vomitus is not bile stained
      d   there is abdominal distension
      e   he has a temperature of 37.2 °C

Knowledge — answers

Paediatric gastroenterology is a relatively small area at undergraduate level.
Questions will be based on symptoms (vomiting, diarrhoea, pain, weight loss,
jaundice, distension) and the common diseases [gastroenteritis, colitis, cystic
fibrosis (CF), hepatitis, coeliac disease, gastro-oesophageal reflux].

1   *The following sections of the gastrointestinal tract are commonly directly affected by the*
     associated conditions
     a   the pancreas and coeliac disease
     b   the rectum and cystic fibrosis
     c   the liver and thalassaemia
     d   the small intestine and rotavirus gastroenteritis
     e   the stomach and Hirschsprung's disease

a   **False.** The pattern of disease involvement reflects the pathophysiology of each
disease and can also be helpful in making a diagnosis. Coeliac disease affects
the areas of the gut exposed to gluten—especially the small bowel including the
terminal ileum. Other features and effects of the disease are discussed further in
question 5.

b   **True.** For a disease that is caused by abnormal ion channel regulator, CF causes
a wide range of effects in various tissues. The gut manifestations include chronic
pancreatitis, biliary obstruction and cirrhosis, meconium ileus and meconium
ileus equivalent, malabsorption, failure to thrive, and rectal prolapse. Diagnosis
is discussed in Respiratory disease, question 9.

c   **True.** Children with thalassaemia have anaemia caused by a high rate of
haemolysis. The demand for red cells is such that synthesis occurs at sites beyond
where blood is normally made (the vertebrae, pelvis, scapulae, ribs, and sternum).
At first other bony sites are used—the bones of the face enlarge in this process
leading to frontal bossing and maxillary hypertrophy. The liver and spleen are
also used as these are the embryological sites of haematopoiesis, causing hepatosplenomegaly.

d   **True**. Infections affecting the gut wall can broadly be divided into those that cause gastroenteritis and those that cause colitis. The gastroenteritis diseases are characterized by a profuse watery diarrhoea with little or no blood and colitis by less diarrhoea volume but by blood and pus in the stool. The small intestine is the site of the majority of water absorption in the gut, and disease of this region overloads the water absorbing capacity of the large intestine.

Rotavirus, *Campylobacter*, *salmonella*, and *shigella* directly invade the small gut mucosa and stops absorption, whereas enteropathogenic and enterotoxigenic *Escherichia coli*, cholera, and shigella cause a toxin-mediated diarrhoea.

e   **False**. Hirschsprung's disease is caused by the failure of migration of ganglionic cells down to the distal gut. Therefore the disease will always affect the most distal part and is less likely to affect increasingly proximal sections. All children with Hirschsprung's will need resection of the aganglionic segment and an operation to allow continence, such as a Duhamel pull through. The larger the segment, the more gut must be resected. Occasionally, the involvement is so extensive short gut syndrome results. Hirschsprung's is also discussed in question 8.

2   *Diarrhoea caused by*
   a   *Rotavirus* is often watery and greenish
   b   *Campylobacter* should not be treated with antibiotics
   c   *salmonella* food poisoning is not infectious
   d   *Giardia* is caused by colonic invasion
   e   *shigella* may contain blood and pus

a   **True**. As indicated in question 1(d), gastroenteritis diarrhoea is watery because insufficient water is absorbed in the small intestine. The green colour results from reduced bile absorption.

b   **False**. Most diarrhoeas are best not treated with antibiotics. Their use may harm the normal organisms of the gut and delay restoration of the usual flora. Also carriage of *salmonella* may be lengthened by the use of antibiotics. Antibiotics are indicated if there is evidence of invasive disease, such as a toxic features or positive blood cultures. Antibiotics are also used in the following situations: *salmonella* under 3 months (ciprofloxacin), *shigella* (cotrimoxazole reduces carriage time), and *Campylobacter* (erythromycin speeds recovery).

c   **False**. Food poisoning may be caused by toxins or organisms. Those mediated by toxins (*Staphylococcus aureus*, *Bacillus cereus*, *Clostridium botulinum*, *Ciguatera* from mackerel) tend to present soon after ingestion, maybe even on the way home from the restaurant! These are usually not infectious. Those mediated by organisms (*salmonella*, *Campylobacter*, *E. coli*) take 1–2 days to present after the contaminated food and are infectious.

d   **False**. *Giardia* invades the small bowel causing watery diarrhoea, nausea, and sometimes chronic malabsorption. It can be treated with metronidazole.

e **True.** *Salmonella*, *shigella*, *Campylobacter*, and *E. coli* can all cause colitis, manifest as a stool containing pus and blood.

3 *Infants with gastro-oesophageal reflux*
  a typically present at 4–6 weeks
  b can be improved by postural manipulation
  c commonly develop an alkalosis
  d are at higher risk of sudden infant death syndrome
  e usually fail to thrive

a **False.** Vomiting in infancy is a very common problem, and may be a symptom of diseases as diverse as gastro-oesophageal reflux (GOR), pyloric stenosis (PS), gut obstruction, sepsis, or an upper respiratory tract infection (URTI). These conditions can usually be differentiated on history and examination alone. The vomiting may be forceful (PS and GOR), may be unrelated to the time of feeds (sepsis, obstruction), or be related to the time of a feed (possetting, GOR, PS) or to a cough (URTI and other respiratory infections). The child may be acutely ill (obstruction, sepsis, PS) or fairly well (URTI, GOR). The abdomen will be distended in most infants with obstruction. If there is long-standing vomiting, GOR or possetting are the only likely causes. The timing of the onset of the vomiting can also be of help, as GOR usually starts soon after birth and worsens as the infant's intake increases and then improves as the infant sits up more and takes more solid food. PS typically presents at 4–6 weeks.

b **True.** Prone posture can be of help in the management of reflux, particularly in the neonatal nursery. Antireflux agents can be of use. The first step is to ensure that the volume of feed is appropriate and that the child is correctly winded after the feed. Next the feed can be thickened using agents such as carobel, or gaviscon can be used to minimize the occurrence and effects of the refluxed acid (see part d). For breast-fed infants and those not responsive to these measures, cisapride can be used. This is a 'prokinetic' that works by increasing the tone of the cardiac sphincter, and promoting stomach emptying; however, its use has recently been questioned as it can cause arrhythmias especially in combination with other drugs, such as erythromycin.

Surgical intervention is of use in refractory reflux, using a Nissen fundoplication.

c **False.** For an alkalosis to develop from vomiting there must be loss of acid in excess of the ability of the kidneys to correct the loss. If the vomiting is caused by obstruction below the duodenum the acid/base disturbance is less severe as the duodenal and pancreatic secretions are alkaline. Unlike PS, GOR is almost never severe enough to cause alkalosis. A baby with PS is discussed in the Nephrology question.

d **True.** Complications of GOR include apnoea, aspiration pneumonia, sudden infant death syndrome, oesophagitis, upper gastrointestinal bleeding, oesophageal stricture, and failure to thrive.

e   **False**. As discussed failure to thrive is unusual in children with GOR.

4   *Hepatitis occurring in children*
   a   is most commonly caused by the hepatitis B virus world-wide
   b   cannot be acquired from a correctly screened blood transfusion
   c   can be congenitally acquired
   d   raises the aspartate transaminase level
   e   usually causes excessive bruising and deranged clotting

a   **False**. Hepatitis is not only caused by infectious viral agents but can also be caused by metabolic and genetic factors. There are now at least four infectious agents that have been identified as causing hepatitis in humans and all can affect children. In the developing world, 5–15% of individuals are carriers for hepatitis B, but in the developed world only 0.1–0.5% carry the disease. Hepatitis A is more common as it is spread by the faecal–oral route, in some countries affecting 90% of the population at some time. Chronic hepatitis A or carrier state is not seen. Hepatitis C may be spread sexually and by blood transfusions. The other infectious cause is the δ virus, but this still leaves an unidentified group. Other viruses, such as Epstein–Barr virus can also cause a hepatitis.

b   **False**. The infectious risk of blood is reduced by screening blood donors (rejecting those who have had hepatitis or jaundice) and testing the blood. However, as it may take 6 months to seroconvert after exposure to hepatitis viruses, it is possible for an individual to be infectious but seronegative. The same is true for HIV. There will also be as yet unrecognized infectious agents that can be transmitted through blood transfusions, and these factors make all blood products potentially dangerous. Fresh frozen plasma, cryoprecipitate, and platelets also carry infectious risk.

c   **True**. Hepatitis B can be acquired from the mother at birth. Intrauterine infection can also occur but is less common. Infants born to women with hepatitis B are given active and passive immunization as outlined in the Community paediatrics and development, question 6.
   Hepatitis in neonates and children may also be caused by metabolic diseases such as α_1-antitrypsin deficiency and Wilson disease.

d   **True**. The laboratory markers of hepatobiliary disease include the 'liver enzymes' aspartate transaminase (AST) and alanine transaminase (ALT). These enzymes are released into the blood when there is hepatocellular damage or inflammation. Alkaline phosphate (ALP) is also released but if there is biliary obstruction there is a disproportionate rise in the ALP. If the child develops liver failure, the synthetic function of the liver becomes inadequate, with deranged clotting, a raised ammonia, and a falling albumin. The metabolic function is also impaired and urea and glucose may be low.

e   **False**. These are signs of fulminant liver failure which is not usual in hepatitis. Types A and B are the commonest infectious causes of fulminant liver failure.

5   Coeliac disease
   a   can be diagnosed on history and examination alone
   b   may present with irritability
   c   is usually accompanied by serum antibodies to gliadin and reticulin
   d   typically presents in the weeks after birth
   e   often causes anaemia

a   **False**. It can be difficult to make the diagnosis of coeliac disease. Although there are suggestive symptoms (see b), and suggestive blood tests (see c), the diagnosis is made by taking jejunal biopsies while on a normal diet and then on a gluten-free diet. In adults a further biopsy is taken after a normal diet is re-introduced. The typical appearance is of villous atrophy with crypt elongation.

Specimens can be taken during duodenoscopy from the distal duodenum or with a Crosby capsule (a spring-loaded biopsy capsule) from the jejunum.

b   **True**. Symptoms of coeliac disease include weight loss, diarrhoea, offensive stool, and irritability. Signs include pallor, abdominal distension, buttock wasting, and clubbing.

c   **True**. These (and others, for example: endomysial) antibodies are present in almost all children with coeliac disease but there are those with the antibodies but no symptoms and a normal biopsy. Antibodies are a useful screening investigation in the malabsorbing child.

d   **False**. Coeliac disease is caused by the reaction to gluten in the diet, and so does not present until wheat products are included in the diet. Current recommendations are that weaning (the introduction of solids) should start at 4 months or later.

e   **True**. In addition to antibodies, children with coeliac disease often have an iron deficiency anaemia and may be folate or in severe cases B_{12} deficient. Serum albumin may be low.

6   When examining a child
   a   spider naevi may be caused by autoimmune hepatitis
   b   clubbing is likely to be associated with cirrhosis
   c   wasting of the buttocks is diagnostic of coeliac disease
   d   a rectal examination should always be performed if there are gastrointestinal symptoms
   e   hepatomegaly is present in over 90% of those with liver disease

a   **True**. Spider naevi are abnormalities characterized by a central feeding arteriole and surrounding venules. They are a non-specific sign of liver disease and can also occur in other conditions in which there is an increase in circulating oestrogens. However, many children have one or two spiders without any disease. Over five in the territory of the superior vena cava is suggestive of liver disease.

If large or unsightly they can be treated with cryotherapy or laser therapy.

b   **False**. Clubbing in children is much more likely to be caused by congenital cyanotic heart disease or CF. Other less common causes in children include pulmonary abscess, tuberculosis or empyema, coeliac disease, and ulcerative colitis.

c   **False**. Wasting of the buttocks implies there is a loss of muscle mass—this will only occur if there is a disease process that is rendering the body catabolic as opposed to a poor diet, where the child will be generally thin with little adipose tissue. Coeliac disease or another cause of malabsorption (e.g. CF, cow's milk protein intolerance) could be responsible, and may also produce a distended abdomen.

d   **False**. A rectal examination is a distressing procedure that should only be performed if there is useful information that is likely to be gained. Indications include rectal bleeding (you might feel the tip of an intussusception or a polyp or see a fissure) and constipation in infancy, where Hirschsprung's is a possibility. Rectal examination will enable the tone of the anal sphincter to be felt and will unplug hard stools.

e   **False**. The definition of hepatomegaly varies with age, with a 3 cm liver being normal in a neonate and a palpable liver abnormal in a 15 year old. Those with an increased liver span may have liver congestion from high venous pressures (e.g. cardiac failure) or may have inflammation of the liver itself (hepatitis), or there may be abnormal storage of substances in the liver in some metabolic diseases (e.g. glycogen storage disease). A large number of children who have had liver disease start with hepatomegaly, but the liver then becomes cirrhotic, small and impalpable.

> 7   *In a patient with malabsorption, the following statements are correct*
>   a   stools that are offensive indicate that there is bacterial overgrowth
>   b   cystic fibrosis causes malabsorption by making the small bowel lining mucus more viscid
>   c   Cotrimoxazole (septrin) will improve children with bacterial overgrowth
>   d   anaemia in coeliac disease is usually caused by iron deficiency
>   e   faecal fat globule estimation can detect fat malabsorption

a   **False**. Malabsorption is a deficiency in the absorption of nutrients from the diet. It may result from a disease in the pancreas, liver, in the gut anatomy or the gut itself. Children with malabsorption should have evidence of defective absorption in that the stools will contain high levels of fat. The fatty acids in the stool make it foul smelling and cause it to float. There may be an osmotic diarrhoea, making the stool bulky. Children will often have evidence of poor nutrient intake and have poor growth, wasting or an anaemia.

Bacterial overgrowth is another cause of malabsorption, usually correctable with surgery. Overgrowth can occur when there is a blind loop or a partial obstruction that causes pooling of the gut contents proximal to the obstruction. The bacteria deconjugate bile salts and so impair the absorption of fat, and consume vitamin B_{12}, leading to anaemia.

b   **False**. Malabsorption can result from any process that interferes with the gut handling of fat. CF causes malabsorption by impairing the function of the exocrine pancreas, which secretes, among other enzymes, lipase. Biliary atresia or other obstructions to bile flow reduces the availability of the bile acids needed to process fat. These acids are also broken down in conditions of bacterial overgrowth. Short gut syndrome (see Growth and nutrition, question 5) reduces the surface area available for absorption and diseases of the mucosa reduce its function.

Children with CF have more viscid secretions because there is insufficient saline secreted along with the proteins in exocrine glands. This is because the defective cystic fibrosis transmembrane protein (CFTR) renders the membrane relatively impermeable to chloride so less water enters the secretions. The viscid secretions are the cause of the chest, biliary, and pancreatic complications of the disease. In the newborn the stickiness of the gut contents can lead to meconium ileus.

c   **True**. For children with malabsorption, treatment is often not possible for the underlying cause, and replacement of deficient bile acids or pancreatic enzymes is needed. However, for those with coeliac disease, a long-term gluten-free diet will allow normal gut function, and for those with bacterial overgrowth antibiotics can be used to temporarily ameliorate the problem while awaiting definitive surgery. Giardiasis can also cause malabsorption, which can be treated with metronidazole.

d   **True**. Anaemia may be caused by deficiency of iron, folate, B_{12}, and copper. In coeliac disease iron or folate deficiency is much more common than B_{12} deficiency, whereas B_{12} deficiency is more common in those with bacterial overgrowth. Those with CF are less likely to be anaemic.

e   **True**. Faecal fat levels can be measured by chemical analysis of the stool, but for screening and diagnostic purposes examination of faeces for fat globules is as useful, and much less difficult. Carbohydrate malabsorption is suggested by the presence of reducing substances in the stool, except in breast-fed infants, where it is a normal finding.

Dynamic tests of gut function can also be helpful. The hydrogen breath test relies on bacteria in the distal gut converting carbohydrate into hydrogen, which is then absorbed and breathed out. High concentrations of hydrogen in the breath imply that there is carbohydrate that is not absorbed by the small intestine. Xylose is absorbed by the proximal intestine, so low blood levels taken after administration of d-xylose indicate dysfunction of this part of the gut. Vitamin B_{12} is mainly absorbed in the terminal ileum, and the Schilling test can be used to evaluate this region. In this test the body is loaded parenterally with B_{12} and then a small test dose of labelled B_{12} administered by mouth. As there is an excess of B_{12} in the body the labelled B_{12} should all be excreted in the urine, but failure to do this indicates a B_{12} malabsorption. This can also be due to deficiency of intrinsic factor (IF), so the test can be performed with and without IF to determine the cause of the malabsorption.

8 *In children with constipation*

  a dietary factors are usually important
  b Hirschsprung's disease can be ruled out if there was no delayed passage of
     meconium
  c a full neurological examination will often reveal upper motor signs in the legs
  d the possibility of child sexual abuse should be considered more than in other
     children
  e urinary tract infections are more common

a **True**. Constipation is such a common problem that it is often treated without properly considering underlying causes. Constipation can be defined as the infrequent passage of hard stools. It occurs when the passage through the rectum is too slow and there is excessive drying of the stool. This may be because peristalsis is slow (Hirschsprung's, opiate use, hypothyroidism, hypokalaemia, antidepressants) or because the sphincters are unable or reluctant to open (spina bifida, behavioural problems). Once the stool is hard, it is difficult for the child to pass the stool and so stool is retained in the rectum. This reduces the effectiveness of the receptors in the rectum which sense when defecation is needed and so further stool accumulates. At this stage, watery fluid from higher up in the large bowel may pass over the hard lumps of stool causing 'overflow diarrhoea'.

Dietary factors are important as the presence of dietary fibre speeds the passage of stool through the rectum and reduces drying. In children without an underlying cause, diet must be altered during treatment or the problem will recur.

b **False**. Hirschsprung's disease is the result of failure of migration of neural crest cells into the distal parts of the gut to form ganglion cells there. Most present with delayed passage of meconium, but many with a short segment of disease do not and present later with chronic constipation.

The neonatal presentation is with gut obstruction, distension, and eventually faecal vomiting. Enterocolitis may develop with fluid and electrolyte loss into the affected bowel.

c **False**. Spina bifida and other spinal cord problems are a statistically uncommon cause of constipation. Those that do have such an underlying cause may be identified by delayed walking, delayed continence, and perhaps a pigmented or hairy patch over the spine. There will be upper motor neurone signs in the legs.

d **True**. In a child without an underlying cause that develops constipation, sexual abuse is an uncommon but important cause to consider and investigate further if there are suspicious factors. This is discussed further in Community paediatrics and development, question 7.

Children also often develop constipation when potty training is started, particularly if there is excessive parental pressure to 'achieve' continence.

e **True**. Constipation may be complicated by abdominal pain, anal fissures, overflow diarrhoea, behavioural problems, and urinary tract infections (UTIs). UTIs are more common because a full rectum prevents the bladder from completely emptying. The UTI needs treatment along with the constipation to prevent recurrence. This is done by first softening the stool (diet, lactulose) and then encouraging peristalsis with senna or picosulphate. If the rectum is overloaded, this may need clearing out from below with enemas or a washout. Once the stool is soft, treatment should be continued for several months to enable the rectum to begin to function normally again.

Data interpretation and reasoning — answers

9   *A child is brought to the family doctor as he has had loose stools for over a month. He has two to seven motions a day, which are sometimes watery and sometimes semiformed*

a   in an otherwise thriving 2 year old intestinal hurry is the most likely cause
b   a history of recent travel would be needed for *Giardia lamblia* to be a potential cause
c   only children with neurological problems are likely to develop overflow diarrhoea
d   lactose intolerance often develops temporarily after a viral gastroenteritis
e   cystic fibrosis is unlikely if his weight is normal

a **True** b **False** c **False** d **True** e **True**

In this question it is particularly important to read each branch of the question with the stem, as information given in one branch does not apply to the other branches. Here is presented a child with a chronic history of loose stools. Acute diarrhoea, that has lasted less than 1 week is most likely to be due to infective gastroenteritis or food poisoning, but longer standing diarrhoea is more likely to be due a problem with gut function. The causes are outlined in Box 10.1.

Diarrhoea may be defined as excessive stool loss that can lead to fluid or electrolyte disturbance. Most children will need to be passing about seven watery stools a day for this to occur. Loose stools are more common and are a frequent cause for consultation.

When evaluating a child with loose stools a good history is particularly important. The number of stools and urine volumes passed and fluid intake will enable the doctor to determine whether the child is or will become fluid depleted as a result of the losses. The consistency is helpful, as small bowel gastroenteritis and to a lesser extent osmotic and secretory diarrhoeas are usually watery whereas dysentery is usually more formed. Colour is unhelpful, except that a stool with blood and pus is good evidence of dysentery.

The medical history may be helpful particularly if the child has thyrotoxicosis or has recently had gastroenteritis. If the latter is the case, the diarrhoea is likely to be due to a temporary lactase deficiency causing lactose intolerance. The infectious gastroenteritis has damaged the gut mucosa and has resulted in protein, fat and carbohydrate malabsorption. Stopping feeds also stops the diarrhoea, identifying

Box 10.1   Causes of diarrhoea

Acute	Viral gastroenteritis
	Dysentery
	Food poisoning
	Post-gastroenteritis lactose intolerance
	Haemolytic–uraemic syndrome
	Intussusception
	Drugs (antibiotics, laxatives, cisapride)
Chronic	Toddler diarrhoea
	Overflow diarrhoea
	Lactase deficiency
	Cow's milk protein intolerance
	Giardial infection
	Coeliac disease
	Inflammatory bowel disease
	Immunodeficiency

it as an osmotic diarrhoea in contrast to a secretory type where the diarrhoea would continue.

If the child is otherwise well, toddler diarrhoea or intestinal hurry is the likely cause. Here the toddler will have loose stools often with identifiable food particles. There are no laboratory abnormalities and all that is required is for the diet to be reviewed and the parents reassured as the condition will resolve.

A travel history should always be taken although most organisms can be found in the developed world. Giardia is to be found world-wide and in children is often spread in day care centres. Following cyst ingestion the organism colonizes the small bowel and causes symptoms of acute diarrhoea, abdominal pain, and malabsorption in about half of those infected. Chronic giardial infection can also result in failure to thrive. Exclusion may require analysis of duodenal fluid or biopsy. It is best treated with metronidazole.

CF is not a usual cause of diarrhoea, instead causing steatorrhoea and malabsorption. It is very unusual for a child with CF not to have abdominal symptoms, whereas it is well recognized that some children with CF have little chest disease.

A history of neurological problems in a child with long-standing diarrhoea is suggestive that there is overflow diarrhoea (see question 8), but children with constipation from other causes such as poor diet or behavioural constipation can also have overflow diarrhoea.

Examination of the child with diarrhoea is helpful mainly to determine the fluid and electrolyte disturbance. Treatment of the diarrhoea is supportive and, if possible, directed at the cause.

10   *A 6-week-old boy is brought to his family doctor because he is vomiting. The doctor*
     thinks that pyloric stenosis is a more likely cause than any other because
     a   he has not gained weight since birth
     b   he vomits every time he coughs
     c   the vomitus is not bile stained
     d   there is abdominal distension
     e   he has a temperature of 37.2°C

a **False**   b **False**   c **False**   d **False**   e **False**

Vomiting at 6 weeks is common and only rarely due to pyloric stenosis (PS), so statistically the child is unlikely to have PS. So this question is looking for features that suggest PS rather than those that are merely consistent with it. These features are projectile non-bilious vomiting soon after a feed, a hungry baby with acute weight loss, and with an olive-shaped tumour palpable in an empty abdomen. Visible peristalsis may also be seen.

Lack of weight gain since birth suggests a serious problem, as discussed in Growth and nutrition, question 5, caused perhaps by a non-gastrointestinal disorder, such as cardiac failure or CF. Vomiting with coughing is common and should prompt examination of the respiratory system. Non-bile-stained vomiting is most likely to be due to gastro-oesophageal reflux, sepsis, or possetting rather than PS. Bile stained vomiting on the other hand is suggestive of intestinal obstruction.

The temperature is normal for a child of 6 weeks and so is not helpful in making any diagnosis.

11 Paediatric surgery

Questions

1 A boy of 7 months is brought to his family doctor because his parents would like him to be circumcised. This should be part of his treatment if
   a he has paraphimosis
   b his foreskin balloons each time he passes urine
   c he has presented with a balanitis
   d he has a poor urinary stream without ballooning
   e he has had two proven urinary tract infections

2 A 2-year-old girl is brought to the emergency department by her parents. She has been vomiting for the last day and has abdominal pain. The paediatric surgeon is called. He would be correct in saying that
   a pneumonia could be the cause of her symptoms
   b she is unlikely to have appendicitis if there is no localization of pain in the right iliac fossa
   c it is possible that these symptoms may be due to abdominal migraine
   d if she has appendicitis white cells may be found in the urine
   e she is too old for a malrotation to present

3 A child with an inguinal hernia
   a is most likely to have an indirect hernia
   b is an increased risk of incarceration
   c is more likely to have been born prematurely
   d will more commonly have hypothyroidism
   e should be observed closely as it may resolve by 5 years

4 A 2-month-old boy is seen by his family doctor because his mother has noticed a swelling in his groin. A hydrocele is more likely than a hernia because
   a the swelling enlarges when he cries
   b his testicle can be felt separately from the swelling
   c it is irreducible

    d   it does not transilluminate
    e   it is usually smaller after sleeping

5   **Undescended testes**
    a   will not undergo malignant change if brought into the scrotum
    b   secrete insufficient levels of testosterone to allow puberty
    c   cannot undergo torsion
    d   include those found at the inguinal ring by definition
    e   should be operated on under 4 months

6   **Abdominal pain**
    a   may be the only presenting symptom of a Meckel's diverticulum
    b   is usually colicky and localized to the left iliac fossa if a child is con-
        stipated
    c   is a common presenting feature of children with diabetic ketoacidosis
    d   is a feature of vesico-ureteric reflux
    e   is often present in children with a sickle crisis

7   **A 10-month-old child presents because the mother has noticed some
    blood passed with a stool. This presentation would commonly be
    associated with**
    a   haemorrhoids
    b   Henoch–Schönlein purpura
    c   intussusception early in the course of the disease
    d   a volvulus
    e   constipation in the preceding week

8   **An antenatal scan at 36 weeks has confirmed the presence of an
    umbilical abnormality involving the gut. Following delivery**
    a   chromosome studies will be needed for infants with exomphalos
    b   a gastroschisis will lose large volumes of fluid
    c   an exomphalos may be found to contain the liver
    d   there is likely to be ischaemia of the gut in an exomphalos
    e   the gastroschisis must be repaired immediately

9   **The following features favour the diagnosis of pyloric stenosis rather
    than another cause of vomiting in an infant of 6 weeks**
    a   the vomiting has gradually worsened since birth
    b   vomiting occurs up to 4 h after each feed
    c   the infant is hungry
    d   the abdomen is distended
    e   weight gain of 900 g since birth

10   *A term male infant of 36 h is admitted to the neonatal unit because of poor feeding. After a normal delivery, with no resuscitation, the infant has fed poorly and has been vomiting yellow-green liquid since about 6 h of age. He has yet to pass meconium. Examination finds a dehydrated infant with a distended abdomen and an umbilical hernia. An abdominal X-ray shows distended loops of bowel. This presentation's cause*

    a is a delayed onset of peristalsis in the majority of cases
    b could be a volvulus
    c is likely to be the umbilical hernia
    d may be pyloric stenosis
    e may well be necrotizing enterocolitis

11   *The following conditions should be operated on urgently*

    a umbilical hernia
    b gastroschisis
    c ventricular septal defect
    d talipes equino-varus
    e laryngeal stenosis

12   *When examining a child*

    a a large olive-shaped mass is easily felt in the epigastrium of children with pyloric stenosis
    b divarification of the rectus abdominalis muscles is normal in a newborn
    c it can be normal for the testes to be impalpable at birth
    d a palpable sigmoid colon is found in children with constipation
    e a rectal examination is useful if intussusception is a possibility

13   *The diagnosis of tracheo-oesophageal fistula*

    a may present as recurrent aspiration
    b may be suspected if there is oligohydramnios
    c usually prevents passage of a gastric tube
    d is suggested in a 'mucusy' newborn
    e is commonly associated with cardiac defects

Answers

Paediatric surgery is a separate speciality from general surgery. Although many principles are the same, the conditions and the approach are different. There are several subspecialties (e.g. paediatric cardiac surgery, paediatric neurosurgery) that do not need to be well understood, but the conditions that a general paediatric surgeon might deal with should be covered. These include hernias, undescended testes, the acute abdomen, and the management of obstruction.

> 1   *A boy of 7 months is brought to his family doctor because his parents would like him to be circumcised. This should be part of his treatment if*
>   a   he has paraphimosis
>   b   his foreskin balloons each time he passes urine
>   c   he has presented with a balanitis
>   d   he has a poor urinary stream without ballooning
>   e   he has had two proven urinary tract infections

a   **False**. Circumcision remains a common operation. Most circumcisions are performed for religious reasons (Jews and Muslims), and this is usually done by a religious representative. Another common reason is for 'hygiene', although there is little scientific support for this indication. The foreskin should be left intact unless it is a site of recurrent infection or it is obstructing the flow of urine.

Phimosis is a narrowing of the outlet of the foreskin and may be congenital or following forcible attempts at retraction. The foreskin may not retract up to 10 years, as the tissue layers gradually separate, so a small opening at 7 months age is normal.

Paraphimosis is a swelling of the glans of the penis following retraction of the foreskin. This obstructs the venous return and causes the swelling. The foreskin can usually be returned to its normal position by gentle squeezing of the glans with appropriate analgesia, but occasionally a circumcision is needed.

b   **True**. Ballooning implies there is some obstruction at the outlet. However, unless there are urinary tract infections (UTIs) or balanitis, circumcision is not always necessary.

As a general principle, as a child grows, obstructions become less severe. This is because the resistance of a tube is related to the fourth power of its radius, so linear growth has a dramatic effect on any stenotic opening, such as a phimosis or tracheal stenosis.

c   **True**. Recurrent balanitis is an indication for circumcision. Balanitis presents with a swollen and erythematous foreskin and a discharge from the outlet of the foreskin. It should be treated with broad-spectrum systemic antibiotics and regular baths. If there is no improvement, an urgent circumcision can be performed.

d   **False**. A poor urinary stream may be caused by obstruction at several levels. The most important ones are at the bladder outlet, where posterior urethral valves (PUVs) can cause antenatal or postnatal urinary tract dilatation that can progress to renal failure. This condition only affects boys. A poor stream may also be caused by a narrow opening to the prepuce. Although parents may often worry about their son's opening, there is usually a good stream, but if the urine only dribbles out with associated ballooning, circumcision would be indicated.

e   **False.** UTIs are caused by many different factors. UTIs caused by obstruction relievable by circumcision are rare and other causes are much more likely (see Nephrology question 2). The infant should be properly investigated for his UTI and started on prophylactic antibiotics as discussed in Nephrology question 8. If there is outflow obstruction, there will be a pool of urine left at the end of micturition that will allow the development of infection. Organisms that are present under the foreskin do not ascend unless there are other urinary problems.

> 2   *A 2-year-old girl is brought to the emergency department by her parents. She has been vomiting for the last day and has abdominal pain. The paediatric surgeon is called. He would be correct in saying that*
>   a   pneumonia could be the cause of her symptoms
>   b   she is unlikely to have appendicitis if there is no localization of pain in the right iliac fossa
>   c   it is possible that these symptoms may be due to abdominal migraine
>   d   if she has appendicitis white cells may be found in the urine
>   e   she is too old for a malrotation to present

a   **True.** One of the problems with paediatric diagnosis is the poor localization of symptoms. At first sight this child sounds as though she must have an abdominal problem, but symptoms such as vomiting and even diarrhoea have may be caused by disease in other systems. Vomiting, for instance, occurs with fevers, coughs, and metabolic disturbances as well as gastrointestinal disease.

Pneumonia is a well recognized cause of upper or central abdominal pain, particularly if the lower lobes are involved. Any child with a cough is likely to vomit as a reflex after the bout, and swallowed sputum may exacerbate the problem.

Viral upper respiratory tract infections are also associated with abdominal pain, as there may be mesenteric lymphadenitis associated with the viraemia. Such children may be differentiated from those with acute appendicitis because they tend to have a softer abdomen and will appear less toxic. Investigations will show no leucocytosis. If there is doubt as to whether a child has appendicitis or another non-specific cause of abdominal pain, a 3–6 h period of observation can be helpful, as those with appendicitis are likely to worsen.

b   **False**. Localization of the pain to McBurney's point is a late feature in the classical presentation of appendicitis and indicates that the inflammation is now affecting the peritoneal wall. A 2 year old would not be expected to localize the pain so well.

c   **True.** One of the many non-surgical causes of abdominal pain is the so-called abdominal migraine. This presents as episodic nausea, vomiting, and abdominal pain with a positive family history of migraine. There may be no associated headache, although this feature may develop as the child grows older.

d   **True**. Local inflammation near the bladder or ureters can also cause a pyuria. A pelvic appendix sits close to the ureters and bladder and so often is associated with a pyuria. Other causes of a pyuria include renal tract infection and inflammation.

e   **False**. Malrotation can present at any age.

When the intestine forms in an embryo, the gradual lengthening leads to twisting to allow it to fit into the abdomen. This puts the duodenum and ascending colon on the right and the descending colon on the left. Malrotation is an embryological abnormality of this process in which the intestines do not return to the abdomen correctly and are incompletely or abnormally rotated.

The most important complication of this is volvulus, where the gut twists on its pedicle and becomes ischaemic. It presents with an acute abdomen and obstruction. Perforation may result. Intermittent volvulus can also occur, or a child may have intermittent abdominal pain, vomiting, failure to thrive, or even be asymptomatic.

3   *A child with an inguinal hernia*
   a   is most likely to have an indirect hernia
   b   is an increased risk of incarceration
   c   is more likely to have been born prematurely
   d   will more commonly have hypothyroidism
   e   should be observed closely as it may resolve by 5 years

a   **True**. Inguinal hernias in children are different in aetiology and management to adult hernias. During fetal life the testicle descends slowly from next to the kidney to the scrotum down the processus vaginalis. This occurs on average by 32 weeks and slightly earlier on the left. The processus then closes. Down this pathway a hernia may form.

Almost all hernias in children are indirect hernias. The only exceptions are direct hernias found when there is a wasted abdominal wall and a high intra-abdominal pressure, as can occur in patients with cystic fibrosis and bronchopulmonary dysplasia (BPD).

b   **True**. Paediatric hernias are also managed very differently to those in adults. The main reason for this is that they are much more likely to incarcerate, obstruct, or strangulate. Hence the aim is to operate as soon as possible (but not as an emergency) even if the hernia can be reduced.

c   **True**. As the processus vaginalis does not close until after testicular descent is finished, premature infants often have undescended testes. Also, because abdominal pressure is frequently raised in premature infants secondary to respiratory disease, abdominal contents are forced into the inguinal canal forming a hernia.

d   **False**. Hypothyroidism can cause a variety of seemingly unconnected signs in an infant. Umbilical hernias, delayed closure of the anterior fontanelle, jaundice, coarse facies, and a coarse cry may all be manifestations of hypothyroidism. This is further discussed in Endocrinology and metabolic disease questions 4, 5, and 14.

e   **False.** This approach would be appropriate for a child with an umbilical hernia, but not an inguinal hernia which needs urgent surgery. Umbilical herniae are not usually a surgical problem, as they usually resolve before school age and almost never develop any complications.

   4 *A 2-month-old boy is seen by his family doctor because his mother has noticed a swelling in his groin. A hydrocele is more likely than a hernia because*
      a   the swelling enlarges when he cries
      b   his testicle can be felt separately from the swelling
      c   it is irreducible
      d   it does not transilluminate
      e   it is usually smaller after sleeping

a   **False.** Swellings in the groin are a common surgical problem that can usually be resolved by careful examination and transillumination. History can also be helpful, particularly concerning variations in the size of the mass during the day and with crying. Crying tenses the abdomen enlarging a hernia but will not affect a hydrocele. Both tend to be smaller after sleeping.

b   **False.** Hydroceles usually are around the testicle so the testicle is often not felt, but there may be a hydrocele of the cord. Hernias on the other hand come from above and so may not have reached the testicle. Even if they have, the testicle can still usually be separated from the hernia.

c   **True.** A hydrocele is caused at this age by a patent processus vaginalis allowing abdominal fluid to collect in the scrotum. Pressure, however, does not reduce it as the processus is closed by 'valves' when pressure is applied. A hernia may be reducible, but not if it is incarcerated, obstructed, or strangulated.

d   **False.** Transillumination is a useful way of differentiating these conditions, as bowel and fluid transmit light very differently. Also useful is to see if the mass can be got above.

e   **False.** Both hernias and hydroceles tend to be smaller after sleeping.

   5 *Undescended testes*
      a   will not undergo malignant change if brought into the scrotum
      b   secrete insufficient levels of testosterone to allow puberty
      c   cannot undergo torsion
      d   include those found at the inguinal ring by definition
      e   should be operated on under 4 months

a   **False.** Undescended testes become dysplastic. They are more prone to seminomas, with up to 10% becoming malignant. Also diagnosis of testicular disorders is more difficult if they are not seen (tumour, torsion). There is some doubt as to whether operating on an undescended testicle changes the rate of malignant change.

b   **False.** Undescended testes do not develop to become sperm synthesizing organs. If they have not become extra-abdominal by the age of 2 fertility will begin to be impaired. Although dysplastic, testosterone is still secreted by undescended testes, and the boy should still go into puberty.

c   **False.** Torsion of the testicle is possible if the testis can rotate around the axis of its blood vessels. It is possible because of laxity in the fixation of some individual's testes, and this may also occur with undescended testes. Torsion in a descended testicle presents with severe pain and tenderness in the hemiscrotum and a high testicle. The diagnosis is clinical but supported by Doppler ultrasound to demonstrate the lack of blood flow in the testis. Surgery to correct the torsion is accompanied by surgical fixation of both testes to prevent recurrence.

d   **False.** A testis that cannot be brought to the base of the scrotum is undescended. Retractile testicles can be brought to the base of the scrotum but also can move up to the inguinal ring.

e   **False.** With all surgery in children, timing is very important for several reasons. First, many surgical problems are congenital and correct with age. Examples include ventricular septal defect, patent ductus arteriosus, vesico-ureteric reflux, cavernous haemangiomas and undescended testes. Secondly, for non-urgent problems, a larger child is technical easier to operate on and will tolerate the procedure better. Thirdly, some operations can be delayed to avoid problems as the child grows, particularly if prosthetic devices are used. For undescended testes, there is no particular advantage with an operation under a year of age so most surgeons operate in the second year.

   6   *Abdominal pain*
      a   may be the only presenting symptom of a Meckel's diverticulum
      b   is usually colicky and localised to the left iliac fossa if a child is constipated
      c   is a common presenting feature of children with diabetic ketoacidosis
      d   is a feature of vesico-ureteric reflux
      e   is often present in children with a sickle crisis

a   **True.** Abdominal pain is another common cause for a surgical paediatric consultation. Features of a surgical cause are listed in the Box 11.1. One of the less common causes of abdominal pain is a Meckel's diverticulum. This is a remnant of the vitello-intestinal duct, where the gut lumen was formerly connected to the yolk sac as an embryo. It may contain gastric mucosa and secrete acid, causing local inflammation and bleeding.

b   **False.** Pain from the colon is typically referred to the suprapubic region because embryologically the gut is a mid-line structure. Similarly, mid-gut pain radiates to the umbilicus and stomach or duodenal pain to the epigastrium. If there

Box 11.1   Features of surgical abdominal pain

Severe, limiting mobility and play
Radiates to the back or away from the mid-line
Associated with bilious vomiting or melaena
Guarding or abdominal rigidity
Abdominal distension
Absent bowel sounds
Associated with other systemic deterioration

is extension of the problem through the layers of the gut wall, then pain is felt at the anatomical site.

c   **True**. Abdominal pain and vomiting may cause confusion in diagnosis (see question 2). Distinguishing clinical features of diabetic ketoacidosis include ketones on the breath (fetor), tachypnoea and polyuria. Diabetic ketoacidosis is discussed in the Endocrinology and metabolic disease questions 3 and 9.

d   **False**. The reflux itself does not cause any pain, but rather an associated UTI if present. Pain in UTIs is suprapubic or in the loins if there is pyelonephritis. But, as with all presentations in children, the younger the child, the more the presentation is likely to be of collapse or irritability with a UTI.

e   **True**. The abdomen is not an unusual site for a sickle crisis, and may involve the gut, other intra-abdominal organs, or the lumbar spine.

   7   A 10-month-old child presents because the mother has noticed some blood passed with a stool. This presentation would commonly be associated with
   a   haemorrhoids
   b   Henoch–Schönlein purpura
   c   intussusception early in the course of the disease
   d   a volvulus
   e   constipation in the preceding week

a   **False**. Common paediatric causes of blood in the stool are listed in Box 11.2. Haemorrhoids are extremely unusual at 10 months or at all in childhood, but are occasionally found in children with portal hypertension with portosystemic shunts.

b   **False**. Although rectal bleeding can occur with Henoch–Schönlein purpura (HSP), it is an unusual manifestation. Abdominal pain and haematuria are much more common. HSP is discussed in Haematology and oncology question 1.

c   **False**. Intussusception at first presents with colicky abdominal pain and pallor. Later, there may be vomiting, shock, and rectal bleeding. Diagnosis is clinical and supported by ultrasound or contrast studies. Barium or air can be used to visualize

---

Box 11.2   Causes of blood in the stool

Anal fissure
Rectal polyp
Intussusception
Meckel's diverticulum
Rectal or oesophageal varices

---

the intussusception and these can also reduce it without a laparotomy. If this does not work, open reduction is necessary.

d   **True.** Volvulus with ischaemia causes rectal bleeding in the same manner as with an intussusception.

e   **True.** Constipation leading to an anal fissure is the commonest cause of this presentation. A fissure may be visible or be within the anal canal. A 'sentinel pile' may also be seen, which is a mound of oedematous skin distal to the fissure. Treatment of the constipation with stool softeners, laxatives, and behavioural changes will lead to healing of the fissure.

> 8   *An antenatal scan at 36 weeks has confirmed the presence of an umbilical abnormality involving the gut. Following delivery*
>   a   chromosome studies will be needed for infants with exomphalos
>   b   a gastroschisis will lose large volumes of fluid
>   c   an exomphalos may be found to contain the liver
>   d   there is likely to be ischaemia of the gut in an exomphalos
>   e   the gastroschisis must be repaired immediately

a   **True.** There are two congenital umbilical abnormalities—gastroschisis and exomphalos. Their differences and similarities are listed in Box 11.3. Thirty-five per cent of infants born with exomphalos have associated abnormalities—mostly cardiac, renal, or chromosomal defects. Gastroschisis is a more serious condition in terms of the surgery and future of the gut, but is usually an isolated defect.

Box 11.3   Gastroschisis and exomphalos

Gastroschisis	Exomphalos
No associations	Associated with chromosomal anomalies
Contains bowel only	May contain other organs
Always on the right of umbilicus	In the cord
Uncovered	Covered by membrane
Rapid development of shock after birth	No major early problems
Antenatal α-feto protein raised	No raised α-feto protein

---

b   **True**. Infants born with a gastroschisis rapidly become cold and shocked because of heat and water loss from the defect as there is no covering membrane for the gut. Before surgery, the lesion should be covered in plastic film to reduce evaporation and heat loss. Colloid should be given.

In contrast, infants with exomphalos will not be similarly compromised as a result of the lesion, because the lesion is covered with the membrane of the cord and peritoneum. This membrane becomes thickened and less permeable rapidly after birth.

c   **True**. Depending on its size an exomphalos may contain gut, liver, or spleen. These structures herniate through the umbilical ring and into the cord in the mid-line. Gastroschisis, however, only ever contains gut and is always on the right of the umbilicus.

d   **False**. The opening into the exomphalos is usually large. With a gastroschisis, it is narrow and there may be obstruction to blood flow leading to ischaemia and infarction of sometimes large segments of gut. This often leads to short gut syndrome or gut motility problems.

e   **True**. Urgent surgery is important to reduce fluid and heat loss and prevent infection, as well as preserving the circulation of the gut. Exomphalos lesions should also be corrected early, but there is not the same urgency.

9   *The following features favour the diagnosis of pyloric stenosis rather than another cause of vomiting in an infant of 6 weeks*
   a   the vomiting has gradually worsened since birth
   b   vomiting occurs up to 4 h after each feed
   c   the infant is hungry
   d   the abdomen is distended
   e   weight gain of 900 g since birth

a   **False**. Infants commonly vomit and there is usually no underlying cause. The commonest aetiologies are overfeeding, gastro-oesophageal reflux (GOR), sepsis, pyloric stenosis (PS), and other causes of obstruction. These can usually be differentiated on history alone.

The onset of vomiting is particularly helpful. A gradual increase since birth is suggestive of GOR or overfeeding, but an acute onset of vomiting suggests sepsis, PS, or obstruction.

Male sex (85%), family history (20%), and being the first child raise the chance of having PS.

b   **False**. How the vomiting relates to feeding can also help. Vomiting soon after a feed suggests GOR, overfeeding, or PS, but vomiting later sepsis or obstruction. A test feed can be given to look for visible peristalsis and observe the vomiting. Babies with PS typically have 'projectile' vomiting, but those with GOR can also have forceful vomiting. Vomiting over the face is probably possetting.

c   **True**. A detailed feeding history (what milk, how much, and how often) is also vital. Poor feeding, with low volumes taken suggests sepsis or obstruction, whereas infants with PS are typically hungry. Large volumes of formula milk will be found in overfed babies. It is almost impossible to overfeed a breast-fed a baby. A normal infant will take about 150 ml/kg per day of feed (6 ml/kg per h) in boluses every 2–4 h.

d   **False**. Children normally have a distended abdomen for the first few years, only developing a more 'adult' flat abdomen after 3 years. This is particularly true in the young infant and due to the small size of the abdomen and the bladder, liver, and spleen are pushed into the abdomen. Infants with PS typically have a scaphoid or empty abdomen. They may also be dehydrated with a hypokalaemic metabolic alkalosis. These results are discussed in Nephrology question 11.

e   **False**. A weight gain about 10 g/kg per day is normal in early infancy, so this child is thriving, and makes any dehydration unlikely. Such a weight gain is against PS, where infants are often losing weight and thin at presentation.

10   *A term male infant of 36 h is admitted to the neonatal unit because of poor feeding. After a normal delivery, with no resuscitation, the infant has fed poorly and has been vomiting yellow-green liquid since about 6 h of age. He has yet to pass meconium. Examination finds a dehydrated infant with a distended abdomen and an umbilical hernia. An abdominal X-ray shows distended loops of bowel. This presentation's cause*

   a   is a delayed onset of peristalsis in the majority of cases
   b   could be a volvulus
   c   is likely to be the umbilical hernia
   d   may be pyloric stenosis
   e   may well be necrotizing enterocolitis

a   **False**. This presentation is strongly suggestive of a surgical cause. Bilious vomiting, no meconium passage (normally passed on the first day), and abdominal distension can be caused by atresiae or stenoses, meconium ileus, Hirschsprung's disease, or malrotation. However, duodenal obstruction does not normally cause abdominal distension and the presentation is a little early for large bowel obstructions to present. Occasionally, a plug of meconium prevents emptying of the bowel, leading to large bowel obstruction.

   Intravenous fluids and gastric aspiration are always needed to support the infant while investigations with plain X-rays and contrast studies are performed.

   X-rays can be characteristic—pneumatosis intestinalis or air in the biliary tree with necrotizing enterocolitis (NEC), and the 'double bubble' in infants with duodenal atresia.

b   **True**. A malrotation progressing to a volvulus is a possible cause of his presentation. This is discussed above in question 2.

c   **False**. In contrast to inguinal or femoral hernias, umbilical hernias very rarely obstruct.

d   **False.** Bile-stained vomitus implies the obstruction is below the pancreas making PS and duodenal atresia unlikely. Also he is too young to present with PS. This typically presents between 3 and 9 weeks. Quite why this is this is not known, although PS has a strong genetic component.

e   **False.** It is only very slight possibility in a term infant. It is a major cause of mortality and morbidity in the infant under 32 weeks. NEC typically presents with abdominal distension and feed intolerance or with circulatory collapse with multisystem failure. It is thought to be caused by gut ischaemia and so is associated with asphyxia, intrauterine growth retardation, and possibly umbilical vessel cannulation. Early feeding with formula milk increases the chance of NEC, while breast milk seems to have a relatively protective effect.

11   The following conditions should be operated on urgently
    a   umbilical herniae
    b   gastroschisis
    c   ventricular septal defect
    d   talipes equino-varus
    e   laryngeal stenosis

a   **False.** For reasons discussed above (question 3), there is no danger in leaving an umbilical hernia to close spontaneously. If it has not closed and the child is becoming embarrassed by it (particularly at school age), surgery can be considered.

b   **True.** As outlined in question 8, early surgery is important in the management of infants with gastroschisis.

c   **False.** Surgery for this condition is delayed until the child is at least 9 months to 2 years if possible. Surgery is considered earlier if the baby is unable to thrive despite maximal diuretic therapy and if pulmonary hypertension is developing. This condition is discussed in Heart disease question 2.

d   **False.** Here, surgery to correct this abnormality is often avoided by strapping the ankle so that bony growth correct the defect. This is further discussed in Rheumatology and orthopaedics question 6.

e   **False.** Again time improves this lesion as the infant grows.

12   When examining a child
    a   a large olive-shaped mass is easily felt in the epigastrium of children with pyloric stenosis
    b   divarification of the rectus abdominalis muscles is normal in a newborn
    c   it can be normal for the testes to be impalpable at birth
    d   a palpable sigmoid colon is found in children with constipation
    e   a rectal examination is useful if intussusception is a possibility

a   **False.** It is difficult to feel the typical olive-shaped mass, and if felt it is usually in the right upper quadrant. By administering a test feed visible peristalsis can be seen and the vomiting can also be observed. However, an empty abdomen makes the mass easier to feel.

b   **True.** In the same way that its mother's rectus abdominalis muscles separated during pregnancy to accommodate the uterus, so the infant is born with separated recti. When a newborn cries, a bulge can be seen in the mid-line in the epigastrium. This closes during the first months.

c   **False.** It is not normal, and such an infant should be closely followed. This is discussed further in question 5.

d   **True.** As in constipated adults, the sigmoid colon thickens and enlarges when it is overfilled with hard stool. This can easily be felt in the left iliac fossa. Constipation is discussed in Gastroenterology question 8.

e   **True.** Rectal bleeding is an indication for a rectal examination as the tip of an intussusception or a polyp may be felt. Other abdominal signs of intussusception include an empty right iliac fossa and a sausage-shaped mass in anywhere except the right iliac fossa and the umbilical region.

13   *The diagnosis of tracheo-oesophageal fistula*

a   may present as recurrent aspiration
b   may be suspected if there is oligohydramnios
c   usually prevents passage of a gastric tube
d   is suggested in a 'mucusy' newborn
e   is commonly associated with cardiac defects

a   **True.** Tracheo-oesophageal fistula (TOF) is a disorder of the separation of the trachea and oesophagus as an embryo. There are five different subtypes (see Box 11.4), and their presentation depends on the exact anatomical defect. The most unusual type is the 'H-type' TOF, where there is a small fistula between otherwise normal trachea and oesophagus. The only problem that this abnormality causes is feed aspiration when the infant swallows or refluxes.

b   **False.** TOF is one cause of polyhydramnios (other causes include twin pregnancy, diabetic mother, Down's syndrome, and neuromuscular disorders affecting

---

Box 11.4   Types of tracheo-oesophageal fistula (TOF)/oesophageal atresia (OA)

1	OA	distal TOF
2	OA	no TOF
3	no OA	H-type TOF
4	OA	proximal TOF
5	OA	proximal and distal TOF

swallowing). This is because fetuses with TOF usually have disordered swallowing or oesophageal atresia. The inability to swallow leads directly to polyhydramnios.

Oligohydramnios is associated with poor urine production by the fetus—found when there is renal tract anomalies or severe placental insufficiency.

c **True**. A 'mucusy' baby has bubbly mucus in its mouth after delivery that continues to reaccumulate despite suctioning. This suggests that the oesophagus is not allowing the swallowing of saliva. Such a baby must have the possibility of a TOF excluded, although a neuromuscular problem is another possibility.

Before any definitive procedure to close the TOF or anastomose the oesophageal atresia, unswallowed saliva needs to be removed continually using Replogle tube, which can sit in the oesophageal pouch. As it has a double lumen, one lumen can be on low pressure continuous suction while the other is open to the air, so that the catheter does not get stuck to the oesophageal wall.

d **True**. Failure of a gastric tube to pass is a useful bedside test for a TOF, although the 'H-type' fistula will of course not obstruct the gastric tube. By using a radio-opaque tube, a chest X-ray can be performed with the gastric tube as far down as possible. This confirms that the tube is in the oesophagus and demonstrates the level of obstruction.

e **True**. Although it may be an isolated defect, it also forms part of the VATER (Vertebral anomalies, Anal anomalies, Tracheo-Esophageal fistulae, Renal, and Radial) and other associations. Both of these incorporate ventricular septal defects (see Heart disease question 13i).

12 Dermatology

Questions

1 **Atopic dermatitis (eczema)**
   a commonly the affects the cheeks of infants
   b is commonly associated with asthma
   c depigments the skin of Afro-Caribbean children
   d may be complicated by staphylococcal superinfection
   e rarely presents under 1 year of age

2 *A girl of 4 is brought to her family doctor because of her itchy skin. Her mother says she is always scratching at her elbows and behind her knees, and it keeps her awake at night. Examining her, the doctor finds that she has scaly, excoriated, and lichenified erythematous areas in both antecubital fossae and popliteal fossae. It would be appropriate for the doctor to*
   a prescribe emollients for the bath
   b start her on oral steroids
   c advise that pets be removed from the house
   d bandage the affected areas at night
   e prescribe chlorphiramine to help nocturnal symptoms

3 *A 3-year-old boy is examined by the community medical officer as he has itchy skin. After examining him, the doctor decides that*
   a because he has asthma, eczema is more likely
   b as the rash has been present for only a week, it is likely to be urticaria
   c he has involvement of the face, which makes chickenpox unlikely
   d the excoriated papules and erythema on the hands and feet are suggestive of scabies
   e he should be treated with topical steroids whatever the diagnosis

4 **Cavernous haemangiomas**
   a are also known as port wine stains
   b may not develop until after birth
   c may cause thrombocytopenia
   d can be treated with laser therapy
   e occur predominantly in the sacral area

5   *Seborrhoeic dermatitis (cradle cap)*
   a can be treated with aqueous cream
   b typically presents at about 6 months
   c often causes nappy rash
   d can become superinfected
   e can be treated with topical steroids

6   *A 3-month-old infant has nappy rash. It is likely that*
   a he has candidal involvement because there are satellite lesions
   b he has ammoniacal dermatitis as there is mainly involvement of the creases
   c there will probably be scarring
   d if there is a severe rash with bleeding he is likely to be iron deficient
   e there will be improvement will barrier cream if the rash predominantly affects the buttocks, but spares the creases

7   *The paediatrician is called to see a newborn baby, born at 42 weeks gestation, now 14 h old. The mother is concerned about abnormalities on her baby's skin. The doctor would be correct in saying that*
   a it is not erythema toxicum because the baby is otherwise well
   b the capillary haemangiomas around the bridge of the nose are likely to fade
   c it is too young for eczema to present
   d the white spots on the nose are probably milia
   e cracks in the skin of the hands and feet require moisturizing cream to aid resolution

8   *Henoch–Schönlein purpura*
   a is caused by platelet deficiency
   b typically affects the buttocks, arms, and legs
   c is associated with parvovirus B19
   d needs follow-up because there may be long-term arthropathy
   e should be treated with corticosteroids

Answers

There are several very common conditions peculiar to paediatrics in this sub-speciality. Rashes and blemishes are also a particular focus of concern by the parents and a common cause of consultation. So revising for dermatology must combine a knowledge of the clinical features and appropriate management of the common conditions: atopic dermatitis or eczema, the rashes associated with infectious diseases, nappy rash, and birth marks. Those associated with infectious disease are covered in that chapter (Immunology and infectious diseases), but the other topics are included here. As a quick guide, some of the rashes are listed under various categories in Box 12.1.

Box 12.1   Common rashes

Erythematous
Acute	Measles, rubella, erythema infectiosum, exanthem subitum
	Scarlet fever, staphylococcal scalded skin syndrome
	Early meningococcal septicaemia
Acute with vesicles	Varicella, herpes
Non-infectious	Juvenile rheumatoid arthritis
	Kawasaki disease
Chronic	Eczema
	Psoriasis
	Fungal infection
	Scabies
	Contact dermatitis
	Urticaria

Purpuric
Acute	Henoch–Schönlein purpura
	Meningococcal septicaemia
	Vasculitis
	Venous obstruction (pertussis, strangulation)
Chronic	Immune thrombocytopenic purpura and other causes of low platelets

---

1 Atopic dermatitis (eczema)
  a commonly the affects the cheeks of infants
  b is commonly associated with asthma
  c depigments the skin of Afro-Caribbean children
  d may be complicated by staphylococcal superinfection
  e rarely presents under 1 year of age

a **True.** Eczema (atopic eczema or atopic dermatitis) affects different areas of the body depending on the age of the child. It is rare for eczema to present under the age of 2 months, although it is often confused with seborrhoeic dermatitis. At first there is involvement of the cheeks and the nappy area, progressing to the extensor surfaces of the limbs and finally the flexures after about the age of 2.

b **True**. Eczema has several well known associations with other atopic conditions (asthma, hay fever, urticaria). In all of these conditions, IgE levels will be high and there will be a reaction to a number of common allergens (house dust mite, pollen).

c **True**. Post inflammatory depigmentation affects all races, but it is more noticeable in dark-skinned children, and persists for many months after the initial problem. This may be commonly noticed after eczema exacerbations, impetigo (*Staphylococcus aureus* skin infection), and chickenpox.

The other changes found in the skin of children with atopic eczema are lichenification, a thickening due to scratching, excoriation, and dryness, affecting most of the body.

d **True**. The skin of children with eczema is conducive to bacterial growth. There are breaks in the epithelial layer allowing the entry of organisms and exudates that provide a nutrient medium. Skin swabs from children with eczema often grow *Staph. aureus*, *streptococcus*, and other organisms. These often do not cause any problems, but can cause a severe skin infection. Eczema herpeticum is another superinfection of eczema, caused by *herpes simplex* and varicella herpetiformis, which is chickenpox in a child with eczema. These conditions require admission and antimicrobial agents.

e **False**. Asthma tends not to present before 12 months and eczema not before 2 months. Hay fever presents after 4 years. The reason for this difference in timing is not known.

2 *A girl of 4 is brought to her family doctor because of her itchy skin. Her mother says she is always scratching at her elbows and behind her knees, and it keeps her awake at night. Examining her, the doctor finds that she has scaly, excoriated, and lichenified erythematous areas in both antecubital fossae and popliteal fossae. It would be appropriate for the doctor to*

a prescribe emollients for the bath
b start her on oral steroids
c advise that pets be removed from the house
d bandage the affected areas at night
e prescribe chlorphiramine to help nocturnal symptoms

a **True**. In this question, the doctor is asked to manage the eczema with a particular emphasis on her nocturnal itching. Eczema is almost always associated with dry skin. This helps distinguish it from other forms of dermatitis, such as contact dermatitis. The first step in managing a patient with eczema is moisturising their skin. This may be achieved by using bath oils (e.g. Balneum), aqueous creams, and ointments, which are more waxy. Creams are easier to apply, but the effect is more short lived. At this stage, avoidance of soaps, detergents, and of clothes made of wool next to the skin should be discussed.

b **False**. Oral steroids would be effective at reducing the inflammation, but inappropriate. The commonest indications for oral steroids in paediatrics are nephrotic syndrome, malignancy, and during asthma exacerbations.

Topical steroids, however, are of great benefit. Agents such as 1% hydrocortisone should be used sparingly on inflamed areas, and a lower strength used for the face. More potent steroids can be used during exacerbations.

c   **False**. If skin allergen testing is undertaken, there is usually an excessive reaction to a number of ubiquitous allergens, so this rarely helps management. Although pets may produce some of these allergens, their removal is very unlikely to improve the eczema but will certainly cause much distress to the child. The only indication for this advice is when there is a clear history of asthma exacerbation due to the pet.

There has been some debate on the importance of exposure to cow's milk protein to eczema. Some children have found benefit from a cow's milk protein-free diet, but many others have not. If this is considered a dietician needs to be involved to maintain adequate nutrient intake. There is no conclusive evidence that breast feeding reduces the incidence of eczema.

d   **True**. Occlusive dressings can be useful to break the cycle of itchiness causing scratching leading to further itchiness. The pathophysiological basis for this is in cytokine (especially histamine) release from mast cells. Other occlusive measures include using tight fitting clothes and soft gloves for sleeping.

e   **True**. For any chronic illness, there must be a balance between effective treatment and side-effects. For a non-life-threatening condition such as eczema, topical agents are thus preferred or those relatively free of side-effects.

In eczema an exception to this principle are antihistamine agents. Chlorpheniramine (Piriton) is available over the counter in many countries as it is an effective antihistamine and its only side-effect (drowsiness) can be quite useful. In children with eczema the nocturnal itch keeps the child and parents awake, and this agent can be of great benefit. The only other time the oral route is used for eczema is when there is super-infection.

   3   *A 3-year-old boy is examined by the community medical officer as he has itchy skin. After examining him, the doctor decides that*
      a   because he has asthma, eczema is more likely
      b   as the rash has been present for only a week, it is likely to be urticaria
      c   he has involvement of the face, which makes chickenpox unlikely
      d   the excoriated papules and erythema on the hands and feet are suggestive of scabies
      e   he should be treated with topical steroids whatever the diagnosis

a   **True**. Itchy rashes in childhood may be either infective or 'allergic'. For the skin to become itchy, the must be a release of cytokines, especially histamine in the skin. This may be either directly from mast cells as occurs in eczema and urticaria, or from another cell type as in contact dermatitis. Inflammation in the skin from another cause, such as infection or even scratching itself can also cause itch. Chickenpox and scabies are good examples of this, but other lesions, such as staphylococcal skin infections and cellulitis are less itchy.

Identifying the cause of the itch is vital to its treatment. Clues may be obtained from the family history (atopy), contacts (chickenpox and scabies), past medical history (atopy), and social history (as scabies is associated with deprivation).

b   **False**. Urticaria typically comes and goes over minutes and hours. Large and dramatic weals may appear and are itchy. Atopic individuals are affected. There may be a history of the weals being triggered by some foodstuff, such as eggs and peanuts. Apart from avoidance of a causative substance, no specific treatment is usually appropriate as the lesions are too short lived, although if persistent, anti-histamines can be used.

c   **False**. Chickenpox particularly affects the face and trunk, and less so the arms. The characteristic of the rash is that it may appear as vesicles, pustules, and crusting all in the same area. It is also very itchy and so is excoriated. This needs no specific treatment in immunocompetent children, but zoster immunoglobulin and acyclovir should be given to immunocompromised children to reduce mortality. Calamine lotion is effective at reducing itch, and antihistamine sedatives can help sleep.

d   **True**. Scabies is caused by a burrowing insect. It avoids the head, except in infancy, and prefers the skin between the fingers and toes, in the groin and axillae, although it can be found anywhere. There may be characteristic burrows and the offending organism can be isolated from skin scrapings and viewed under a microscope. To treat effectively, the whole family need to be bathed in a medical insecticide and all the bedding and clothes in the house washed at once. As it is a very infectious disease, reinfection around the family is common, and it is more common in situations of poverty and overcrowding.

e   **False**. Steroids are not always appropriate for skin disorders! The main paediatric indications for topical steroids are eczema, seborrhoeic dermatitis, and ammoniacal nappy rash when the condition has not responded to first-line treatment.

4   *Cavernous haemangiomas*
   a   are also known as port wine stains
   b   may not develop until after birth
   c   may cause thrombocytopenia
   d   can be treated with laser therapy
   e   occur predominantly in the sacral area

a   **False**. One of the problems with skin lesions is that they are often known by several different names. A port wine stain is a large capillary haemangioma, and if in the correct area, be part of the Sturge—Weber syndrome. This is discussed in Neurology question 6. 'Stork marks' are also capillary haemangiomas but smaller, found on the back of the neck or around the eyes. Those around the eyes typically fade as the child ages, but those on the neck usually persist. Strawberry naevi are cavernous haemangiomas. Milk spots are better known as milia and are white papules on the nose and face. Miliaria are white vesicles on a red background on the face and upper trunk.

b   **True**. A few cavernous haemangiomas are present at birth and the rest develop later. Whenever they present, they are sure to grow larger relative to the infant over the first 9–12 months, during which time they are bright red (strawberry) in colour. They then gradually infarct causing them to become darker and in the centre, paler. They then gradually shrink relative to the child and eventually disappear by the age of 5 leaving no scar. As they infarct there may be ulceration in the centre.

c   **True**. This is one of the complications of cavernous haemangiomas, caused by platelet consumption within a large lesion. Large or multiple cavernous haemangiomas can cause high output cardiac failure being full of arteriovenous shunts. Smaller lesions, if critically placed also lead to complications, and would merit surgical removal. This would be if they obstruct vision causing amblyopia (where the cortical pathways for vision do not develop secondary to lack of visual stimulus), or if a haemangioma obstructs the airways. Systemic steroids are also used to reduce the size of the lesions.

d   **False**. As outlined above, these lesions rarely require any treatment. Laser therapy can only be used to treat superficial lesions—capillary haemangiomas in particular.

e   **False**. They can be found anywhere on the body, whereas Mongolian blue spots, hairy patches, and pigmented areas are found more frequently in the sacral area.

   5   *Seborrhoeic dermatitis (cradle cap)*
         a   can be treated with aqueous cream
         b   typically presents at about 6 months
         c   often causes nappy rash
         d   can become superinfected
         e   can be treated with topical steroids

a   **True**. Seborrhoeic dermatitis is a skin condition in which there are thick greasy flakes on an erythematous background. It predominantly affects the scalp. This may give the appearance of dryness. At first simple emollient creams can be used and then mild corticosteroids. It is not always necessary to treat this rash as it always resolves with time and rarely causes any problem for the infant as it does not itch.

b   **False**. The timing of various skin lesions appearance is useful in making a diagnosis. Birth marks (see Box 12.2) are either present at birth or appear soon after, such as cavernous haemangiomas. There are various rashes and skin conditions that appear in the neonatal period and fade soon after, such as erythema toxicum. Eczema does not usually present until 2 months of age at the earliest.

Box 12.2   Birth marks

Milia
Milaria
Capillary haemangioma
Cavernous haemangioma
Mongolian blue spot

---

c   **True.** This is one of the four common causes of nappy rash as discussed in question 6. Other sites that are commonly affected include the scalp, forehead, face, and axillae.

d   **True.** Cracks between the flakes can open up the skin and allow organisms into the skin. There will be an exudate with crusting and erythema. Local lymph nodes may become enlarged especially around the ear. Antibiotics will be required.

e   **True.** Topical steroids are only of use on their own if there is inflammation without infection. In children this mainly means eczema, seborrhoeic dermatitis, and resistant ammoniacal nappy rash.

6   *A 3-month-old infant has nappy rash. It is likely that*
    a   he has candidal involvement because there are satellite lesions
    b   he has ammoniacal dermatitis as there is mainly involvement of the creases
    c   there will probably be scarring
    d   if there is a severe rash with bleeding he is likely to be iron deficient
    e   there will be improvement will barrier cream if the rash predominantly affects the buttocks, but spares the creases

a   **True.** There are four common types of nappy rash. *Candida* can cause a severe rash, which typically has satellite spots just outline the edge of the main area of involvement. This is not a manifestation of immunodeficiency (although the neonate is relatively immunodeficient), rather, the moist environment of the nappy allows the infection to develop. It is treated with topical antifungal agents, such as nystatin or miconazole (Daktarin). There is often oral candidiasis in the same baby, which will also need treatment.

b   **False.** This is the commonest type of nappy rash. Ammoniacal, or irritant nappy rash is caused by the effect of ammonia produced by urea-splitting bacteria on the skin. The rash is worst at the sites of contact with urine, on the buttocks, and other convex areas under the nappy. The creases are spared. This rash is exacerbated by prolonged contact with urine, and is associated with neglect. It is treated by separating skin and urine, which can be achieved with barrier cream or by keeping the nappy off.

c   **False**. Scarring occurs if the epidermis is entirely obliterated in an area. Therefore, nappy rash will not scar unless it is extremely severe.

d   **False**. Zinc deficiency causes a widespread rash, worse in the nappy area. On the other hand, Iron deficiency will cause anaemia, and is also thought to cause intellectual defects even before anaemia develops.

Much more common are the other types of nappy rash, associated with seborrhoeic dermatitis and eczema. These are worse in the creases and there are signs elsewhere on the body of the disease. After encouraging frequent nappy changing and periods without a nappy, they can be treated with emollients and mild topical steroids.

e   **True**. This is suggestive of ammoniacal dermatitis, and so barrier cream should work.

> 7   *The paediatrician is called to see a newborn baby, born at 42 weeks gestation, now 14 h old. The mother is concerned about abnormalities on her baby's skin. The doctor would be correct in saying that*
>
> a   it is not erythema toxicum because the baby is otherwise well
> b   the capillary haemangiomas around the bridge of the nose are likely to fade
> c   it is too young for eczema to present
> d   the white spots on the nose are probably milia
> e   cracks in the skin of the hands and feet require moisturizing cream to aid resolution

a   **False**. Despite its worrying name (also called toxic erythema and erythema toxicum neonatorum), this is an entirely benign condition. It typically appears in the first few days of life. It is found on the trunk and limbs and there are diffuse erythematous areas with central white spots. These very much look like pustules, hence the name of the condition. The characteristic feature of this condition is that the lesions may come and go over several hours. No treatment is required.

b   **True**. However, haemangiomas on the back of the neck are likely not to fade.

c   **True**. This disease will not be present at birth.

d   **True**. Milaria and milia are both present on the skin of the newborn. Milia are the white spots on the nose and face whereas milaria are white vesicles with an erythematous background on the upper part of a baby's body. This is further covered in question 4.

e   **False**. Although often used, these creams are of no benefit. The skin of a postmature neonate has no vernix and is very dry superficially. There is cracking of the skin, particularly of the hands and feet and there may be bleeding. The problem usually resolves in the first 2 weeks.

8   *Henoch–Schönlein purpura*

   a   is caused by platelet deficiency
   b   typically affects the buttocks, arms, and legs
   c   is associated with parvovirus B19
   d   needs follow-up because there may be long-term arthropathy
   e   should be treated with corticosteroids

a   **False.** Henoch–Schönlein purpura (HSP) is, as its name suggests a purpuric skin rash, and is caused by a vasculitis. It is found most on the buttocks and legs, but may spread to other areas. Its distribution may help distinguish it from the purpura associated with meningococcal disease. HSP lesions are unlikely to be large and the affected child will not be as ill.

b   **True.** These are the main sites of involvement. Box 8.2 lists the common rashes and their characteristic features.

c   **False.** There are several rashes that are thought to perhaps have an infectious aetiology, which has yet to be identified. This group includes HSP and Kawasaki disease. HSP often occurs after an upper respiratory tract infection, and is more likely to occur in contacts than other children. Kawasaki disease can occur in epidemic from and there is some evidence that it may be related to bacterial toxins. Parvovirus B19 causes aplastic crises in sickle cell disease and erythema infectiosum (see Immunology and infectious diseases question 5).

d   **False.** Apart from the rash, HSP frequently causes abdominal pain and joint pain. Arthralgia with joint swelling may develop but long-term arthritis is very unusual. Intussusception can also occur as a complication of HSP. Nephritis may develop and be asymptomatic or present with hypertension, haematuria, or proteinuria. The nephritis usually resolves without specific treatment, but a proportion go on to have renal failure. Other than these problems, the disease has a benign course and can be treated conservatively. HSP is discussed in Haematology and oncology question 1.

e   **False.** Unless a complication develops, no specific treatment is needed.

13 Growth and nutrition

Knowledge—questions

1 **It is correct that**
   a human milk has a higher fat content per litre than cow's milk
   b cow's milk protein intolerance is best treated by reintroducing breast feeding
   c human breast milk contains less iron than the infant's requirements
   d the sodium concentration of formula milk is much higher than in breast milk
   e postenteritis lactose intolerance is best treated by delaying reintroduction of milk feeding

2 **When assessing a child who may have a growth disorder**
   a the supine height should be used until 2 years
   b determination of pubertal stage is not needed unless there is growth delay
   c early morning growth hormone levels should be measured in a short child
   d the bone age can be determined from the appearance of the distal radius
   e weight should only be measured before a feed

3 **Breast milk**
   a is chosen in preference to a preterm formula for infants under 30 weeks gestation
   b should be avoided during episodes of gastroenteritis
   c contains IgA
   d has a lower phosphate content than cow's milk
   e helps prevent gastroenteritis

4 **The following conditions are usually associated with normal linear growth**
   a Edward's syndrome
   b Noonan's syndrome
   c neurofibromatosis type 1
   d renal tubular acidosis
   e Sturge—Weber syndrome

5   **Failure to thrive**

   a   usually is found in infants with cyanotic heart disease
   b   is defined as a weight under the third percentile
   c   may be the presenting feature of vesico-ureteric reflux
   d   is invariable if there is less than 50% of gut length remaining after resection
   e   always occurs in patients with cystic fibrosis

6   **Feeds**

   a   supplemented with fat and carbohydrates are appropriate for infants with ventricular septal defects
   b   providing energy to 150% of recommended daily allowance improves prognosis in cystic fibrosis
   c   with a high proportion of complex carbohydrates are recommended for diabetic children
   d   should be supplemented with iron in children with sickle cell disease
   e   in children with nephrotic syndrome should be supplemented with albumin

7   **Starting an infant on solid feed**

   a   should occur early if there is breast milk insufficiency
   b   is important to prevent iron deficiency anaemia
   c   should occur after the eruption of the first teeth
   d   should be avoided if the child has a neurological swallowing problem
   e   will improve gastro-oesophageal reflux

8   **The parents of a short 7-year-old boy have been referred to the growth clinic and request that he is started on growth hormone. It is true that**

   a   the benefits of treatment must be balanced against the risk of Creutzfeldt–Jacob disease
   b   growth hormone must be given in pulses if it is to work effectively
   c   growth hormone will increase sitting height more than limb length
   d   the shorter he is the more difference growth hormone will make
   e   treatment would not be indicated unless his growth velocity were reduced

Data interpretation and reasoning—questions

9   *A 5-year-old girl has been referred to the paediatrician because she is shorter than her class peers. She was born at 39 weeks with a birth weight of 2 kg (under the third centile) and with a normal length and*

head circumference. Her weight was monitored during the first 6 months, during which time her weight crossed from the third to the 50th centile. She was then not seen again until at her school entry medical, where she was found to have a height below the third centile and weight between the 10th and 25th centiles. She is otherwise well except for asthma, which is treated with twice daily inhaled budesonide and bricanyl

a   her asthma treatment may be the cause of her poor growth
b   growth hormone deficiency is unlikely as her weight is over the 10th centile
c   intrauterine growth retardation has reduced her growth potential
d   a delayed bone age would be consistent with hypothyroidism
e   this pattern of growth is typical for Turner's syndrome

Knowledge — answers

Growth and nutrition is a particularly 'paediatric' topic that is not only very important but also a favourite for examiners. Understanding of the physiology and endocrinology of growth is vital as well as a working knowledge of how to approach a child who is too short or too tall. Fortunately, the basics are quite simple and only a few conditions need be known in detail. Adequate nutrition is required for growth, and although most children have no problem deciding how much this is, paediatricians are required to know various facts about normal nutrition. Dietary management in disease states [cystic fibrosis (CF), diabetes] has now been shown to be important in outcome, so should be understood in outline.

1   It is correct that
  a   human milk has a higher fat content per litre than cow's milk
  b   cow's milk protein intolerance is best treated by reintroducing breast feeding
  c   human breast milk contains less iron than the infant's requirements
  d   the sodium concentration of formula milk is much higher than in breast milk
  e   postenteritis lactose intolerance is best treated by delaying reintroduction of milk feeding

a   **True.** One of the areas of confusion concerns the differences between the different types of milk. This is compounded by the detail that all milk composition tables are in and the various different brands of milk that are similar but have different names. Box 13.1 hopefully helps this confusion a little. Essentially there are only four types of milk—cow's, electrolyte modified cow's, electrolyte and protein modified cow's milk, and human milk. There are also special milks such as soya milk and elemental milks. As can be see from the box cow's milk is much higher in sodium, calcium, and phosphate than human milk. Cow's milk has more protein and the protein is more casein than whey. This may be because the human infant has a relatively slow growth rate when compared with other species. Instead human milk is higher in fat and carbohydrate. Modified cow's milk attempts to make it more suitable for the human infant, first by altering the electrolyte load and then altering the casein/whey ratio.

Box 13.1   Milk types and composition

Type	$Na+$ mmol/l	$Ca2+$ mmol/l	PO_4^{3-} mmol/l	Casein %	Protein g/100 ml	Fat g/100 ml	Examples
Cow's	23	30	30	70	3.4	3.9	
Electrolyte-modified	6–10	10–15	5–7	70	1.5	3.6	SMA white cap, follow-on formulas
Electrolyte- and protein modified	6–10	10–15	5–7	40	1.5	3.6	SMA gold cap, Cow and Gate premium
Breast	6.5	8.8	4.6	40	1.3	4.2	

The fat content of human milk gradually increases during the feed, and it is thought that this leads to 'fullness' at the end of the feed. Therefore, breast-fed babies tend to have smaller and more frequent feeds than bottle-fed babies. Also the breast-fed infant can regulate its water intake by either having short watery feeds or longer fatty feeds. In hot weather this helps prevent dehydration. The bottle-fed infant should be offered water in such a situation.

b   **False**. Even though designed for the infant there are some problems with breast feeding. One problem is that unless milk is demanded, production of milk slows down and eventually stops. This can be a problem if the baby is premature, has a temporary illness, or undergoes surgery, but regular expression of milk can maintain flow.

Cow's milk protein intolerance is thought to affect 1% of infants and may present with acute or chronic diarrhoea that may be bloody, and weight loss. There may be gut protein loss. A biopsy will often show patchy villous atrophy. However, by the time it is diagnosed it will not be possible to reinitiate breast feeding as supply will have ceased. Instead a cow's milk protein-free milk such as soya milk can be used. The intolerance is usually temporary.

c   **True**. During the first 3 months there is a dramatic fall in haemoglobin and the iron liberated is used in other cells as they divide. Breast milk has little iron content and is unable to supply demand in this period. The body is also poor at absorbing the iron during this period, even when it is added artificially as is the case with formula milk. By 6 months of age the child will have exhausted most of its iron stores and then will need an alternative dietary supply. That is why solid feeds (high in iron) should be introduced before this age. Iron deficiency anaemia is further discussed in Haematology and oncology, question 10.

d   **False**. As has been discussed in (a) the sodium content is altered to make cow's milk formulae suitable for infants. This is needed because the infant's kidney cannot excrete large amounts of sodium until later in life. Current recommendations are that cow's milk should not be introduced until the child is 1 year old.

The high sodium content of cow's milk also makes it dangerous to give to a child with acute diarrhoea. Hypotonic fluid is lost in diarrhoea and rehydration with cow's milk will render the child hypertonic. The management of an infant's feeds in dehydration is further discussed in question 3.

e   **True**. Lactose is a disaccharide found in milks. Lactose intolerance commonly develops after an episode of viral gastroenteritis and lasts days to weeks. There is also developmental lactose intolerance, which is much more common in certain populations, such as Afro-Caribbeans. Both are caused by absent or low levels of lactase in the gut mucosa and as a result the gut cannot break down the lactose into glucose and galactose. The lactose is, therefore, left in the bowel lumen where it acts as an osmotic laxative. There will be diarrhoea for as long as there is lactose in the diet and stools will be positive for reducing substances.

This condition is treated by avoidance of milk or use of lactose-free milk. If the condition is temporary, they can be reintroduced later.

   2   *When assessing a child who may have a growth disorder*
       a   the supine height should be used until 2 years
       b   determination of pubertal stage is not needed unless there is growth delay
       c   early morning growth hormone levels should be measured in a short child
       d   the bone age can be determined from the appearance of the distal radius
       e   weight should only be measured before a feed

a   **True**. Assessment of growth requires accurate and reproducible measurements of height, weight, and head circumference. There may also be the need for other measures such as skinfold thickness and standing/sitting height.

The length of a child is difficult to measure. Under the age of 2 the child lies supine on a scale and with one operator holding the head to the top of the device, the distance to the foot is measured. Over the age of 2 the child must stand upright, looking forward. Pressure is applied under the mastoid processes and the height measured. A 2 year old measured lying down is about 2 cm longer than the same child standing up.

Reproducibility is the key to measurement—the same operator for a given child is much more accurate than different ones. Also, as children grow slowly, measurement more often than every 4 months is not useful.

Head circumference is routinely measured under the age of 1, and is useful to diagnose those with hydrocephalus or poor brain growth. The largest circumference of 3 attempts is taken when the tape is tightly applied around the child's head from the frontal to the occipital regions.

Both of these measures and the weight should be plotted on a growth chart to determine the pattern of growth, which is more important than the current size of the child (see question 5).

b   **False.** Following the fast growth rate during the period *in utero* and in the first year, the growth of a child slows down until puberty. During puberty there is considerable linear and muscular growth and then the epiphyses fuse. It is always important to determine the pubertal stage (see question 6 and 11 of the Endocrinology section) as growth must be interpreted in its light. For instance a short 13 year old may have delayed puberty and have plenty of growth potential or may have had a premature puberty and has now stopped growing.

c   **False.** Growth hormone (GH) and to a lesser extent triiodothyronine (T3) are the most important hormones promoting growth in the period from after 1 year to puberty. Under the age of 1 year insulin (directly stimulated by dietary intake) and also T3 are most important.

GH is not easy to measure. In common with cortisol, GH levels fluctuate during the day, and most GH is released in pulses at night. A single level will not be of great diagnostic value. A profile is better with samples every half hour, but of most practical use is the stimulation test. GH is stimulated by clonidine, hypoglycaemia (induced with insulin) and glucagon and the levels of the GH measured to see if the child has a normal response to the stimulus. Insulin stress tests are most dangerous as hypoglycaemia must be induced for the test to work.

d   **False.** The bone age is a useful investigation in the short child. It is measured by comparing the radiographic appearance of the small bones of the patient's wrist with the normal. The ossification centres appear at predictable times in normal children and so the bone age is the apparent age of the wrist bones. In a short child whose the bone age is less than the real age of the child will not have constitutional delay of growth and instead may have hypothyroidism, GH deficiency, or a medical cause for the poor growth. Catch-up growth will be possible if the problem is corrected. Conversely, if the bone age is normal for the child, a treatable cause is unlikely.

The radial head X-ray is used to diagnose and monitor the progress of children with rickets.

e   **False.** In a neonate the weight may vary by up to 100 g depending on whether the baby has just had a feed or opened its bowels or bladder. However, it is impractical to always measure a weight in the same condition. Also it should not matter. Growth takes place slowly, so if the weight is measured more often than weekly and the length more often than every 4 months changes are likely to be smaller than the errors and so be unreliable.

3   Breast milk

a   is chosen in preference to a preterm formula for infants under 30 weeks gestation
b   should be avoided during episodes of gastroenteritis
c   contains IgA
d   has a lower phosphate content than cow's milk
e   helps prevent gastroenteritis

a   **True.** There are several advantages of breast milk for pretermers and only one disadvantage, that it may be insufficient in sodium and energy content. However, breast milk will contain immunoglobulins to diseases the mother has been exposed to, and other immunologically active substances (lactoferrin, lysozyme, and the bifidus factor). Breast milk is associated with a lower incidence of necrotizing enterocolitis and also probably helps prevent other neonatal infections. Establishing breast milk feeding even for a baby who cannot suck (under 34 weeks) requires the mother to express the milk herself and many parents like participating in the care of their infant in such a direct way. When the infant begins to suck, the nipple can then be offered.

b   **False.** When a child has gastroenteritis the diarrhoea is usually due to the lack of reabsorption of intestinal juices and may also have secretory and osmotic components. The lack of reabsorption is due to direct mucosal damage, the secretion component by toxins (e.g. *Vibrio cholerae*, enteropathogenic *Escherichia coli*) and the osmotic component by lack of absorption of solutes in the diet.

Therefore, when a child has gastroenteritis, intake must aim first to replace the water and electrolytes lost in the diarrhoea. Substances that require mucosal action to digest (e.g. disaccharides) should be avoided. Instead mixtures have been developed (e.g. Electrolade, oral rehydration solution, Dioralyte) that contain sodium, potassium, and glucose with water. The glucose aids sodium absorption through the glucose – sodium cotransporter and provides energy for the mucosa.

If an infant is breast fed and develops gastroenteritis, which is less likely anyway, breast feeding should continue. The baby will alter its intake to increase the water content of the feed and decrease the fat. Additional electrolyte solution may also be needed. Antibodies and other immune substances also speed recovery.

c   **True.** This is the major immunoglobulin found in mucus secretions, and acts to prevent viral binding to the intestinal wall.. Also in breast milk are other antibacterial substances (see a), lymphocytes, and macrophages.

d   **True.** Other differences are discussed in question 1.

e   **True.** Owing to a variety of immunological factors and improved hygiene possible with breast feeding, gastroenteritis is statistically less likely in breast-fed than bottle-fed infants. This difference is particularly important in the developing world. Here the overall mortality for breast-fed infants is much lower than bottle-fed infants. This is due to a large number of factors including lack of clean water to make up a bottle, hygiene, insufficient funds to make bottle feeds to full strength, and immunological components in the breast milk. For this and other reasons, the marketing of formula feeds in the developing world is felt to be ethically un-acceptable.

4 *The following conditions are usually associated with normal linear growth*
   a Edward's syndrome
   b Noonan's syndrome
   c neurofibromatosis type 1
   d renal tubular acidosis
   e Sturge–Weber syndrome

a **False**. This question looks as though you would have needed to memorize the growth potential of all the likely syndromes that you may encounter, but if a little is known about the condition, many of the complications and the growth potential can be deduced. In general, syndromes either do nothing to your growth or reduce it. There are only a few exceptions—Marfan's and homocysteinuria, Beckwith–Weidermann (see Endocrinology questions 1 and 12), Klinefelter's, and Soto's syndrome. The latter is identified by the combination of mental retardation and excessive stature.

All chromosomal abnormalities except Klinefelter's reduce growth, as in Down's, Turner's, Edward's (trisomy 18), and Patau's (trisomy 13) syndromes. Heart defects are also usual, and there are often other characteristic features, such as the polydactyly of Patau's and the short sternum of Edward's. The characteristic of poor growth caused by a genetic defect is that it starts early *in utero* as opposed to placental nutrition deficiency, which causes late-onset intrauterine growth retardation.

b **False**. Noonan's syndrome is often thought of as 'male Turner's', but this is wrong. For a start there are females with Noonan's and the features are dif-ferent. Downsloping palpebral fissures, mild intellectual impairment, pectus excavatum, and right-sided heart lesions occur in Noonan's, whereas Turner's girls have a normal face and intelligence and the heart lesions are left sided (co-arctation and aortic stenosis). These two syndromes share a webbed neck and short stature.

Noonan's is inherited in an autosomal dominant fashion.

c **True**. Unless there is associated scoliosis, those with neurofibromatosis type 1 have normal growth. This autosomal dominant condition affects the skin (café-au-lait patches, neurofibromas), the iris (Leish nodules), and there is a tendency towards malignancy.

d **False**. Renal tubular acidosis (RTA) presents with growth failure, anorexia, and vomiting. There may also be rickets. The characteristic of RTA is an in-appropriately acidic urine in the face of a systemic acidosis. In proximal RTA, the defect is in the proximal tubule bicarbonate reabsorption and when the serum bicarbonate is low enough, the distal tubule can reabsorb the filtered bicarbonate, making the urine acid. In distal RTA this is not possible and the urine is always alkaline. Treatment is with correction of the acidosis.

e **True.** Sturge – Weber syndrome is a neurocutaneous disorder caused by meningeal angiomas and associated facial haemangiomas involving the skin of the ophthalmic division of the trigeminal nerve. There is consequently atrophy of the underlying brain with convulsions. The condition may cause reduced growth in the contralateral limbs, but overall growth is unaffected.

5 *Failure to thrive*
   a usually is found in infants with cyanotic heart disease
   b is defined as a weight under the third percentile
   c may be the presenting feature of vesico-ureteric reflux
   d is invariable if there is less than 50% of gut length remaining after resection
   e always occurs in patients with cystic fibrosis

a **False.** There is no reason why congenital cyanotic heart disease should cause failure to thrive. Growth is dependent on nutrient supply and insulin levels and not on oxygen delivery. For example, the fetus has a oxygen saturation of only about 70% and this is the period of the fastest growth.

On the other hand acyanotic congenital heart disease often impairs growth. This is discussed in Heart disease question 5.

b **False.** 'Failure to thrive' is a useful concept because it implies that the child is not reaching its growing potential. For it to have a useful definition it must not encompass those who are genetically small and are under the third centile for height or weight but growing parallel to this centile. It must also exclude those who have an acute disease that is self-resolving that can cause weight loss, such as gastroenteritis. Therefore, the most useful definition is the steady crossing of two major centiles. So a child who was just under the 97th centile for weight would be failing to thrive when he crossed the 50th centile.

c **True.** Vesico-ureteric reflux (VUR) predisposes to urinary tract infections (UTIs). In infants UTIs are difficult to diagnose and may present as diarrhoea, fever with no localizing signs, vomiting, jaundice, or failure to thrive. Most chronic paediatric conditions can present with failure to thrive, especially those involving the gut (reducing absorption), those causing recurrent infection (leads to a catabolic state and reduces intake) such as CF and immunodeficiency, those causing loss of nutrients such as protein losing enteropathy and malignancy.

However, almost half of children failing to thrive do so for psychosocial reasons, ranging from incorrect feed mixing, poor feed timing, or just neglect.

When assessing a child failing to thrive a detailed history and examination is required. A detailed feed history (type, volume, frequency, infant's behaviour) is obtained along with information about vomiting, diarrhoea, and other known disorders.

For those with a possible organic cause, a urine culture, stools for ova, cysts, and parasites, and blood for haemoglobin, iron, folate, and thyroid-stimulating should be taken with other appropriate investigations depending on the clinical assessment. If a psychosocial cause is suspected and it does not respond to advice, admission to hospital for observed feeding is usually successful at increasing weight gain.

d   **False**. Short gut syndrome is usual if the gut is less than 25% of the normal length after resection. However, some gut function is restored in the 2 years after resection and children with gut as short as 15 cm with an intact ileocaecal valve or 30 cm without it can grow normally with a special diet.

e   **False**. As with most 'always' answers, this is false, even though most children with CF do malabsorb, have a high energy expenditure and poor intake, and so fail to thrive. Some individuals are now being identified with positive sweat tests without major gut dysfunction. However, a child with chest disease that is not failing to thrive is unlikely to have CF.

6   *Feeds*
   a   supplemented with fat and carbohydrates are appropriate for infants with ventricular septal defects
   b   providing energy to 150% of recommended daily allowance improves prognosis in cystic fibrosis
   c   with a high proportion of complex carbohydrates are recommended for diabetic children
   d   should be supplemented with iron in children with sickle cell disease
   e   in children with nephrotic syndrome should be supplemented with albumin

a   **True**. Infants with acyanotic heart disease may fail to thrive because they have a poor intake (tachypnoea), poor absorption (gut oedema), and increased energy expenditure (tachypnoea, tachycardia). Diuretics can reduce these problems, but for the child to grow big enough to undergo a safe operation, energy supplementation is needed. Fat is the most concentrated feed in terms of energy content and potential effects on the heart of a high fat diet are not important in this context.

b   **True**. One of the recent advances in the care of children with CF is the improvement in their diet. If child with CF loses weight, the ability to fight the next infection is reduced and so the infection takes longer to get over. In turn this means a longer time during which the child is catabolic and not eating.
   To stop this problem developing children with CF have a high energy diet and overnight often receive gastrostomy feeds. Vitamins, particularly the antioxidant vitamin E are usually used.

c   **True**. Although it may seem wrong to give a patient with impaired carbohydrate handling a high carbohydrate diet, this is better than a fatty diet as diabetic children are likely to develop arterial disease when older. Refined sugars should be avoided as they enter and leave the circulation rapidly, and it is difficult to give insulin to balance this. Complex carbohydrates are absorbed more slowly and can be more easily matched with insulin.

d   **False**. Children with sickle disease become iron overloaded if they have repeated transfusions. The same is true of thalassaemics and results in haemosiderosis. Iron can be chelated with desferrioxamine, preventing the onset of cirrhosis, heart failure, diabetes, and other endocrine dysfunctions.

e   **False.** As discussed in Nephrology question 4, those with nephrotic syndrome lose certain proteins (albumin, complement) in the urine. The diet for such children should be low in salt and moderately water restricted. Although albumin is wasted in the urine, it cannot be replaced in the diet as protein is broken down before absorption.

> 7   *Starting an infant on solid feed*
>   a   should occur early if there is breast milk insufficiency
>   b   is important to prevent iron deficiency anaemia
>   c   should occur after the eruption of the first teeth
>   d   should be avoided if the child has a neurological swallowing problem
>   e   will improve gastro-oesophageal reflux

a   **False.** The World Health Organization (WHO) recommends that infants are breast fed for 2 years, but in the developed world this rarely happens. Weaning is the process of changing a baby form breast to another form of nutrition, be it bottled formula or solids. Although breast and bottle offer similar nutrition, solid feeds change the type of energy received (less fat, more carbohydrate), increase the iron intake and allow the baby independence from its mother.

Breast milk insufficiency is a rare (1% of mothers) disorder, but commonly the mother feels that her milk supply is not meeting the child's demands. This may be due to a variety of factors, such as poor attachment or positioning of the infant, stress or illness in the mother, and anatomical factors in the infant, such as cleft palate.

If the breastfeeding problems do not resolve with advice on positioning and technique, a bottled formula can be started as supplementation. Solid feeds should not be started until 3–4 months of age but certainly by 6 months.

b   **True.** As breast milk contains little iron and formula milk iron is not well absorbed, solid feeds are important to prevent iron deficiency anaemia. This is further discussed in question 10 of the Haematology section.

c   **False.** The first teeth to erupt are the lower first incisors, that arrive at about 6 months, to be followed by the upper first incisors at 9 months. These teeth are not needed to eat the sloppy feeds that infants are offered, but useful to chew finger foods, such as biscuits. At this time an infant is mouthing—putting everything it picks up into its mouth to feel and taste it. This process will dissolve or soften many foods.

d   **False.** Many generalized neurological problems affect swallowing. This process is mediated by cranial nerves IX and X, and is impaired in children with cerebral palsy, muscular dystrophy, and congenitally absent cranial nerves (e.g. Möbius syndrome).

Neurological swallowing problems affect both liquid and solid feeds, and often solid feeds are better tolerated than liquid ones. If the swallowing problems are such that the child is failing to thrive, a gastrostomy tube can be inserted to allow overnight feeding.

e   **True**. Gastro-oesophageal reflux is improved by prone position, thicker or more solid feeds, smaller feeds and a tighter cardiac sphincter, which can be developed with cisapride or surgery.

> 8   *The parents of a short 7-year-old boy have been referred to the growth clinic and request that he is started on growth hormone. It is true that*
>   a   the benefits of treatment must be balanced against the risk of Creutzfeldt–Jacob disease
>   b   growth hormone must be given in pulses if it is to work effectively
>   c   growth hormone will increase sitting height more than limb length
>   d   the shorter he is the more difference growth hormone will make
>   e   treatment would not be indicated unless his growth velocity were reduced

a   **False**. The GH now available is not the cadaveric hormone used up to the 1980s for the treatment of this disease but made biosynthetically.

b   **False**. Although endogenous GH is secreted in pulses particularly at night, exogenous hormone is still effective when given in a daily bolus. This is in contrast to some hormones secreted in a pulsatile fashion, such as gonadotrophin-releasing hormone (GnRH). Excess GnRH can be given to suppress the secretion of follicle-stimulating hormone and luteinizing hormone and delay the onset of precocious puberty. GH is given by subcutaneous injection.

c   **False**. GH directly causes an increase in blood glucose and the breakdown of lipids. Its main actions are indirect, acting via somatomedins synthesized in the liver such as insulin-like growth factor 1 (IGF-1). The somatomedins increase protein synthesis and cell division.

In terms of the effect on growth, the limb length is affected more than the spine length, whose growth is dependent particularly on the pubertal growth spurt.

d   **True**. As soon as GH deficiency is diagnosed, treatment should be started. This is because the increase in growth velocity brought about by the treatment will have more time to increase the final height. Also the most effect of exogenous hormone is seen when the levels are lowest—so the shortest children are likely to have the greatest effect. This is termed an asymptotic response. There is little effect on final height for short children with no GH deficiency.

e   **True**. The growth velocity is the rate of height increase per year. So at the very least two measurements 4 months apart are needed to calculate this measure. It can be used to monitor growth during childhood and when on treatment. It will distinguish between the small child growing at a normal rate and the child growing at a slow rate that may benefit from intervention. This measure is also useful in assessing thyroxine replacement treatment in hypothyroid children. A low rate of growth indicates insufficient hormone and a high rate excessive replacement (once catch-up growth is complete).

In recent years the indications for GH have broadened, perhaps related to the wider availability of the hormone. It is now thought to increase final height in Turner's syndrome, and it is being evaluated in Noonan's syndrome, intrauterine growth retardation, and chronic renal failure. It is also being used in the treatment of children with burns.

Data interpretation and reasoning—answers

9 *A 5-year-old girl has been referred to the paediatrician because she is shorter than her class peers. She was born at 39 weeks with a birth weight of 2.0 kg (under the third centile) and with a normal length and head circumference. Her weight was monitored during the first 6 months, during which time her weight crossed from the third to the 50th centile. She was then not seen again until at her school entry medical, where she was found to have a height below the third centile and weight between the 10th and 25th centiles. She is otherwise well except for asthma, which is treated with twice daily inhaled budesonide and bricanyl*

   a her asthma treatment may be the cause of her poor growth
   b growth hormone deficiency is unlikely as her weight is over the 10th centile
   c intrauterine growth retardation has reduced her growth potential
   d a delayed bone age would be consistent with hypothyroidism
   e this pattern of growth is typical for Turner's syndrome

a **False** b **False** c **False** d **True** e **False**
This child has several potential reasons for her short stature hinted at in this scenario. She was born well below the 10th centile (the definition for IUGR), but the length and head circumference are both normal. This is suggestive of placental insufficiency rather than a genetic cause for the low weight at birth, which is confirmed by the period of what appears to be catch-up growth until 6 months of age. She now presents with a low height but normal weight. This is suggestive of an endocrine cause and makes a systemic disease unlikely, as systemic diseases tend to affect weight before height. Her pattern of growth is also abnormal and constitutional delay or Turner's syndrome are unlikely. Small doses of steroids do not affect growth and such a level of topical steroids will not be causing her short stature. Furthermore, keeping her asthma under control will help her maintain growth when correctly treated. Likely causes include hypothyroidism and idiopathic GH deficiency.

Physical assessment should be used to exclude Turner's and thyroid function tests to eliminate hypothyroidism. If these are negative, a GH stimulation test can be performed. Bone age would confirm that there is an underlying disorder and would be delayed in hypothyroidism and GH deficiency

14 Community paediatrics and development

Knowledge—questions

1 *Mortality in children is*

   a most common in the first 28 days after birth
   b unlikely to be due to trauma in the 1–4 age group
   c now rarely caused by sudden infant death syndrome
   d almost never caused by congenital malformations after the age of 4
   e more likely to be due to infections than neoplasia in the first year

2 *At 3 years of age, an average child can*

   a copy a circle
   b run
   c recognize three colours
   d give their first and last name
   e take off their clothes

3 *The distraction test*

   a identifies hyperactive children
   b requires little cooperation from the child
   c should not be used in an unwell child
   d is useful from 3 months as a screening tool
   e requires three adults

4 *The following conditions are usually associated with normal neurodevelopment*

   a treated phenylketonuria
   b a balanced translocation of chromosome 21
   c Turner's syndrome
   d Marfan's syndrome
   e the VATER association

5 *The diphtheria/pertussis/tetanus vaccine*

   a is a live vaccine
   b can be given at the same time as the *Haemophilus influenzae* type B vaccine

    c should not be given to a coryzal child without a fever

    d requires further doses to increase immunity

    e should not be given to HIV-positive children

6 *A child is brought for immunization. It would be appropriate to*

    a delay administration of the vaccine because the child has a febrile illness

    b give the MMR vaccine orally

    c give BCG, MMR, polio, and diphtheria/pertussis/tetanus immunizations at the same time

    d give oral paracetamol if there is a fever after the immunization

    e administer hepatitis B vaccine to a newborn child of a woman seropositive for hepatitis B surface antigen

7 *Child sexual abuse*

    a more commonly involves boys than girls as the victim

    b often presents with deterioration in school performance

    c is the commonest cause of anal fissures

    d may present with a urinary tract infection

    e is suggested by vulval soreness

8 *Children who have been abused or neglected are more likely to be*

    a not known to health and social services

    b developmentally delayed

    c exhibiting 'frozen watchfulness'

    d born to parents who are socially disadvantaged

    e failing to thrive

9 *In a multidisciplinary child development team*

    a psychologists mainly deal with behavioural problems

    b social workers are not involved unless there are child protection issues

    c physiotherapists aim to limit deformity caused by hypertonia

    d speech therapists help manage feeding problems

    e portage is used to improve mobility

10 *School refusal*

    a is synonymous with truancy

    b often presents with abdominal pain

    c is best treated by a combination of graded return to school and anxiolytics

    d may be precipitated by an adverse life event

    e if often a manifestation of separation anxiety

11   Children in low socio-economic groups are more

a   likely to have been born prematurely
b   likely to suffer from eczema
c   likely to live in the country
d   often injured in an accident in the home
e   often breast fed

12   Current UK legislation holds that

a   children with a 'statemented' disability must attend a special school
b   children under 16 are unable to give informed consent legally
c   the child's wishes are always to be followed
d   children must never be separated from their parents
e   a child cannot be admitted against the wishes of the parents before a case conference is held

13   Routine screening of children

a   prevents amblyopia
b   is first carried out for congenitally dislocated hips at the 9-month check
c   is recommended for those at risk of iron deficiency anaemia
d   is carried out on all Afro-Caribbean infants at birth for sickle cell disease
e   for cystic fibrosis is carried out with the Guthrie card on all infants

14   The UK government's 'Health of the Nation' (1992) targets to improve the health of children include

a   reduction of the smoking prevalence in the 11–15-year-old group
b   increase uptake of *Haemophilus influenzae* type B and diphtheria/pertussis/tetanus immunizations to over 85%
c   reduce social inequality and its impact on children's health
d   reduction of the death rate from accidents in those under 15 years
e   lowering the proportion of obese children under the age of 5 years

15   In the UK, immunization

a   levels for pertussis successfully prevent disease transmission to those under 2 months
b   against polio is now not recommended
c   can prevent most secondary cases of meningococcal septicaemia
d   uptake for measles vaccine (as MMR) is only about 50%
e   is recommended at 2, 3, and 4 months for the *Haemophilus influenzae* type B vaccine

16   Toilet training children

a   is usually accomplished earlier in boys
b   is accomplished in 90% of individuals by 2 years of age in the UK

c may lead to constipation
d requires the child to speak
e is affected by spina bifida

Data interpretation and reasoning—questions

17   *A 7-year-old boy is sent for a medical review by the school doctor. His teachers are concerned that there may be a physical reason why he cannot read as well as his peers. He is good at ball sports and works well with numbers. In the past he learnt to walk at the age of 11 months but did not talk in sentences until he was over 3 years. It is possible that his problem is related to*

a global developmental delay
b cerebral palsy
c a latent squint
d his father being slow to read
e visual impairment

18   *A 5-year-old boy is seen by a community paediatrician in an enuresis clinic. He usually wets his bed two or three times each night, but has been dry during the day since he was 3 years old. A developmental inquiry reveals that he started to walk at 11 months and began to speak in sentences at the age of 3. To manage his nocturnal enuresis*

a tricyclic antidepressants can be of use
b a star chart is an effective intervention
c if he is not treated the problem is unlikely to resolve
d urinalysis will be of value to identify those with renal pathology
e a pad and bell must wake him up to be effective

19   *An 11-month-old girl is seen in the developmental clinic following delivery at 30 weeks gestation. She sat at 8 months, but is unable to crawl or pull to stand. Her mother says that she can turn to sounds and babbles 'dadadada' and 'mamamama'. She is seen to have a pincer grip and transfers cubes well, but is unable to cast objects. She can hold her own bottle, but cannot feed herself with a spoon*

a she has delayed gross motor milestones
b she should be able to understand her own name
c it will not be necessary to perform a distraction test

    d she may have Down's syndrome
    e she will not be able to pick up a raisin offered to her

20   *An 8-month-old boy has a distraction test. Although his mother reports that he understands his name and is babbling, he does not turn to the rattles during the test. A full enquiry shows that otherwise there are no areas of developmental concern. Possible explanations for these findings include*

    a the rattles used for the test were too quiet
    b the room used for the test had become too noisy
    c gentamicin therapy as a neonate
    d serous otitis media
    e kernicterus

21   *The following tests and results suggest the associated problems*

    a fragile X chromosome may explain learning difficulty in males
    b periosteal reaction suggests a previous fracture
    c Guthrie test will demonstrate a high serum phenylalanine
    d Barr bodies are diagnostic of Down syndrome
    e *Candida* on a vulval swab suggests sexual abuse

22(i)   *A 2-month-old girl is taken to the emergency department by her mother at 11 p.m., who is concerned that her child is less alert than normal, and has not fed since lunchtime. In the past she has been seen twice times in the department, with a bruise to her eye and a severe rash to her nappy area. Although she has no temperature, she seems pale and lethargic. Because of her previous admissions, there is concern that this presentation might be due to non-accidental injury. This suspicion is increased by*

    a a bruise on her forehead
    b a torn frenulum
    c retinal haemorrhage
    d a focal convulsion during examination
    e a sunken fontanelle

22(ii)   *The girl has all of these features. It would now be appropriate to*

    a arrange urgent retinal photocoagulation to prevent worsening of the retinal bleed
    b arrange an urgent outpatient appointment to coincide with a case conference
    c send the child for a head CT scan to look for a subdural haematoma

d arrange a skeletal survey
e involve the police

Knowledge — answers

This section aims to cover several different areas—development and the developmentally delayed child, immunization, screening, and child protection as well as (in the interpretation and reasoning section) look at decision making in this field. From an MCQ topic point of view, immunization must be thoroughly understood, and key developmental milestones known. As much of the work of community paediatricians involves the child with special needs or a potentially abused child, an approach to these situations should be prepared.

1 Mortality in children is
  a most common in the first 28 days after birth
  b unlikely to be due to trauma in the 1—4 age group
  c now rarely caused by sudden infant death syndrome
  d almost never caused by congenital malformations after the age of 4
  e more likely to be due to infections than neoplasia in the first year

a **True**. Reduction in morbidity and mortality can be achieved at three levels. Primary prevention prevents the disease in the first place, by immunization, prophylactic treatment, and social measures, such as reducing poverty. Secondary prevention treats the disease, minimizing its prevalence and spread and tertiary prevention reduces the effects of the disease and its complications.

The commonest time for a child to die is in the first week of life, and after that the next 3 weeks. The main causes are respiratory, prematurity, and congenital malformations, and the neonatal mortality rate (deaths under 28 days per 1000 live births) is about 5/1000 for England and Wales (1986) overall, but varies from area to area.

b **False**. In the 1—4 year group, overall mortality is 1/1000. Major causes are trauma, congenital malformations, infection, and neoplasia.

c **False**. The infant mortality rate (IMR) is the death rate under 1 year per 1000 live births and is about 9/1000 (England and Wales, 1987). This is a good indicator of the level of social disadvantage within a country, and in some developing countries is as high as 110/1000 (Pakistan, 1987). The most common causes are sudden infant death syndrome (SIDS), causing up to 25% of deaths, congenital malformations, infections, and neoplasia. A reduction in the IMR is expected following the 'back to sleep' campaign.

d **False**. Congenital malformations continue to play an important part in mortality, although after the age of 4 trauma and neoplasia are more common causes. Some congenital malformations are incompatible with life for more than a few days (e.g. Potter's syndrome, Edward's syndrome) while others only cause death after several years (e.g. storage disorders).

e   **True**. Neoplasia is an uncommon cause of death in the first year as this group of diseases usually takes some time to advance to a life-threatening stage.

The implication of these statistics is that in order to reduce childhood mortality, the most important efforts currently possible will in reducing childhood poverty, which is associated with deaths from SIDS, trauma, and infections.

2   *At 3 years of age, an average child can*
a   copy a circle
b   run
c   recognize three colours
d   give their first and last name
e   take off their clothes

a   **True**. When approaching a developmental question, the wording should be closely observed. Here the word 'average' is used, which means the mean of the population. 'Normal' is usually taken to mean within the normal range of the population. Usually, the question asked will be so clearly true or false at undergraduate level so that the different definitions of normal are unimportant.

A developmental question will often be split into the developmental 'systems' —gross motor, fine motor/vision, hearing/speech, and social. When faced with developmental data, one needs to evaluate each system separately to see if there is specific or global delay. Specific delays are usually caused by a specific problem (e.g. blindness, muscle disease), but global delay by a central brain or genetic problem. Some useful milestones are listed in Box 14.1.

All developmental milestones are simply skills along the road of gradually increasing command a child acquires over their environment. This starts by control of the proximal before the distal (eyes, then head, then arms, then trunk, then legs) before moving on to the space around (crawling, walking, running, climbing stairs, riding a bicycle, as well as communicating). Any new skill requires other skills to have already been learnt. The ability to draw a person is only acquired after the baby has learnt to fix and follow, grasp objects, and then develop a pincer grip and finally a pencil grip. Similarly, trunk and proximal muscle control will have to have been developed to allow a fine motor task to be possible. Also the timing of development in different systems is sensible—for instance an infant develops closer attachments to its carers and stranger wariness at a time when its increased mobility could get the infant into trouble.

Once a child has a pencil grip, it seems a slow process for the child to learn to draw. Copying a shape tends to occur about 6 months before the child can do the task independently. A vertical line can be copied by $2\frac{1}{2}$ years and a circle by the age of 3. Complexity also increases with age in a predicable fashion, so much so that the 'Goodenough draw-a-man' test can be used to assess development.

Box 14.1   Useful milestones (25th–75th centiles)

No head lag	3–5 months
Sitting	5–7 months
Crawling	8–10 months
Walking	11–14 months
Hopping	3–4 years
Turns to sound	4–6 months
Single words	12–15 months
Combined words	14–23 months
Fixes and follows 180°	1–3 months
Reaches for objects	3–5 months
Transfers	5–7 months
Pincer grip	7–9 months
Uses pen	18–26 months
Smiles	0–6 weeks
Stranger wariness	5–9 months
Feeds self with spoon	13–18 months
Dresses self	2–3½ years
Separates easily	2–3½ years

b   **True.** Boys tend to learn to walk and run earlier than girls. Conversely, speech and social skills are acquired faster for girls than boys. If a child is not walking by 18 months there is a reasonable chance that they have either muscle disease (Duchenne muscular dystrophy, metabolic myopathy) or a neurological problem (cerebral palsy)

c   **True.** Most children will recognize more than three colours by the age of 3, but this (and many other 'learnt' skills) depends on parental input.

d   **True.** Language development is particularly dependent on interaction with adults. The average child can say individual words by the age of 1 and put two together by 2 years. Speech then develops more rapidly. By 3 years the first and last name will be known as well as the meaning of abstract nouns like cold and tired.

Speech delay may be caused by a hearing problem (serous otitis media, sensori-neural deafness, middle ear disease) a neurological problem or a familial speech delay (see question 17).

e   **True.** Social skills are also acquired by interaction. By 18 months an average child can remove clothes, but it is another year before any are put back on and a further year (3½) before they are put on correctly!

   3   The distraction test
      a   identifies hyperactive children
      b   requires little cooperation from the child

     c should not be used in an unwell child
     d is useful from 3 months as a screening tool
     e requires three adults

a   **False.** The distraction test is used to screen for children with impaired hearing in the general population. This has a prevalence of about 3/1000 (1/1000 children are congenitally deaf), whereas in premature infants it is about 1/100 (aminoglycosides, asphyxia, meningitis). The aim is to identify those with either treatable ear disease, especially serous otitis media and those who require hearing aids. By using the distraction test, hearing disorders can be identified before a child presents with speech delay.

Hyperkinetic children are distractible and the test may not be possible for them. This term is less subjective than 'hyperactive', the description often given to boisterous children by their carers. Hyperkinetic features children include a short attention span, inability to finish a task, poor relationships with peers, and distractibility. This is similar to the term 'attention deficit disorder' (ADD) or 'attention deficit hyperactivity disorder' (ADHD). These disorders are treated by a combination of 'stimulants', such as dexamphetamine and behavioural therapy.

b   **False.** Performing a distraction test is not easy. First, you need a very quiet room, a fairly settled child and two adults in addition to the mother. The room should ideally be relatively free of visual distractions. First, the child is distracted by a silent toy held in front of him which is then hidden behind the 'distracter's' back. While the child is looking to see where the toy has gone, the 'tester' makes sounds 1 m away from the child's ear on one side or the other and on the level of the ear, but without allowing the child to see what is making the noise. The child should turn immediately to the side of the noise to pass the test. Carefully selected noises are used to evaluate the hearing as fully as the test allows. Nuffield or Manchester rattles give specific volumes and frequencies, and 'OOOOO' and 'SSSSS' sounds can also be used to evaluate the response to low and high frequency speech, respectively.

Because of these considerations, the child is required to cooperate with the test. If this is not going to be possible, or the hearing of an at-risk neonate is to be evaluated, other techniques can be used, such as auditory evoked responses (AER). This test measures the electrical response in the brainstem using skin electrodes following pulsed sounds delivered to the ear. Oto-acoustic emissions (OAEs) also check the function of the ear and its neural pathways without the need for cooperation. The organ of corti is an active sensory organ in that it has muscles that contract in response to sounds of different frequencies. This contraction is transmitted back through the middle ear and can be picked up using a sensitive microphone in the external canal. So OAEs can confirm the integrity of the conductive and sensory pathways.

c   **True.** An unwell child is less likely to turn reliably to the sounds and will give a false positive result. So too will a child with otitis media, where there is a temporary reduction in hearing.

d   **False.** To respond to a distraction test, an infant must be able to sit up supported and have full head control. Not all infants of 3 months can do this (see Box 14.1). Also the test is designed to identify those who cannot lateralize sounds (perhaps because of a treatable hearing problem). Again, most infants at 3 months will not be able to turn to sounds.

e   **True.** See part b.

> **4   *The following conditions are usually associated with normal neurodevelopment***
> a   treated phenylketonuria
> b   a balanced translocation of chromosome 21
> c   Turner's syndrome
> d   Marfan's syndrome
> e   the VATER association

a   **True.** Wherever possible developmental delay should be anticipated, enabling early intervention and maximization of developmental potential. Some conditions are easy to predict—for instance Down's or Edward's syndrome will always have delayed development. However, development is dependent on a variety of factors in addition to the diagnosis.

Phenylketonuria is an inherited (autosomal recessive) defect either in the enzyme phenylalanine hydroxylase or its cofactor used in the conversion of phenylalanine to tyrosine. This leads to accumulation of phenylalanine in the blood and this is excreted as phenylpyruvic acid in the urine. This leads to severe mental retardation if treatment is not instituted. If the disease is diagnosed early (using the Guthrie card) normal neurodevelopment can be expected. Treatment involves exclusion of phenylalanine from the diet (in protein). After the age of 5 years the diet can be relaxed in some patients until a pregnancy is planned by the patient.

The other cause of developmental delay dependent on early treatment is hypothyroidism. This affects 1/4000 infants, whereas phenylketonuria only affects 1/10 000. Hypothyroidism is further discussed in Endocrinology and metabolic disease questions 4, 5, and 14.

b   **True.** Trisomy of chromosome 21 produces Down's syndrome. Also 5% of children with Down's have a unbalanced translocation of a part of 21 to another of the chromosomes, in addition to the two normal chromosome 21s. This results in the Down's phenotype. About half of these are new mutations but 50% are born to developmentally normal mothers with a balanced translocation of a part of chromosome 21. This means that a part of one chromosome 21 has been moved to another chromosome (typically 13, 14, or 15) and a part of that chromosome returned to 21. As the complement of genetic material is normal, there are no features of Down's. However, during meiosis, the chromosomes can separate to produce gametes that either have too much chromosome 21, too little, are normal, or also carry the translocation. Those with too much chromosomal material develop as children with Down's syndrome.

Features of Down's syndrome are listed in Box 14.2.

Box 14.2   Features of Down and Turner's syndromes

Down's	Turner's
Epicanthic folds	
Upslanting eyes	
Brushfield spots	Webbed neck
Flat nasal bridge	Wide-spaced nipples
Low set simple ears	
Microcephally	
3rd fontanelle	
Protruding tongue	
Hypotonic	
Single palmar crease	Lymphoedema of the feet and hands
Sandle gap in toes	Wide carrying angle
Septal anomalies in heart	Coarctation and AS
Gut atresia	Horseshoe kidney
Short stature	Short stature

---

c   **True.** Turner's syndrome is usually associated with normal intelligence and development. Other features are listed in Box 14.2.

d   **True.** Marfan's syndrome is a disorder of connective tissue. Paediatric manifestations include the characteristic body shape (wide span, tall, arachnodactyly, high arched palate, hypermobile joints) and the cardiac manifestations (aortic regurgitation, thoracic aortic aneurysmal dilatation, and aortic rupture).

e   True. The VATER association is associated with normal neurodevelopment. It consists of Vertebral defects, Anal atresia, Tracheo-oEsophageal fistula, and Radial limb anomalies. It is discussed in the Heart disease section, question 13(i).

> 5   *The diphtheria/pertussis/tetanus vaccine*
>   a   is a live vaccine
>   b   can be given at the same time as the *Haemophilus influenzae* type B vaccine
>   c   should not be given to a coryzal child without a fever
>   d   requires further doses to increase immunity
>   e   should not be given to HIV-positive children

a   **False.** There are several ways in which vaccines can be prepared to give immunity but not let the recipient suffer the disease.

Live attenuated organisms can be used. These have the disadvantage of sometimes being infectious to other individuals but usually offer good immunity.

Also, this type in often unsuitable for those with severe immunodeficiencies, on immunosuppressive drugs or on chemotherapy. MMR, Sabin (oral polio vaccine), BCG, varicella (not used in the UK), and yellow fever are all live vaccines.

Killed vaccines can be used safely where transmission of disease would be a problem, such as in a special care nursery and can also be used in those with immunodeficiency, although immunity may not develop. This group includes pertussis, hepatitis A, and the Salk (injectable polio) vaccine.

Toxins or proteins from the surface of the infecting particle can also be used to generate immunity. Diphtheria, tetanus, typhoid, meningococcus types A and C, pneumococcus, hepatitis B, and *Haemophilus influenzae* type B (HIB).

Killed or toxoid vaccines are often given with an immunogenic substance such as aluminium hydroxide to increase immune activation at the time of administration.

b   **True**. The UK immunization schedule requires the administration of HIB, diphtheria/pertussis/tetanus (DPT), and oral polio all at the same time. The schedule is shown in Box 14.3.

Box 14.3   UK immunization schedule

Birth	BCG or hepatitis B if at risk
2, 3, 4 months	Diphtheria, pertussis, tetanus, polio (oral), and HIB
12–18 months	Measles, mumps, and rubella
3–5 years	Diphtheria, tetanus, polio
5+ years	Measles and rubella
10–14 years	BCG if not in infancy, diphtheria, tetanus, polio

---

c   **False**. Although this may be the commonest reason for not giving a vaccine, it is not a recognized contraindication. Contraindications may be general or specific to a vaccine. Generally, a child should be well at the time of vaccination, without an intercurrent illness or fever. They should have no evidence of allergy to the vaccine or its constituents. For pertussis this might manifest as excessive screaming, a large local swelling or a high fever after a previous dose of the vaccine. As MMR is prepared with neomycin, allergy to this or kanamycin is a contraindication, but allergy to egg (it is prepared in egg) is only a relative contraindication.

d   **True**. The requirement is for three doses of DPT at 2, 3, and 4 months followed by a preschool booster of DT. This is to maximize generation of immunity, as under 70% become immune after the first dose.

e   **False**. HIV antibody positivity does not mean that immunity is impaired and vaccines can be safely given. Immunization with MMR and Sabin (polio) is recommended for HIV-positive children even if they have active disease but not BCG, as there have been several cases of invasive BCG following vaccination. HIV disease is further discussed in Immunology and infectious diseases, question 11.

6 *A child is brought for immunization. It would be appropriate to*
   a   delay administration of the vaccine because the child has a febrile illness
   b   give the MMR vaccine orally
   c   give BCG, MMR, polio, and diphtheria/pertussis/tetanus immunizations at the same time
   d   give oral paracetamol if there is a fever after the immunization
   e   administer hepatitis B vaccine to a newborn child of a woman seropositive for hepatitis B surface antigen

a   **True**. As discussed above, acute febrile illness is a contraindication for all vaccination.

b   **False**. Vaccines can be given into the deep subcutaneous space, intramuscularly and intradermally. BCG must be given intradermally and cholera, typhoid, and rabies vaccines can be given intradermally. All other vaccines can be given intramuscularly or deep subcutaneously. The usual site chosen is the anterolateral aspect of the thigh, although the deltoid muscle or gluteus maximus can be used for some vaccines.

c   **True**. Both thighs can be used at the same time to administer vaccines as well as the oral route. Killed or toxoid vaccines can be given at any appropriate time, but after one live vaccine has been given 3 weeks should elapse before another vaccine is given.

d   **True**. Even newborn infants tolerate paracetamol well at a dose of 10 mg/kg. Following a normal vaccination, the infant may become febrile and irritable and will experience pain from the site of the injections. These symptoms can be relieved with paracetamol.

e   **True**. Hepatitis B is the commonest cause world-wide of cirrhosis and carcinoma of the liver, and most cases are acquired at delivery from the mother. As there is a long incubation period (2–6 months) immunization at birth, with further doses at 4 weeks and 6 months can prevent transmission of this disease.
   There is often confusion about the serology and its meaning. Hepatitis B surface antigen (HBsAg) with HBe antibodies means the patient is a carrier and has low infectivity. HBeAg (i.e. no antibodies) indicates active hepatitis, and that there is high infectivity. Carrier status in the mother should prompt hepatitis B immunization, but active hepatitis in the mother should lead to immunization and administration of hepatitis immunoglobulin to the baby.

7 *Child sexual abuse*
   a   more commonly involves boys than girls as the victim
   b   often presents with deterioration in school performance

c   is the commonest cause of anal fissures
d   may present with a urinary tract infection
e   is suggested by vulval soreness

a   **False.** There is no typical victim of child sexual abuse (CSA), but girls are victims more often than boys. The perpetrator is usually well known to the child, either the father, mother's partner, a relative, or neighbour.

b   **True.** Diagnosis is difficult as CSA victims usually do not disclose what has happened, so any disclosure should be taken seriously, even if later retracted. Signs of CSA include inappropriate sexualization by the child, changes in behaviour or school performance, and physical features, as discussed below.

c   **False.** The commonest cause of fissures is constipation. Typically (but not always), fissures caused by constipation are in the mid-line, while those cause by anal penetration are not. When the fissure has healed there will still be a scar. Bruising around the anus is seen in the days after penetration.

The reflex anal dilatation test is used when assessing the anus of a child suspected of being a CSA victim. The buttocks are held apart and the anus watched. It should close in a normal child, but opens to give a 'positive' test. This may mean the child has been abused, but false positives are common in children especially if constipated.

d   **True.** Urinary tract infection (UTI) may occasionally be a presenting symptom in an abused girl, but other causes are much more common. These are discussed in Nephrology, question 3.

e   **False.** A full protocol for CSA evaluation is suggested in Box 14.4, and includes examination of the vulva. Vulval tears, bruising, and the state of the hymen are useful findings. Vulval soreness is a common symptom and not strongly associated with CSA.

Box 14.4   A protocol for investigation of child sexual abuse

Gather all relevant parties (social worker, CSA consultant, police)
Take history, using dolls, pictures, etc.
General physical examination
Evidence of genital or anal trauma—knee chest, or lithotomy position
Presence of blood or semen (Wood lamp can be used)
Vaginal or mouth swabs
     sperm
     STD screen
     sperm antibodies
Police may take samples of hair or from under nails

8 *Children who have been abused or neglected are more likely to be*
  a not known to health and social services
  b developmentally delayed
  c exhibiting 'frozen watchfulness'
  d born to parents who are socially disadvantaged
  e failing to thrive

a **False**. Many children who are neglected or abused have usually already been seen by medical services for a variety of injuries and illnesses. It is thought about 10% of the injuries resulting in attendance to the emergency department in children are due to non-accidental injury (NAI). Also, review of the patient records of those later found to be abused often reveals previous suspicious events.

It is therefore important that suspicious incidents are properly investigated. In the history, there may be vagueness or inconsistencies in the story or developmentally unlikely feats (e.g. a 3-week-old child rolling out of a crib). Also the story may not fit the injuries. In non-accidentally injured children there is often a delay in presentation, whereas most parents will attend promptly if there has been an accident. Lastly, the reaction of the parent is commonly inappropriate to the situation, and they often insist that the child must not be admitted even when clearly medically necessary.

b **True**. Several risk factors make a child more likely to suffer NAI. In the child, these include developmental delay, twins, premature delivery, and being fostered. In the social situation, the mother is more likely to be young, unemployed, single or have a history of mental illness or abused themselves in the past. There are often difficult relationships in the family, either between parents or between parent and child.

However, these are factors that also make a situation most stressful and deserving of support.

Developmental delay can result from neglect, as interaction with adults is required for development especially of social, speech, and fine motor skills.

c **True**. 'Frozen watchfulness' is relatively rare even in abused children. It describes a child sitting inappropriately impassively and still, as if waiting to be hit, unable to prevent or escape that fate. It is usually only found when there has been severe long-standing abuse. Abused children may also be unusually clingy or be indistinguishable from other children in their behaviour.

d **True**. As discussed further in question 11, social disadvantage makes a variety of diseases and problems more common, including abuse and neglect.

Most of the risk factors for abuse are associated with socio-economic deprivation. Aside from measures to reduce economic disparity within society, education, resources, and services can be directed towards families with young mothers, single mothers, children with medical problems, and with other reasons for making child care especially stressful and difficult. The health visitor and social worker are best placed to offer this.

e **True.** Failure to thrive is reviewed in Growth and nutrition question 5. One of the commoner causes has been labelled as 'non-organic failure to thrive', and this is associated with NAI and neglect. This means that there is no medical problem with the child causing the failure to thrive, and admission to hospital for regular (hospital) meals allows a normal weight gain. The poor weight gain at home is due to inappropriate or insufficient food being presented to the child in a way that the child cannot take, either because of poor timing or because the child cannot feed itself.

   9 In a multidisciplinary child development team
      a psychologists mainly deal with behavioural problems
      b social workers are not involved unless there are child protection issues
      c physiotherapists aim to limit deformity caused by hypertonia
      d speech therapists help manage feeding problems
      e portage is used to improve mobility

a **True.** Children with developmental delay are usually managed by a multi-disciplinary team. This is because there are often complicated problems that no specialist can deal with on their own. A community paediatrician co-ordinates the team, arranging assessment and treatment by other personnel, as well as ensuring there is continuity and communication between other team members. Psychologists assess cognitive development and can advise on suitable education. Behavioural problems are also common and they will treat these.

b **False.** Social workers can help advise on and arrange benefits, other resources, schools, and special housing. They also keep a record of children with special needs.

c **True.** Physiotherapists are important in the treatment of any child with neuromuscular disease, such as cerebral palsy. Their aim is to maximize the performance of the body by improving flexibility, preventing contractures, and helping children learn efficient ways of using the muscle function they have to mobilize and play.

d **True.** Speech therapists specialize in speech and swallowing. They can advise and instruct parents on how to feed a child with feeding difficulties, and also aid communication either using sounds, signed language (e.g. Makaton) or symbol boards.

e **False.** Portage is a scheme that plans and implements structured play for children with developmental delay with the aim of improving developmental progress.
   Other members of the multidisciplinary team are occupational therapists, community nurses, and health visitors. The family doctor must also be kept fully informed of the team's activities.

   10 School refusal
      a is synonymous with truancy
      b often presents with abdominal pain

    c   is best treated by a combination of graded return to school and anxiolytics
    d   may be precipitated by an adverse life event
    e   if often a manifestation of separation anxiety

a   **False**. Children will often not want to go to school. Where it is persistent and accompanied by psychological problems, this can be termed school refusal. Truancy is where a child goes somewhere else instead. School refusal is mainly due to separation anxiety or to school phobia.

b   **True**. Many physical manifestations including abdominal pain accompany school refusal. The common feature of all of these is that they are worst in the morning of schooldays only, improving by lunchtime. Recurrent abdominal pain may also be caused by abdominal migraine, be surgical, or related to constipation, chest or renal disease.

c   **False**. Whatever the cause, a gradual return to school must accompany any treatment. If separation anxiety is the main problem, independence must be encouraged. If there is a phobia about some aspect of school (e.g. bullying) then this needs to be addressed in conjunction with the return to school. 'Anxiolytics' such as benzodiazepines should only be used for short-term sedation in children and are inappropriate for psychological conditions.

d   **True**. Unconnected events such as a death, moving house, or parental health problems may provoke psychological changes.

e   **True**. This is more common in the younger school refusers, whereas phobias are said to be more common in older children.

   11   Children in low socio-economic groups are more
      a   likely to have been born prematurely
      b   likely to suffer from eczema
      c   likely to live in the country
      d   often injured in an accident in the home
      e   often breast fed

a   **True**. Lower socio-economic groups have an increased incidence of almost all ailments. The reasons for this are not always clear, although for some situations (e.g. accidents) it easier to see why. Other diseases are commoner in lower socio-economic groups because of life-style associations with those groups (e.g. there is a higher rate of lung cancer that can partially be explained by increased smoking). Another important factor is economic disparity between the richest and poorest in society, which itself worsens the health of the poor, compared with another society without such a disparity. This may relate to the ability to access health care.

   Children are affected indirectly by socio-economic class in several ways. Lower socio-economic groups have increased levels of single parenting, poorer housing, have more unemployed or younger parents, more children per family, and higher rates of disability in the family. Parents are more likely to live in an inner city in more cramped conditions. The parents are more likely to suffer from psychiatric illness, and drink alcohol excessively or smoke. Often these factors combine to increase disease in the children.

There is an excess of premature births in lower socio-economic groups, perhaps because of the increased rate of genital and urinary infections in this group.

b **False**. Eczema is one of the few diseases more common in higher socio-economic groups. Other examples include anorexia and malignant melanoma. Atopy is also more common in children of higher socio-economic status. The differences may relate to reduced exposure to viral infections in higher socio-economic groups and because wealthier families will have more carpets and less ventilated (better insulated) houses, increasing the levels of house dust mites. Asthma is, on the other hand less common, especially if severe.

c **False**. Living in inner cities is much more common in lower socio-economic groups. This reduces the access to safe playing areas and exposes the child to crime, accidents, and increased pollution.

d **True**. Accidents in the home are more common because there are on average more children, fewer parents to look after them and more cramped conditions. Scalds, electrical burns, and falls are the events that particularly occur in the house.

e **False**. In the UK, only 40% of children are still breast fed at 6 weeks. The lowest rates are in the lowest socio-economic groups. Breast feeding is reviewed in Growth and nutrition, questions 1 and 3.

12 *Current UK legislation holds that*
   a children with a 'statemented' disability must attend a special school
   b children under 16 are unable to give informed consent legally
   c the child's wishes are always to be followed
   d children must never be separated from their parents
   e a child cannot be admitted against the wishes of the parents before a case conference is held

a **False**. A statement of special educational needs is acquired under the 1993 Education act. A child with educational difficulties is formally assessed and, based on the conclusions, given extra resources to enable the child to maximally access the curriculum. This may require a special school (e.g. for those with developmental delay or for the deaf), but instead could be carried out in a mainstream school, perhaps with a helper, mobility aids, or something as simple as a special desk.

b **False**. It was ruled in the 'Gillick' case that a child is able to give consent under the age of 16 if they have sufficient understanding of the issues to enable the consent to be informed. This ruling was given in the case of contraception, where it was held that parental consent was not absolutely necessary for contraception.

c **False**. Children's wishes are to be respected according to the Children Act 1989 and the UN Convention on the Rights of the Child 1989, now ratified in the UK, but the wishes are not always rational or possible to fulfil. The other key points in these documents recommend privacy and support from carers be available at all times. They state that a child has the right to health information, support if disabled, and their own culture. They also lay out legal pathways for custody and protection, as discussed in question 22.

d **False**. These recommendations also state that children should always be allowed to be with their parents. There are some ages when this is particularly important—from when attachments are formed (after 9 months) to 18 months.

On the other hand, the newborn does not seem to mind if its parents are present or not, but bonding of the parents to the child can be interrupted if they are not able to be together after birth. This is a common problem for premature infants, as they may be confined to an incubator and clinically unstable or ventilated. Also mothers who have had Caesarean sections may find it difficult or painful to feed, change, or cuddle their babies. These factors can all disrupt attachment.

e **False**. When NAI is suspected and the parents refuse to allow the child to be admitted for a 'medical' indication on the advise of the doctor, a child can be put in a 'place of safety' under a police protection order. This provision under the Children Act 1989 allows assessment of the child for 72 h. After this, an emergency protection order must be sought, which lasts 8 days and extends parental responsibility to the local authority and allows a case conference to take place.

A child may be then placed on the child protection register. Here they may be placed under a care order and removed from the parents, or under a supervision order, whereby the child is monitored at home. Conversely, the decision may be taken to place the child under no order.

13 *Routine screening of children*

    a   prevents amblyopia
    b   is first carried out for congenitally dislocated hips at the 9-month check
    c   is recommended for those at risk of iron deficiency anaemia
    d   is carried out on all Afro-Caribbean infants at birth for sickle cell disease
    e   for cystic fibrosis is carried out with the Guthrie card on all infants

a **True**. Screening is a topic that comes up in most specialities. For something to be worth screening for, it must have a latent phase during which treatment will alter outcome. A practical and effective, preferably non-invasive test must also exist. Ideally, a screening programme will reduce total health expenditure.

Children are routinely examined at birth, 4 days, 6 weeks, 3 months, 9 months, 3 years, and at school entry. Their eyes are also tested and growth measured regularly while at school.

The timing of these tests is designed to screen for certain conditions. At birth and at 4 days, major congenital abnormalities and syndromes, skull deformities, cataracts, cleft palate, cardiac disease, respiratory distress, herniae, undescended testes, congenital dislocation of the hips, and ankle deformities are particularly looked for. At 6 weeks, in addition to the above, growth is measured and cardiac abnormalities are particularly focused upon. Fixing and following is observed to see if the baby's visual pathways are developing correctly and that there is no major visual problem. Any delay in fixing and following beyond 6 weeks should prompt an ophthalmic review and could be caused by retinopathy of prematurity, cataracts, neurological problems, congenital glaucoma, or retinoblastoma.

Amblyopia is the lack of cortical pathways for handling visual stimuli that develops from a sensory defect, be it a cataract or a refractive error. Even if the eye defect is corrected, acuity will never be restored. Early diagnosis and treatment of eye disorders prevents amblyopia. Also, by patching the good eye after the vision of the lazy eye is restored enable improvement of acuity in the lazy eye and restoration of binocular vision.

Vision is assessed throughout childhood. At 9 months, fine motor skills are observed and demonstrate acuity. A strabismus is looked for. If there is a concern about acuity, this can be tested for using balls of various size, thrown across a child's field of vision at a specific distance. The 3 year check includes a refractive assessment, matching shapes or letters on a table placed in front of the child with identical ones of decreasing size a set distance away from the child. At school, Snellen charts can be used.

b   **False**. Congenitally dislocated hips are first screened for in the newborn examination, using Barlow (does it dislocate) and Ortolani (does it relocate) manoeuvres.

At 9 months, congenitally dislocated hips will now be fixed into a dysplastic acetabulum, located posteriorly and superiorly to the normal one. Barlow's and Ortolini's tests will therefore be negative. These are the tests that should have picked up that the hips were dislocated under 6 weeks of age. By 9 months the signs of limited abduction, extra skin folds, and an apparently short thigh will be seen. This topic is further discussed in Rheumatology and orthopaedics, question 3.

Instead of looking primarily for hip problems, the 9 month check allows a review of the child's growth and development. The distraction test is also used to assess hearing formally for the first time.

c   **True**. Iron deficiency anaemia affects about 25% of infants, but low ferritin levels are found in far more infants. Although most (term) infants are born with good stores of iron, acquired in late gestation, this is rapidly used as the child grows. Even without iron deficiency, haemoglobin falls dramatically during the first 3 months of life reaching a trough at 4 months. Various factors make iron deficiency worse—delayed weaning, poor intake of solids, and prematurity.

As anaemia may be difficult to recognize unless severe, and iron deficiency even anaemia may cause intellectual or cognitive problems, screening for at-risk groups can be justified.

d   **False**. Almost all sickle cell disease occurs in Afro-Caribbean infants. However, as early treatment does not improve outcome, there is no justification for screening for the disease. Sickle cell disease is discussed in Haematology and oncology, question 2.

e **False**. The Guthrie card is currently used in all areas to measure thyroid-stimulating hormone (TSH; detecting children with an abnormal thyroid gland but a normal pituitary) and phenylalanine (to detect phenylketonuria). In some areas the Guthrie card has been used to measure immunoreactive trypsin, which allows early intervention in those with cystic fibrosis. This has not been carried out on a wider scale because there is doubt as to whether the small benefit of starting early flucloxacillin and physiotherapy is outweighed by the cost of the programme.

14 The UK government's 'Health of the Nation' (1992) targets to improve the health of children include
   a   reduction of the smoking prevalence in the 11–15-year-old group
   b   increase uptake of *Haemophilus influenzae* type B and diphtheria/pertussis/tetanus immunizations to over 85%
   c   reduce social inequality and its impact on children's health
   d   reduction of the death rate from accidents in those under 15 years
   e   lowering the proportion of obese children under the age of 5 years

a **True**. In attempting to make an impact on the mortality statistics, certain key areas were identified by the UK government—coronary heart disease, strokes, cancers, sexually transmitted diseases, accidents, and mental illnesses. In looking for ways to reduce incidence of these diseases, targets were set. The most important of these is the reduction of smoking in the under 15 age group by 6%. As the majority of smokers have started smoking by the age of 18, this age group is the most important. Increased penalties for those selling cigarettes to children, bans on advertising, and health campaigns can all help to achieve this target.

b **False**. Current immunization rates run at 95% for HIB and DPT in the UK. High rates have been encouraged by funding arrangements between the UK government and family doctors. In other countries, access to benefits (France) and school (USA) is made more difficult for unimmunized children, so increasing the vaccination rate.

c **False**. Although this is probably the most important way to reduce disease and its effects in a country, this is not one of the 'Health of the Nation' targets. This is further discussed in question 11.

d **True**. Accidents are the leading cause of death from age 4 to 15, and can be reduced by improved design of roads and traffic control measures. In the home, advice by health visitors, as well as better housing and residential areas can also decrease accidents.

e **False**. Adult obesity is one of the targeted areas in 'Health of the Nation', and those who are obese as adults frequently become so during childhood. However, a high weight in infancy is associated with reduced cardiovascular death in later life.

15 *In the UK, immunization*
   a levels for pertussis successfully prevent disease transmission to those under 2 months
   b against polio is now not recommended
   c can prevent most secondary cases of meningococcal septicaemia
   d uptake for measles vaccine (as MMR) is only about 50%
   e is recommended at 2, 3 and 4 months for the *Haemophilus influenzae* type B vaccine

a **False**. Immunization not only protects those who have been immunized, but, as there are then less children who can have the disease, it reduces transmission to the unimmunized. This is 'herd immunity'. The currently level of pertussis vaccination is about 95% in the UK, but in other countries such as Spain is only 70%. During the 1970s, due to fears over the neurological sequelae of the vaccine, immunization uptake fell to 30%. There was then an epidemic in which 200 000 children were infected with whooping cough.

The disease is most serious for those under 6 months and can cause death from anoxia or bronchopneumonia and weight loss from vomiting. As far as the risks of the vaccine are concerned, there have never been enough cases to confirm if the vaccine is responsible for permanent neurological damage or not. Even if it did, the rates would be far lower than those caused by the disease. In addition to this possible risk with the vaccine, it also commonly causes fever, crying, and occasionally episodes of limpness and pallor as well as local redness and swelling.

Contraindications for the DPT vaccine are an acute febrile illness, and a severe local or generalized reaction to a previous dose. Allergy, epilepsy, or a family history of these are not contraindications.

b **False**. There have been no cases of wild-type polio in the UK in non-immigrants for 10 years, but, because immigrants or travellers from abroad could import the virus, vaccination is still recommended to maintain immunity.

The oral polio vaccine (Sabin) itself is not without problems. Being a live vaccine, it multiplies in the gut and vaccinated children will excrete live attenuated virus for several days after the dose. This is rarely a problem, but about one in a million recipients develop vaccine poliomyelitis. Furthermore, as viral particles are in the stool for up to 6 weeks after vaccination, the virus can be transmitted to other unimmunized infants, in a setting such as a creche or special care nursery. The killed form (SALK) is recommended in special care nurseries and careful hygiene should be observed when changing nappies in recipients.

The vaccine is given with the DPT and HIB injections at 2,3, and 4 months and with the DT booster before school entry in the UK guidelines (see Box 14.3).

Contraindications are acute febrile illness, vomiting, or diarrhoea, and as with all live vaccines, immunosuppression and pregnancy, although this should not interfere with the UK schedule!

c **False**. In the Western world, most cases of meningococcal disease are caused by *Neisseria meningitidis* type B. In other areas, type A (India) is more common and type C can cause epidemic disease. There is no vaccine available for type B, but a polysaccharide vaccine is available for types A and C. This can be given to contacts of index cases with these strains of the bacteria. For these and type B, rifampicin antibiotic prophylaxis must be offered to close contacts. This is discussed further in of the Immunology and infectious diseases question 1.

d   **False**. Previously, when measles vaccine was given alone, uptake was only about 50%, and so cases and deaths from measles were more common. Uptake of MMR is now over 90%, and the death rate has fallen to one per year in the UK. Bronchopneumonia, encephalitis, and subacute sclerosing panencephalitis (SSPE) are the complications most likely to lead to death. The vaccine is given to all children without contraindications (see question 5) at between 12 and 18 months.

MMR vaccine is not without complications. These, to some extent, mimic the diseases themselves. Commonly about 1 week after the infection, the child may develop a fever, a rash, and occasionally swollen parotid glands.

e   **True**. The HIB vaccine is given at these times to prevent the quite considerable mortality (about 20 children a year in the UK) and long-term morbidity from HIB disease before the introduction of the vaccine. This was from meningitis (60%), epiglottitis (15%), and septicaemia.

The vaccine is a conjugate polysaccharide–protein preparation, and is recommended for all infants without contraindications (acute illness, severe reaction to the first dose). The only common side-effect is local swelling and redness at the injection site.

16   Toilet training children
    a   is usually accomplished earlier in boys
    b   is accomplished in 90% of individuals by 2 years of age in the UK
    c   may lead to constipation
    d   requires the child to speak
    e   is affected by spina bifida

a   **False**. Toilet training in the requires the child to maintain sphincter tone and then relax the sphincter tone at a socially appropriate time. In some countries (e.g. UK and USA) it is expected that the child must appreciate the meaning of the sensation when the rectum or bladder are full and then request the potty, whereas in other countries carers will put the child on the potty at regular times and allow the child to pass stool or urine. This approach is less demanding on the child and so is accomplished earlier.

Boys are usually a little slower than girls at acquiring these skills.

b   **False**. Here a distinction must be made between daytime and night-time continence, as different neurological pathways are required for each. Night-time continence usually lags many months behind daytime continence. On the other hand continence of faeces and urine comes at about the same time.

In the UK most parents will not initiate toilet training until 2 years and most children are continent in the daytime by 3–4 years. About 1% have daytime enuresis over the age of 6 years, but about 20% of children at 6 regularly have nocturnal enuresis.

c **True**. Toilet training may fail if there is an organic problem (see part e) or if there is stress in the family, perhaps relating to the toilet training. The child may resist sitting on the potty, or be unable to relax the necessary sphincters when there, resulting in constipation. In this situation, a period back in nappies is needed as well as treatment for the constipation.

d **False**. Non-verbal communication is sufficient for toilet training.

e **True**. An organic problem is much more likely if there is secondary enuresis (UTI, chemical urethritis, diabetes), but again this may be caused by stress in the home (moving house, new baby, etc.). Primary enuresis may be caused by neurological problems, such as spina bifida or cerebral palsy, or urinary tract anomalies, such as ectopic ureter, posterior urethral valves, or a pelvic mass. Overall, organic pathology accounts for only about 5% of cases of primary enuresis.

Data interpretation and reasoning — answers

17   *A 7-year-old boy is sent for a medical review by the school doctor. His teachers are concerned that there may be a physical reason why he cannot read as well as his peers. He is good at ball sports and works well with numbers. In the past he learnt to walk at the age of 11 months but did not talk in sentences until he was over 3 years. It is possible that his problem is related to*

a   global developmental delay
b   cerebral palsy
c   a latent squint
d   his father being slow to read
e   visual impairment

a **False** b **False** c **False** d **True** e **False**
A review of the developmental history given with this scenario indicates that this boy has normal development except in the area of language. Reviewing his developmental systems, his gross motor development can be seen to be normal from his walking at 11 months and enjoying ball sports. Fine motor and vision are likely to be normal as evidenced by his proficiency at ball games and ability to work with numbers. There is no information on his social development, but he does seem to have delayed speech milestones (not speaking in sentences until the age of 3) and now has another delayed language milestone as evidenced by the teachers concern over his reading.

This is therefore a specific language delay, not a global developmental delay. Cerebral palsy may also cause a language delay, but this will, by definition, be in conjunction with a motor problem, causing delayed gross motor milestones.

Visual impairment or a latent squint are not likely causes of his reading delay, as there is no evidence of any other visual problem. A latent squint is not present when both eyes are looking at an object, but a strabismus revealed when one eye is covered in a cover test. As the cover is removed, the covered eye moves to take up fixation on the object the other eye is already looking at.

This scenario may be caused by a variety of problems, including middle ear disease and a specific language delay. This is a disorder that is much more common in boys and that runs in families.

18 *A 5-year-old boy is seen by a community paediatrician in an enuresis clinic. He usually wets his bed two or three times each night, but has been dry during the day since he was 3 years old. A developmental inquiry reveals that he started to walk at 11 months and began to speak in sentences at the age of 3. To manage his nocturnal enuresis*

   a tricyclic antidepressants can be of use
   b a star chart is an effective intervention
   c if he is not treated the problem is unlikely to resolve
   d urinalysis will be of value to identify those with renal pathology
   e a pad and bell must wake him up to be effective

a **True** b **True** c **False** d **True** e **True**

When answering a question on the development of continence in children, there are a few key terms and concepts. Primary enuresis (or encopresis) means the child has yet to acquire control of bladder or bowels. It is to common up to the age of 3.

Secondary enuresis or encopresis describes the situation when a formerly continent child becomes incontinent, and is much more likely to be due to an organic problem (see question 16). Daytime bladder and bowel control is often acquired at the same time, but night-time control usually follows months behind. Hence nocturnal enuresis is much more common than daytime enuresis.

Urinary continence requires different mechanisms during the day and during the night. Nocturnal enuresis is night-time incontinence in a child who is continent during the day. It affects 20% at 6 and about 8% at 10 years. The natural history of the problem is that it will improve with time, but many children and parents want the process hastened.

The first measures for nocturnal enuresis are simple. A urine dipstix test to exclude kidney disease (proteinuria, haematuria), diabetes (glycosuria) and urine infection is appropriate. Then reducing night-time fluid intake can help. Next, a behavioural approach can be used. A star chart rewards a child for each dry night and can be surprisingly effective. A water-sensitive pad placed under the child triggers a bell that wakes the child after the episode of incontinence. Soon, however, the child learns to wake before passing urine to allow for a trip to the toilet. Drug therapy also has its role, especially for special occasions, such as going to stay at a friend's house. DDAVP intranasally or tricyclics can be used, although relapse is very common when the drug is stopped. Overall, about 70% of children can be successfully treated, with a 15% relapse rate.

> 19 *An 11-month-old girl is seen in the developmental clinic following delivery at 30 weeks gestation. She sat 8 months, but is unable to crawl or pull to stand. Her mother says that she can turn to sounds and babbles 'dadadada' and 'mamamama'. She is seen to have a pincer grip and transfers cubes well, but is unable to cast objects. She can hold her own bottle, but cannot feed herself with a spoon*
>
> a she has delayed gross motor milestones
> b she should be able to understand her own name
> c it will not be necessary to perform a distraction test
> d she may have Down's syndrome
> e she will not be able to pick up a raisin offered to her

a **False** b **True** c **False** d **False** e **False**

This developmental data question is complicated by the child's premature birth. As the child has been born 10 weeks early the milestones should come 2–3 months later than those for a child born on its due date. Although this is not always so, and some milestones may come earlier than expected, it is a useful yardstick for the first year.

When her premature delivery is taken into account, her corrected age is about $8\frac{1}{2}$ months. Using the milestones in Box 14.1, it can be seen that this child has no features of developmental delay. Delay in this context does not mean slower than the average, but outside the normal range for age to acquiring the skill. Developmental delay is always present in Down's syndrome, although its degree may be variable. IQ in Down's children has a mean of 50, ranging from 25 to 75. By contrast, children with Turner's syndrome have a normal IQ. Mental retardation is defined as an IQ below 70, severe mental retardation less than 50, and profound less than 20.

A developmental check should always be a mixture of history (the mother's observations) and what you see as the child plays in front of you, with your age appropriate toys. The mother's observations often show the child to be more advanced than your observations, due to the foreign nature of a developmental check and maternal optimism. At 9 months you should ask if the child can recognize their name and if they will come when called from the next room. In the gross motor developmental system you should ask about sitting, crawling, and pulling to stand. Fine motor questions could include asking if there is a pincer grip, and enquiring if there is a hand preference. Under 2 years a hand preference implies that there is a problem (neuromuscular or visual) with the non-preferred side. Social skills that should have been acquired include smiling, playing peek-a-boo, being able to hold and eat a cracker, and perhaps some stranger wariness.

To examine a child at this age developmentally, first the child must be closely observed during play with some coloured 1 inch cubes. This will demonstrate the grip, transfers, and if there is a problem with one side of the body. Smaller objects such as raisins can be picked up if the child has a pincer grip. In older children hundreds and thousands can be used. As the hearing assessment is an important part of the 9 months check, it is still necessary to do a distraction test (see question 3). This can be done at this stage in the examination if the room is quiet enough and there is enough time. The gross motor section of the examination is best left until the end as many children dislike it. However, starting with the child lying supine, you can see turning over or crawling or sitting. Pulling the child up into the sitting position tests for head lag and the ability to sit. Then pulling to stand demonstrates the tone in the legs and balance. Lifting the child up and suspending in the prone position allows you to look at the neck tone and the parachute reflexes (saving reflexes needed for walking). Lowering the child down to lie prone, a crawling posture may be adopted or the child may raise itself up on its elbows in the sphinx position.

20 *An 8-month-old boy has a distraction test. Although his mother reports that he understands his name and is babbling, he does not turn to the rattles during the test. A full enquiry shows that otherwise there are no areas of developmental concern. Possible explanations for these findings include*
   a   the rattles used for the test were too quiet
   b   the room used for the test had become too noisy
   c   gentamicin therapy as a neonate
   d   serous otitis media
   e   kernicterus

a **False** b **True** c **True** d **True** e **True**

In this question, a child has failed a distraction test but is otherwise developmentally normal, even in the hearing and speech developmental system according to the mother. This either means the test has given a false positive result, or the child has a mild hearing problem, perhaps only affecting one ear, or the mother has overestimated her son's abilities.

Question 3 discusses the requirements for a distraction test. A noisy room might well unexpectedly reduce a child's ability to distinguish the sound of a rattle and give a false positive result, but as the test prescribes a certain rattle volume, this cannot be a cause for failing to turn to the noise. Medical causes for apparent hearing loss during the first year can be divided into conductive loss (impacted cerumen, serous otitis media, acute otitis media, perforated tympanic membrane) and sensorineural loss (hypoxic brain damage, following meningitis, kernicterus, and gentamicin therapy)

Further assessment will involve pure tone audiometry or if a middle ear disease suspected, tympanometry.

21 *The following tests and results suggest the associated problems*
   a   fragile X chromosome may explain learning difficulty in males
   b   periosteal reaction suggests a previous fracture
   c   Guthrie test will demonstrate a high serum phenylalanine
   d   Barr bodies are diagnostic of Down's syndrome
   e   *Candida* on a vulval swab suggests sexual abuse

a **True** b **True** c **True** d **False** e **False**

Tests are used in community paediatrics in two main situations: to help decide if a child has been physically or sexually abused and in developmental delay. This is important to do as there are treatable causes of developmental delay (e.g. hypothyroidism, phenylketonuria, social deprivation, deafness, and blindness), and a diagnosis enables informed genetic counselling and a prognosis. Much of the treatment available for developmentally delayed children is, however, based on the problems rather than the underlying diagnosis (see question 9).

Blood is also taken once in a every child's life for screening using the Guthrie card. Drops of capillary blood taken from the heel of babies over the age of 7 days are put on a card and sent to a testing laboratory. Routinely serum phenylalanine and TSH is measured to detect infants with phenylketonuria and congenital hypothyroidism. These conditions are discussed in question 4 and Endocrinology and metabolic disease question 5, respectively.

In investigating developmental delay, there may be a chromosomal abnormality. A karyotype looks at the chromosomes, but special conditions are sometimes required to demonstrate the 'fragile X' chromosome. Barr bodies are X chromosomes found in the cells of the buccal mucosa and is a good test for female genotype.

Other than Down's syndrome, there are many chromosomal deletions that present with abnormal facies, developmental delay and sometimes malformations of other systems. Examples include Wolf syndrome (4p−) and Cri du Chat syndrome (5p−). Fragile X is an X-linked disorder affecting about 1 in 1500 boys. There are prominent ears and macrocephaly. It is the second most common cause of learning difficulties and there are frequently behavioural problems, such as a short attention span. Other causes of developmental delay are shown in Box 14.5.

History and examination with photographic support is needed initially in evaluating children in whom abuse is suspected. Investigations can be useful to support these findings. The 'skeletal survey' involves X-rays of the whole skeleton

---

Box 14.5   Common causes of developmental delay

Specific delay	Language
	Blindness
	Deaf child
Global delay	Chromosomal
	Genetic, e.g. Hurler syndrome
	Intrauterine adverse event
	Birth asphyxia
	Infection
	Trauma to head
	Social deprivation

to identify undisclosed fractures, old fractures, and evidence of fractures at different stages in healing. Different aged fractures suggest physical abuse over a period of time. A periosteal reaction is a finding consistent with a healing fracture in a young bone, and is often present even if no break can be seen. Other fractures are rarely acquired accidentally, for instance long bone fractures before an infant can walk. A radioisotope bone scan is said to be more sensitive at identifying multiple fracture, but gives less information about the age of the fractures. In suspected physical abuse, confusion can be caused by osteogenesis imperfecta or copper deficiency, both of which predispose to fractures and clotting disorders.

Vulval or vaginal swabs are used in the evaluation of child sexual abuse. *Candida* is commonly found in normal children, but chlamydia, gonococcus, or other sexually transmitted organisms are strongly suggestive of sexual abuse.

22(i) *A 2-month-old girl is taken to the emergency department by her mother at 11 p.m., who is concerned that her child is less alert than normal, and has not fed since lunchtime. In the past she has been seen twice times in the department, with a bruise to her eye and a severe rash to her nappy area. Although she has no temperature, she seems pale and lethargic. Because of her previous admissions, there is concern that this presentation might be due to non-accidental injury. This suspicion is increased by*

a   a bruise on her forehead
b   a torn frenulum
c   retinal haemorrhage
d   a focal convulsion during examination
e   a sunken fontanelle

a **True** b **True** c **True** d **True** e **False**

The history must be used in conjunction with the examination in children who may have been physically abused. This is discussed in question 8. Here a young infant is brought in at a late hour, with a delayed presentation. Multiple attendances to the emergency department are suspicious. A severe nappy rash might occur if the nappy is not changed frequently enough, as is usual in neglect. Also the previous bruise is suspicious. How did a baby of 2 months bruise its eye? Before a baby can turn over, it cannot damage itself. Some bruises may occur accidentally to the face, particularly the forehead when a child is walking and almost all children have bruised shins. Bruises on the trunk, not over bony prominences, near the eye or on the buttocks should always raise the question of NAI. A torn frenulum in a baby is almost pathognomonic of NAI, being caused by a bottle, dummy, or finger being forced into a closed mouth.

This presentation is with a quiet and pale child. This may be caused by sepsis, but it this context the 'shaken baby' syndrome is more likely. Holding an infant around the chest and shaking backwards and forwards vigorously will tear the bridging cerebral vessels causing a subdural haematoma. Evidence for this can be a bulging fontanelle or retinal haemorrhage. Direct damage to the brain may also occur and result in convulsions. Permanent brain damage is common after this injury.

22(ii) *The girl has all of these features. It would now be appropriate to*
  a arrange urgent retinal photocoagulation to prevent worsening of the retinal bleed
  b arrange an urgent outpatient appointment to coincide with a case conference
  c send the child for a head CT scan to look for a subdural haematoma
  d arrange a skeletal survey
  e involve the police

a **False** b **False** c **True** d **True** e **True**

Having seen a possible abused child, the first priority is to ensure the child does not return home, and instead to admit the child until her injuries have been fully investigated. If the parents will not allow this for medical reasons, a police protection order can be used to make the ward a 'place of safety', and an emergency protection order sought to allow time for assessment and a case conference. This is discussed further in question 12. The police can be involved directly or via the social workers who will now have to investigate the child and family situation to find a safe place for the child to go to when discharged. It is always the aim to try and keep the child with the natural parents, and this may be possible if they receive psychological or financial help (e.g. counselling, education on parenting, alcohol detoxification). The child can be placed on the child protection register and will then be closely followed by the social services. Criminal proceedings against the parents may also be undertaken by the police.

Investigations for a possibly abused child are listed in Box 14.6. Here a skeletal survey would be needed to investigate the physical abuse possibility, and a head CT scan to determine if neurosurgical intervention is necessary.

Box 14.6   Investigations of use in physical abuse

Skeletal survey
Radioisotope bone scan
Bleeding and clotting studies
Photographs
Head trauma/shaken baby—CT scan
Abdominal trauma—liver enzymes, urinalysis for blood

Note: page numbers in **bold** refer to questions, those in normal type refer to answers